Introduction to Health Care Quality

INTRODUCTION TO HEALTH CARE QUALITY

Theory, Methods, and Tools

Yosef D. Dlugacz

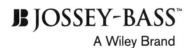

A Wiley Brand

Published by Jossey-Bass
A Wiley Brand
One Montgomery Street, Suite 1000, San Francisco, CA 94104-4594—www.josseybass.com

Jossey-Bass books and products are available through most bookstores. To contact Jossey-Bass directly call our Customer Care Department within the U.S. at 800-956-7739, outside the U.S. at 317-572-3986, or fax 317-572-4002.

Wiley publishes in a variety of print and electronic formats and by print-on-demand. Some material included with standard print versions of this book may not be included in e-books or in print-on-demand. If this book refers to media such as a CD or DVD that is not included in the version you purchased, you may download this material at **http://booksupport.wiley.com**. For more information about Wiley products, visit **www.wiley.com**.

Library of Congress Cataloging-in-Publication Data

Names: Dlugacz, Yosef D., 1947- author.
Title: Introduction to health care quality : theory, methods, and tools / Yosef D. Dlugacz.
Description: First edition. | Hoboken, New Jersey : Jossey-Bass & Pfeiffer Imprints, Wiley, [2017] |
    Includes bibliographical references and index.
Identifiers: LCCN 2016020039 (print) | LCCN 2016020736 (ebook) |
    ISBN 9781118777916 (pbk.) | ISBN 9781118779576 (epdf) | ISBN 9781118779590 (epub)
Subjects: | MESH: Quality of Health Care—organization & administration |
    Health Care Reform—methods | Patient Safety | Quality Control |
    Health Information Management—methods | United States
Classification: LCC RA971 (print) | LCC RA971 (ebook) | NLM W 84.4 AA1 |
    DDC 362.1068—dc23
LC record available at https://lccn.loc.gov/2016020039

Cover Design: Wiley
Cover Images: © duncan1890/iStockphoto, © Tsyhun/iStockphoto,
© sturti/iStockphoto

Printed in the United States of America
FIRST EDITION

PB Printing   10 9 8 7 6 5 4 3 2 1

To Doris, whose love,
intelligence, compassion,
and humor have accompanied
me for the past 45 remarkable years

CONTENTS

LIST OF FIGURES AND TABLES

Figures

Tables

PREFACE

When I began to think about revising the outdated *Quality Handbook for Health Care Organizations: A Manager's Guide to Tools and Programs* (Jossey-Bass, 2004), my goal was to introduce and explore the many changes that have made an impact on health care in the last decade. I quickly realized that I couldn't simply revise the book for a second edition; too much had changed. An entirely new book introducing quality management was needed if I wanted it to be of value to health care professionals and students. This *Introduction to Health Care Quality: Theory, Methods, and Tools* seemed necessary.

Even the change in titles is revealing. Quality is no longer the sole purview of managers. To the contrary, now everyone—clinicians, administrators, executives, patients—involved in health care services needs to work within a quality framework and be familiar with quality management processes. Students who hope to work in health care, whether in the clinical, administrative, or policy-making roles, need to know the fundamentals of quality management to succeed. Physicians, nurses, pharmacists, and public health policy makers all need to involve themselves in performance improvement activities and understand how to transform data into useful information in order to take action. Administrators and executives have to meet the goals of specific quality measures set by government agencies in order to be reimbursed for the delivery of care and medical services.

My books are designed to be of practical use to students and professionals and are based on my experience working in the field of quality management for decades and teaching fundamentals of quality all over the world. I have the good fortune of being part of a vast health care system that encompasses the entire spectrum of health care services—21 hospitals, the Feinstein Institute for Medical Research, the Krasnoff Quality Management Institute, the Center for Learning and Innovation, rehabilitation and skilled nursing facilities, a home care network, a hospice network, and progressive care centers—offering a range of outpatient services; ambulatory facilities; psychiatric care; long-term nursing care; and children's organizations. Thus I have direct and immediate access to the issues that most concern administrators and executives, floor and unit managers, clinicians, policy makers, IT professionals, and others. Writing from personal experience gives me the opportunity to share practical issues of quality in action and relay the direct application of quality management theory, methods, and tools.

I have always been a champion of quality and I like to think an advocate for patients' rights and patient safety. I have worked diligently to ferret out gaps in care and potential gaps in safety to improve performance, and further communication and accountability across the hospital and the continuum of care. I followed this path because I believe in the tenets of quality management; I believe in the objectivity of data to make a case for good or poor care. I believe in numbers, in measurements, in tracking improvements and interventions over time using reliable and valid data.

But it was not until I myself became a patient that my theoretical expertise quickly became of immediate and practical concern. As a patient, I found myself vulnerable to issues of safety and communication failures that I had written about and spoken about but had never directly experienced. Although I had always understood the importance of patient identification, for example, until I was receiving chemotherapy and the nurses made absolutely sure that I was getting the correct dose of the correct medications in the correct manner, and asked me multiple times to confirm my name, I didn't realize how reassuring it was to know that the procedures developed to ensure proper patient identification were in place and being followed. When I needed my MRI results to be transmitted to my oncologist in a timely fashion, I didn't want any failures of communication to take place. Ensuring quality care became deeply personal.

And although I am probably better educated than most about dealing with health care data, I found that when I was confronted with three very different plans of care from three very highly regarded physicians, I needed to understand mortality rates and complications from treatment, numbers, variation, and evidence in a new way. How many patients with my particular very rare cancer had each doctor treated and with what outcome? I realized how valuable my experience as a quality professional was. I knew what questions to ask. Quality care is, of course, a goal for organizations to strive for, but it is also for everyone. I realized that everyone—health care professionals, patients, and potential patients—should be quality managers. This book, then, is for everyone.

New models of health care are so-called patient-centered, making patients central to the care plan and treatment process. Again, to me, this is no longer theory. It is in fact critical that patients understand what is happening to them, why they are having the treatment they are having, what the predicted outcomes will be, and what complications might occur. All these issues, basic to quality management, were now basic to me. All patients should indeed be treated holistically. We are not defined by our disease or our illness; we are people with psychosocial experiences and needs, some of us more capable than others or simply luckier than others in being able to take good care of ourselves.

Everyone should be a quality manager. Everyone will have occasion to interact with a health care delivery system of one kind or another, either for themselves or for family and loved ones. Everyone needs to be schooled about quality, how to assess care, what to look for, what is expected, what should not be tolerated. Everyone should be an advocate for quality care. I hope this book will be useful to professionals and nonprofessionals alike.

ACKNOWLEDGMENTS

I want to thank the many people who have made this book possible. Thanks to Dr. William Tap, and the extraordinary team of health professionals at Memorial Sloan Kettering, where I received good care: the intelligence and compassion, professionalism and expertise that every patient deserves and so few receive. I can't thank you enough. And thanks to Dr. Samuel Kenan, of Northwell Health, whose surgery skills and oncology knowledge saved my life.

Thanks to the many people, present and past, who have worked to make the North Shore–LIJ Health System, now Northwell Health, excel in quality. Abraham Krasnoff, John Gallagher, and Lawrence Scherr believed in quality management and in me. The chair of the board of trustees, Mark Claster, has been a champion of quality for many years and has been instrumental in shaping quality concepts for the board and for the health system. Michael Dowling, the CEO of Northwell Health, has trusted me and supported me in establishing the Krasnoff Quality Management Institute and is committed to building the best-quality health system possible. His executive team of Mark Solazzo, David Battinelli, MD, Gene Tangney, and others have made quality a priority and have recognized its importance in establishing and maintaining outstanding care.

To the entire Krasnoff team, especially Debi Baker for her support with graphics and careful perusal of the manuscript; Megan Smith for her constant support with everything; Marcella De Geronimo, Kevin Masick, Eric Hamilton, Rosemarie Linton, Larry Lutsky, Anne Marie Fried, and the rest of the group for their generous willingness to offer their expertise; and everyone else who has shared their professional smarts with me in the writing of this book, many many thanks. Thanks also to my friend and colleague Alice Greenwood for her commitment and support and editorial prowess, whose contributions have made a real difference in this book. Her capacity to translate complex ideas into accessible language for a broad audience has helped to make my books not only successful but a pleasure to write.

Thanks to the wonderful folks at Jossey-Bass, including the late Andy Pasternack, who encouraged this new volume; to Seth Schwartz and Melinda Noack for their intelligence, good humor, and support; to the people at Wiley, Patricia Rossi, Monica Rogers, Jeevarekha Babu, and the copyeditor, Debra Manette, for shepherding the book into publication; and to the rest of the team: You made the production of this book a real pleasure.

And as always to my wonderful family—my children, Adam, Stefanie, Hillel, Stacey, James, and Stacy—and my extraordinary grandchildren—Kylie, Lila, Jack, Nico, and Amber—your love carried me through this chapter of my life, and your faith in me has been inspiring.

To my wife, Doris, to whom I owe everything!

ABOUT THE AUTHOR

Yosef D. Dlugacz, Ph.D., is the Senior Vice President and Chief of Clinical Quality, Education, and Research of the Krasnoff Quality Management Institute of the Northwell Health system. The goal of the institute is to bridge the gap between theoretical knowledge learned in the academic setting and the realities of applying quality management methods in today's health care reform environment. Dr. Dlugacz's research focuses on developing models that link quality, safety, good clinical outcomes, and financial success for increased value and improved efficiencies.

Dr. Dlugacz's methodologies have been praised nationally and internationally, and he has appeared in numerous teleconferences promoting quality and safety. Many of the best practices that have resulted from the quality management performance improvement process he has established have been published by The Joint Commission as standards for the entire industry.

His academic appointments have included: Associate Professor of Science Education at the Northwell Hofstra School of Medicine; Adjunct Professor of Information Technology and Quantitative Methods at the Hofstra University Frank G. Zarb School of Business; Visiting Professor to Beijing University's MBA Program; and Professor at Baruch Mt. Sinai, MBA program, City University of New York.

Dr. Dlugacz has published widely in health care and quality management journals on a variety of clinical care and quality topics. The Healthcare Financial Management Association published his article "High-Quality Care

Reaps Financial Rewards" in its Strategic Financial Planning publication. His book *The Quality Handbook for Health Care Organizations: A Manager's Guide to Tools and Programs* (Jossey-Bass, 2004) has been praised as a valuable text for new quality professionals. His book *Measuring Health Care: Using Quality Data for Operational, Financial, and Clinical Improvement* (Jossey-Bass, 2006) helps to educate professionals about the relationship between quality care and financial success. *Value-Based Health Care: Linking Finance and Quality* (Jossey-Bass, 2010), which explores the relationship between quality care and organizational efficiency, was selected for a 2010 Bugbee-Falk Award from the Association of University Professionals in Health Administration and nominated for the ACHE/Hamilton Book of the Year Award. Dr. Dlugacz was invited to write two chapters for *Error Reduction in Health Care: A System's Approach to Improving Patient Safety*, edited by Patrice Spath (Jossey-Bass, 2011).

Dr. Dlugacz received his PhD in sociology from the Graduate Center of the City University of New York.

INTRODUCTION

Health care is changing—its delivery, its structures, even its underlying philosophy. Wellness, rather than sickness, is now the focus of government concern. The patient experience of health and well-being, rather than the physician's interpretation, is now central, and patient expectations are measured, communicated, and meaningful for financial success. Smaller health care organizations are banding together to become larger health care systems because financial efficiencies dictate such collaborations. Data are abundantly available to track various aspects of care. All these changes encourage new ways of thinking about health care and the organizations that deliver that care; those professionals who hope to understand and thrive in this new environment require quality tools, techniques, information, and education.

Introduction to Health Care Quality: Theory, Methods, and Tools is designed to familiarize health care professionals and students, administrative and clinical leaders, and policy makers with contemporary issues in quality management in the new health care reform environment. In addition, due to the rapidly changing technology for tracking medical information, such as the electronic health record, quality managers and health professionals will need to have increased familiarity with database development, data analytics and statistics, the role of measurements in monitoring quality, and performance improvement methodologies if health organizations are to succeed in the increasingly competitive marketplace. Because government agencies are linking quality variables to financial success, health professionals today are required to communicate information accurately and transparently and meet newly established benchmarks for the delivery of care. This book is designed to help professionals meet these needs.

Quality professionals, indeed all health care professionals, are required to work within new models of health care delivery, such as the patient-centered medical home, accountable care organizations, value-based purchasing, bundled payments, and pay for performance. Community programs that encourage wellness and prevention are now reimbursed whereas under the older models, hospital services and patient volume controlled financial outcomes. It is a new health care world, and those involved in it require new information and new skills.

The purpose of this book is to provide just that: to give professionals and students the tools they need to work effectively within the increasingly data-driven health care environment. Quality data provide the foundation of care decisions, performance improvement initiatives, prioritization of resources, documentation about meeting expectations, analyzing market competition, and understanding the patient experience. Physicians and other clinicians are expected to work within the quality framework, collect data, report outcomes, collaborate in multidisciplinary teams, and develop communication strategies as never before. Inpatient hospital, ambulatory centers, and health care system leadership have to become involved in quality data and measurements in order to administer effectively and maximize reimbursements. Patients, who are the health care consumers, are more able than ever before to access comparative information about different care facilities and providers and make informed choices about where they spend their health care dollars.

This book addresses these quality issues from the point of view of my personal experience as a quality professional for the past 30 years. It offers experiential, practical, and applied examples of hands-on implementation of how the fundamentals of quality management can improve efficiency and effectiveness of organizational and clinical processes, based on my career as the Senior Vice President of Quality Management and as the Executive Director of the Krasnoff Quality Management Institute, for Northwell Health (formerly the North Shore-LIJ Health System), one of the largest integrated health systems in the United States. My goal is to show quality management in action, offering theoretical information and practical examples within each chapter. The exercises at the end of each chapter, "Quality Concepts in Action," are designed to reinforce the quality concepts discussed in that chapter in applied situations. The references, suggestions for further reading, and useful websites at the end of each chapter provide students of health care quality with rich resource material for further exploration of the quality concepts and ideas in the chapter.

The material in the chapters not only exposes interested professionals to quality management fundamentals but also attempts to provoke creative ways of thinking about the provision of care. In addition to offering new material, each chapter reinforces and integrates previous discussions. I have taken examples from my experience, and although for privacy issues they are hypothetical, the examples are entirely realistic. The first five chapters review quality management theory and fundamentals and the changes necessary to the new reform environment. Chapters 6 through 9 show the application of quality theory with the tools and techniques used for performance improvement. Chapter 10 reviews and concludes the issues highlighted in the previous chapters.

Chapter 1 outlines the basics or fundamentals of quality management, introducing the most influential quality theorists, from Nightingale through Donabedian, and organizations concerned with quality, among them The Joint Commission, the Centers of Medicare and Medicaid Services, and the Institute of Medicine. A discussion of how to develop quality indicators for performance improvement is offered.

Chapter 2 highlights the changes and new models of care required by the health care reform bill, the Accountable Care Act, such as accountable care organizations, bundled payments, pay for performance, value-based purchasing, the patient-centered medical home, and so on. In this chapter the role of health information technology is discussed, including the pros and cons of electronic health records. Improving communication between physician and patient, encouraged in the health care reform environment, has led to innovative practices, such as narrative medicine, which is being taught in medical schools to increase professional awareness of how to elicit information.

Chapter 3 introduces in general terms the changing paradigms involved in providing safe quality care in different settings, such as the inpatient hospital and the community. It also stresses the importance of quality measurements in the reform environment and of effective leadership in making productive change. Various techniques to improve multidisciplinary communication, such as huddles, are outlined. The importance of health literacy in improving patient safety is also discussed in this chapter. An example of developing effective structures for moving information throughout a health system is offered, as is the role of quality data and measurements in promoting change for performance improvement.

Chapter 4 examines new challenges for health professionals that the reform environment promotes, such as the importance of statistical information and quality measurements in monitoring quality of care and patient satisfaction. Dashboards of measurements are discussed for their value in assessing care and improving processes, especially for issues involved in chronic disease management. Health information technology and various data sources are also reviewed for appropriateness in monitoring care. Improving communication across the continuum, using microsystems, macrosystems, Lean, TeamSTEPPS, SBAR, and checklists, is discussed.

Chapter 5 stresses the role of administrative and clinical leaders in improving patient safety and how metrics and measurements should be used by leaders to monitor the processes of care and patient safety. Principles of High Reliability Organizations are shown to address patient safety issues in a proactive paradigm. The role of quality management, nursing leaders, and the medical staff in promoting a safety culture is outlined. Examples of effective ways to report data for business intelligence and for decision making are presented. Prioritization issues and the role of dashboards in determining priorities are discussed, as well as how to interpret gaps in care, errors, and leaders' role in monitoring adverse events.

Chapter 6 shows how to work with quality tools and methods to manage problems, identify gaps in care, and target errors with such quality management tools as root cause analysis, failure mode, effects analysis, cause-and-effect diagrams, flowcharts, and other graphical displays of information. Basic statistical concepts involved in using data for analysis and quality research are presented. The value of using clinical pathways to improve communication and standardize the process of disease management is argued. Improving performance methodologies, such as the Plan-Do-Study-Act cycle, is defined.

Chapter 7 continues the discussion of the role and challenges of working with quality data to evaluate care and the difference between using data for regulatory compliance and for performance improvement. Issues involved in extracting data from the electronic health record are discussed. Case studies are offered to show the application of data to real-life hospital situations, such as the appropriate assignment of end-of-life patients, chronic disease management, readmission, and working with aggregated data to make improvements. Examples offered include variation from the standard of care and variance analysis, which are monitored by control charts.

Chapter 8 discusses issues involved in using quality measurements to understand and improve care from the points of view of the clinician, administrator, and patient. Process and outcomes measures are used as examples. Measures used for the value-based purchasing or pay-for-performance paradigms as well as patient satisfaction measures are presented. Examples of dashboards of measures, developed so that leaders have ready access to importance quality information, are offered. This chapter also includes using safety and environment of care measures to improve patient safety.

Chapter 9 shows how to use the quality tools, such as throughput, queuing theory, and APACHE data for ICU efficiency, to manage efficiencies, and explains how to develop protocols and algorithms of care to optimize efficiency and safety for various procedures, such as bariatric surgery and more global issues, such as understanding mortality, from a clinical and administrative point of view. This chapter delves into the complex problems attached to patient-centered care, working in teams, and delivering the message of change throughout the organization.

Chapter 10 concludes with the challenges health care professionals will face in the future, regardless of the composition of staff or distinctions among health care organizations, since quality metrics and principles of teamwork and performance improvement underlie all levels of care. The chapter summarizes the previous chapters' exploration of the role of leaders, the use of quality data and measurements in performance improvements, and identifying barriers to effective change.

Introduction to Health Care Quality

PART ONE

QUALITY MANAGEMENT FUNDAMENTALS

CHAPTER ONE

FOUNDATIONS OF HEALTH CARE QUALITY

Chapter Outline

Defining Quality
Contributions of Quality Theorists—Nothing New under the Sun
Quality Management Methodologies
Organizations Making an Impact on Quality and Safety Standards
Centers for Medicare and Medicaid Services
Institute for Healthcare Improvement
Agency for Health Research and Quality
National Quality Forum
The Leapfrog Group
Data: The Foundation of Quality Management
Summary
Key Terms
Quality Concepts in Action
References
Suggestions for Further Reading
Useful Websites

Key Concepts

- Understand issues involved in defining the concept of quality in health care.
- Introduce important quality theorists.

- Describe quality methodologies.
- Explain the role of agencies and groups that have an impact on health care quality.
- Review the role of data as the foundation of quality management.

Quality, which is easily recognized—and even more easily recognized in its absence—is surprisingly hard to define. One knows it when one experiences it, be it in a car, a restaurant, or a health care organization, and one knows when it is missing. It can be considered an attitude or orientation, a dedication of individuals in an organization to strive for excellence, or quality can be based on an individual's perception and his or her value system.

Perhaps the least controversial definition of quality was proposed in 1990 by the Institute of Medicine (IOM), an independent, nonprofit organization that advises decision makers and the public about health care issues: "Quality of care is the degree to which health services for individuals and populations increase the likelihood of desired health outcomes and are consistent with current professional knowledge" (Lohr, 4). It should be noted that "desired health outcomes" are difficult to define and measure, and may be dependent on knowing the population and the community served. To understand quality, it is useful to know the history of how quality management has evolved, the significant thinkers and theorists who have contributed to defining quality, and the organizations that have influenced how health care is delivered in the United States.

Defining Quality

Quality standards are not fixed entities but rather should be thought of as a moving target, going between better quality or worse quality, defined by the expectations of customers. If customer expectations are met, quality is considered to be high. However, meeting customer expectations is complicated because customers themselves may not even be aware of or able to articulate their expectations regarding quality. For this reason, many organizations conduct satisfaction surveys and analyze complaints in order to better understand what customers want from their health care experience.

In fact, health care quality has to meet the expectations of many groups of customers: patients and their families, physicians, organizations, regulators, payers, and communities. Each of these customers may have different expectations of quality, such as access to care (do customers/patients get the care they need?) and effectiveness of care (are they better?). Medical outcome expectations, or effectiveness, are usually set through professional organizations and adopted as standards of care. Today, patients and payers have information and opinions about their care that is eroding the primacy of physicians to be the sole setters of expectations. Patients, communities, governmental agencies, and payers are setting standards in addition to physicians.

Contributions of Quality Theorists—Nothing New under the Sun

Many of the early quality theorists defined methods, tools, and techniques that are still being used today in health care settings. Many of the problems identified by these quality thinkers still exist today. Many of the solutions they proposed are still being discussed today. Each of these prominent theorists contributed something to our understanding of what quality means and how to provide quality outcomes. A brief introduction to some of the highlights of their work in quality follows.

Florence Nightingale

In thinking about medical quality, the place to start is with Florence Nightingale (1820–1910), an English social reformer and statistician. She is considered to be the founder of modern nursing and became famous for her nursing skills with wounded soldiers during the Crimean War. However, her work encompassed more than improving nursing practice and broadening nursing education. In addition, she was an advocate for health care reform and wrote works to educate laypeople about medical knowledge. Nightingale was also a social reformer, especially of women's rights and hunger relief. She had the good fortune to be born into a wealthy family to a progressive-thinking father who encouraged her education, especially her exceptional mathematical and analytic skills.

Nightingale can be credited with creating the framework for quality management, using data as the bases for graphics about monthly improvements in mortality associated with her sanitary reforms. She understood the association among overcrowding, sanitation, infection, and mortality. In this way, she linked cause with effect. She pioneered the visual representation of statistical information, using the pie chart (see Figure 1.1) and the histogram (see Figure 1.2) to illustrate sources of patient mortality.

These figures reveal the same information in different formats. Both, however, make it clear at a glance that the majority of deaths (60 percent) were the result of poor hygiene and sanitation, double the number of deaths from battle wounds. Graphical displays are powerful representations of information.

Nightingale's comprehensive statistical analysis of rural India's sanitation was instrumental in reform. In 1873, she reported that mortality among the

FIGURE 1.1. CAUSES OF PATIENT MORTALITY PIE CHART

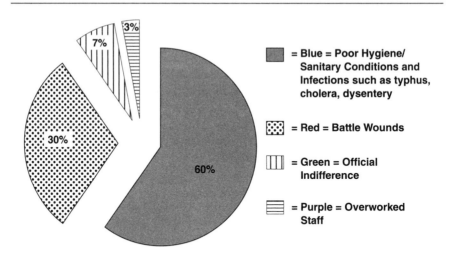

FIGURE 1.2. CAUSES OF PATIENT MORTALITY HISTOGRAM

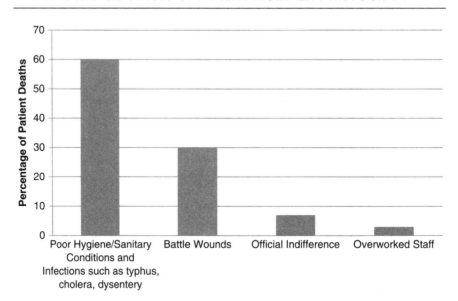

soldiers in India had declined from 69 to 18 per 1,000. She knew that "statistics of a hospital ought to include not only the nominal list of the dead, but the cause of death" as well (Joint Commission on Accreditation of Health-care Organizations [JCAHO] 1999, 146). Today, 150 years after her work, the health care community sees the value of using **outcomes measurements** (data describing a patient's health state) in identifying quality care and cost effectiveness. Nightingale "realized that if judgments of outcomes were to matter, it would require attention to accurate data collection and accurately defined measures" (Batalden and Mohr 1999, 11).

In addition to understanding and exposing cause and effects and promoting outcomes measurements based on creditable data, Nightingale also understood that problems could be caused not by individuals alone but by systems. She understood the structures, processes, and waste in health care organizations; she set standards for staffing. All these ideas are still being discussed in quality management departments today. Many people think they are discovering new ideas, but Nightingale was using these ideas, and most productively, long ago.

Ernest A. Codman

Like Nightingale, Ernest Amory Codman (1869–1940) was a medical reformer who sought to improve medical care by analyzing outcomes, or what he called **end results.** He tracked his patients on end-results cards, noting demographic data, diagnosis, treatment, and outcomes—data that health care organizations are still attempting to accurately collect and analyze today. Codman worked to standardize care and reduce variation in order to create efficiency as well as good outcomes. He was the first physician to promote the study of outcomes and **evidence-based medicine** (making judicious use of the most current research and information to make medical decisions); before Codman, only Florence Nightingale had concerned herself with these ideas.

Codman believed that physicians should be held accountable for the success of their care, and if their patients did not have good outcomes, physicians should question why not and change their practice accordingly. Codman's idea was straightforward: "The common sense notion that *every* hospital should follow *every* patient it treats, long enough to determine whether or not the treatment has been successful, and then to inquire, 'If not, why not?' with a view to preventing similar failures in the future" (Codman 1934, Preface).

The surgeons who were his colleagues at Massachusetts General Hospital were not eager to embrace this level of accountability, and in frustration Codman quit and opened up his own End Result Hospital, where he was able to practice what he preached, using performance measurements to evaluate care and make improvements. This concept of end results was a forerunner of what is today termed *evidence-based medicine.* At his hospital, between 1911 and 1916, of the 337 patients who were discharged, Codman recorded 123 errors. Not only did he record these results but he published them to promote what we now call **transparency** (access to reliable accurate information about care). Codman believed physicians should admit to and learn from their mistakes.

Codman was concerned with the types of medical errors that might prevent good results and developed a classification system for errors: lack of technical skill, poor surgical judgment, and lack of diagnostic skill or failures in equipment. Today we talk about "waste" and "value," concepts that Codman was concerned with decades ago. Today we think of waste as overuse, underuse, misuse of medical services, failure of care coordination, administrative complexity, and fraud (Health Policy Brief 2012). Codman's concept of waste involved unnecessary deaths caused by ill-judged operations or poor diagnoses, functions associated with surgeons. He wanted to use the data accompanying the evaluations to publicly rank surgeons. Unsurprisingly, he was not popular with his peers. Even today, physicians are reluctant to work from standards, claiming that it impinges on their individual judgment and promotes "cookbook" medicine. They prefer the evidence of their experience rather than the recorded experience of others.

A tireless crusader for quality, Codman was instrumental in founding the American College of Surgeons and its Hospital Standardization Program, which later became the Joint Commission on Accreditation of Healthcare Organizations (now called The Joint Commission, TJC), a not-for-profit accrediting agency that evaluates quality of care and patient safety. Codman's ideas are promoted today by government and regulatory agencies (such as the Centers for Medicare and Medicaid Services [CMS] and TJC), as well as private professional groups (e.g., Institute for Healthcare Improvement [IHI] and the Leapfrog Group). Remarkably, a century later, Codman's commonsense approach to the evaluation of care is still not universally accepted by the medical establishment.

William Andrew Shewhart

William Andrew Shewhart (1891–1967), a physicist, engineer, and statistician, is another pioneering quality theorist, known for developing **statistical quality control** (using statistical methods to assess and improve quality) and the Shewhart improvement cycle of **Plan-Do-Study-Act** (PDSA). Employed in industry for Western Electric and Bell Telephone, among others, his work highlighted the importance of reducing variation (i.e., changes) in a process and continuously monitoring that process. What now seems obvious, that variation leads to poor quality, was a new idea with Shewhart.

An example of the importance of standardization could be taken from any arena, not just manufacturing or health care. Think of building a house. If the roof is too small, the rain and snow will come in; if a door is too big, it won't close. We expect no variation in our products, not some of the time but all of the time. We want standardization. But health care quality management professionals today are unable to convince clinicians of the importance of standardization and lack of variation. As Dr. Donald Berwick, president emeritus and senior fellow at the Institute for Healthcare Improvement and the former administrator of the Centers for Medicare and Medicaid Services, admonished many years after standardization was first proposed by Shewhart:

"Professionals need to embrace the scientific control of variation in the service of their patients and themselves" (1991, 1212).

Shewhart described how lack of standardization increased variation and degraded quality, and he framed variation as the result of one of two causes, either assignable (or special) cause variation or chance (or common) cause variation. Significantly, in 1924 he described the first **control chart** for distinguishing between the two (see Chapter 7). Control charts launched the idea of statistical process control and quality improvement. Shewhart said that data contained both signal and noise, and it was important to separate the two. He realized that bringing a process into statistical control where there is only a chance cause of variation would enable accurate predictions of future outcomes as well as be efficient economically; in other words, control would reduce waste and improve quality.

Among Shewhart's goals was to help management make good decisions, based on data rather than subjective experience. To combine creative management with statistical analysis, he developed what he called the Learning and Improvement cycle, now known as the PDSA cycle of quality improvement (see Chapter 6). Shewhart believed that constant (re)evaluation of practice would lead to successful outcomes. He worked with and influenced the thinking of Edward Deming and Joseph Juran, and his concept of statistical control led to the development of the **Six Sigma** improvement process (a data-driven methodology to identify and eliminate defects in a process) later adopted by General Electric under Jack Welch, which transformed that organization.

William Edwards Deming

W. Edwards Deming (1900–1993) was also an engineer and statistician who worked with Shewhart and is often associated with his teachings. He was also a proponent of the PDSA cycle of performance improvement (which Deming called the Shewhart cycle and others call the Deming cycle). He worked in Japan after World War II and had a significant impact on improving that country's devastated manufacturing process.

The Japanese had studied Shewhart's techniques, and after the war, as part of their reconstruction efforts, they looked for an expert to teach them about statistical control. Deming trained Japanese managers and business executives in concepts of quality as well as statistical control. His message was that improving quality would result in decreased costs. He believed that variation caused waste. When Japanese businesses applied Deming's philosophy, they were enormously successful. The result of this success was an international demand for Japanese products. Although Deming never used the term, he is credited with developing Total Quality Management.

Deming encouraged business leaders to think about manufacturing as an interrelated system with a common aim rather than as a series of individual pieces. His philosophy was that when the focus of the organization and top leaders was on quality, quality increased, costs were reduced, and market share increased, but when the focus was primarily on costs, over time, costs would rise and quality would suffer.

According to his obituary published in *The New York Times* (Holusha 1993), when he was brought in to Ford to help explain why the sales numbers of Hondas and Toyotas were superior to Ford's, he said: "Can you blame your competitor for your woes? No. Can you blame the Japanese? No. You did it yourself." He exhorted managers to treat workers like partners and encourage them to identify problems in the workplace without fear of reprisals. Today, in the health care setting, we are still wrestling with issues of fear, reprisals, and problem-solving methods.

DEMING'S PHILOSOPHY OF QUALITY

Deming's philosophy of quality is summarized in what he called a System of Profound Knowledge, which is comprised of four key ideas:

1. Appreciation of a system
2. Understanding variation
3. A theory of knowledge
4. Understanding human behavior and psychology

When Deming was hospitalized and he received inefficient care, he realized that health care organizations had serious problems: There were many treatment delays, the showers didn't work, and so on. He blamed leaders. He saw how hard nurses worked and realized that "the design of this system to reduce unwanted variation in care could only be improved by a leadership that was obviously lacking" (Best and Neuhauser 2005, 311). He wanted organizations to be customer-focused and for leaders to be aware of and meet customer expectations. Today, the CMS has developed patient surveys (Hospital Consumer Assessment of Healthcare Providers and Systems [HCHAPS]) to determine whether customer expectations were met or not.

Avedis Donabedian

Avedis Donabedian (1919–2000) was born in Lebanon to Armenian parents who fled to an Arab village north of Jerusalem. He trained as a physician there before moving to America and teaching in medical schools, among them Harvard and the University of Michigan. Often called the father of health care quality, he was very interested in health services research, especially in assessing quality of care. In *Evaluating the Quality of Medical Care* (written in 1966),

Donabedian discusses the importance of evaluating quality through examining structure, process, and outcome, referred to as the Donabedian model of patient safety. The structure, process, and outcome model remains today the dominant paradigm for evaluating health care quality.

Donabedian adopted and adapted the systems approach of industrial quality theorists to the delivery of health care services. His writings lay out seven "pillars" of quality health care: efficacy, efficiency, optimality, acceptability, legitimacy, equity, and cost. Every one of Donabedian's pillars is being discussed today, sometimes as if it was a novel idea. ·

Donabedian had modern and sophisticated ideas about how to assess quality, discussing in his writings issues related to access to care, the importance of measuring and evaluating quality, the completeness and accuracy of medical records, observer bias, patient satisfaction, and cultural preferences in health care, all still relevant today. However, his thinking about quality in health care was also quite personal. He said:

> Systems awareness and systems design are important for health professionals, but are not enough. They are enabling mechanisms only. It is the ethical dimension of individuals that is essential to a system's success. Ultimately, the secret of quality is love. You have to love your patient, you have to love your profession, you have to love your God. If you have love, you can then work backward to monitor and improve the system. (Mullan 2001, 137)

An excellent quality management program includes internalized caring and compassion for the patient.

Joseph M. Juran

Joseph M. Juran (1904–2008), another influential quality theorist, was an engineer and management consultant who also worked in post–World War II Japan, helping to rebuild the country's economy through improved manufacturing practices. Along with Shewhart and Deming, Juran is considered among the three founders of modern quality improvement. His philosophy involves three managerial processes, sometimes referred to as the "Juran trilogy":

1. Quality planning to meet customer expectations
2. Quality control to ensure that processes are working efficiently
3. Quality improvement to optimize results.

Juran was also the first to apply the **Pareto principle**, developed by the Italian economist Vilfredo Pareto, to quality—the idea that 80 percent of a problem is caused by 20 percent of the causes. Therefore, if improvements were focused on the 20 percent, the results would have big effects.

FIGURE 1.3. MEDICATION ERROR RATE PARETO CHART, JANUARY 2011–JUNE 2011

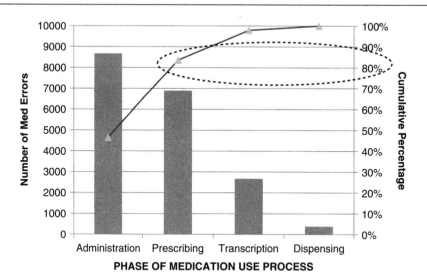

A Pareto chart is basically a bar chart with the highest bar, representing the largest amount of defects or problems, on the left and the shortest bar, representing the fewest problems, on the right (see Figure 1.3). The left vertical axis shows the frequency of the occurrence and the right vertical axis shows the cumulative percentage which is tracked by a line graph.

Figure 1.3 shows that the vast majority of medication errors, in fact 80 percent, occur during the administrative and prescribing phases of the medication use process. Juran was at the forefront of linking quality and cost. One might say that, with a Pareto chart, you know where your buck will return the biggest bang. The chart is useful in prioritizing issues for resource expenditure, in this case improving processes related to medication administration and prescription.

Among Juran's greatest contributions to quality theory was his realization that organizational culture is responsible for the inertia that must be overcome in order to implement change. Juran credited his insight to Margaret Mead's *Cultural Patterns and Technical Change* (1955) (Best & Neuhauser, 2006), which convinced him that only by understanding an organization's cultural barriers to change could change be implemented; change had to conform to the organization's values. Today quality management professionals are still struggling to implement methods to change health care culture to encourage staff to accept and adopt changed practices.

Philip Crosby

Philip Crosby (1926–2001) was a business management expert who contributed to quality theory. His work became popular in the 1970s when American manufactured goods were losing market share to Japanese products because they were superior in quality to American-made products. Crosby is best known for promoting the concept of **zero defects** in a process. In 1979 he published a book, *Quality Is Free*, in which he said that to improve quality, "do it right the first time" (DIRFT), an approach that is surprisingly difficult to implement, as evidenced by unresolved gaps in safety that haunt hospitals today. His writings were popular with the public, especially when he described the cost of poor quality. Crosby, like his contemporary quality theorists, realized that poor quality or good quality was dependent on leaders setting up expectations for quality.

Crosby promoted four fundamental principles of quality:

1. Quality is defined as conformance to product/customer requirements.
2. Quality should involve prevention of errors.
3. The performance standard for quality is zero defects.
4. Quality can be quantified by the price of nonconformance (the cost of non-valued activities).

Issues of conforming to requirements, focus on prevention, zero defects, and understanding the cost of poor quality are still discussed in health care improvement efforts (Creech 1994, 478).

CONTRIBUTIONS OF QUALITY THEORISTS

Florence Nightingale

- Link causes with effects.
- Use data to understand outcomes.
- Analyze problems as flawed systems.

Ernest Codman

- Track end results to understand problems in care.
- Reduce variation to create efficiency.
- Insist that physicians be accountable for the results of their treatments.

William Shewhart

- Use statistical quality control.
- Improve with Plan-Do-Study-Act cycle.
- Monitor variation, which leads to poor quality.
- Understand cause of variation through control charts.

William Deming

- Use statistical quality control.
- Link improved quality with decreased cost.
- Eliminate variation, which causes waste.
- Hold leaders accountable for quality.

Avedis Donabedian

- Analyze structure, process, and outcomes as the basis of quality.
- Maintain the seven pillars of health care quality: efficacy, efficiency, optimality, acceptability, legitimacy, equity, and cost.

Joseph Juran

- Meet customer expectations.
- Link quality and cost.
- Recognize the importance of organizational culture to excellent quality.
- Allocate resources using Pareto chart analysis.

Philip Crosby

- Demand zero defects.
- Focus on error prevention.
- Eliminate variation.
- Link quality and cost.

Quality Management Methodologies

Many methods of managing quality have been proposed and used over the years. Regardless of specifics, they all use data to analyze processes of care and stress effective communication strategies to move information among caregivers and across levels of care.

Total Quality Management

Many of the ideas of prominent quality theorists, such as Crosby, Juran, and Deming, among others, have led to an approach to quality called Total Quality Management (TQM), which shifts the responsibility for quality from a hierarchical and bureaucratic approach to a holistic or decentralized one. TQM is a customer-focused management system that uses data and effective communication techniques to integrate quality into the culture of an organization, congruent with the organization's mission, vision, and goals.

All employees are expected to adopt this customer-focused approach, which targets satisfying customer expectations. If employees are to be empowered to take risks and speak their minds, then there can be no fear of reprisal in the workplace; management and leaders have to support quality efforts and encourage effective communication strategies both among employees and between employees and managers.

TQM stresses processes, which takes inputs from internal or external sources and transforms them, through defined steps, to outputs for customers. Performance measures are used to monitor the process and check for unexpected variation. TQM expects continued assessment and improvement (such as with the PDSA cycle) to meet expectations and lower costs. In addition to leadership commitment, TQM stresses teamwork to realize common objectives of long-term quality improvement.

Continuous Quality Improvement

Continuous Quality Improvement (CQI) is a general theory of quality based on the work of Shewhart, Deming, and Juran. Although the principles of CQI predate these theorists, their recognition of the importance of applying the scientific method to quality contributed to the theory.

In 1989, Dr. Brent James published *Quality Management for Health Care Delivery*, which summarized a multihospital initiative to develop quality monitoring and management tools. He said a successful quality improvement model should ask three questions:

1. Are we doing the right things?
2. Are we doing things right?
3. How can we be certain that it's done right the first time, every time? (13)

These fundamental questions are still being asked today, and attempts to answer these questions seem to be getting ever more complicated. In order to achieve a system that delivers high-quality care and appropriately controls expenses, two principles have to be central:

1. Eliminate inappropriate variation.
2. Document continuous improvements.

Both these principles depend on accurate measurements and a valid database to provide the groundwork for quality management. In addition, health professionals need to translate theory into practice to transform the hospital culture so that quality management theory is internalized and recognized as being more than simply compliance with regulatory standards.

DEFINING QUALITY TERMS

It may be useful to distinguish among terms often used in discussions of quality: *quality assurance, quality control, quality improvement*, and *quality management*.

- *Quality assurance* (QA) is focused on ensuring that the product—in this case, the delivery of health care services—is meeting expectations through the identification of problems or defects in the system, developing solutions, and monitoring the effectiveness of the solutions. QA is used widely by state and federal regulatory agencies, such as state departments of health and The Joint Commission, to reinforce identifying problems in the delivery of care and developing corrective actions to improve them. QA is also focused on compliance with regulatory expectations.
- *Quality control* (QC), often used interchangeably with quality assurance, is a system that monitors the desired level of quality to ensure that specific goals or criteria are met through continuous inspection and that makes corrections when problems are identified.
- *Quality improvement* (QI) is aimed at performance improvements through assessing current conditions and developing strategies for improvements. Unlike QA, which identifies problems, QI is focused on identifying common causes and on processes that require improvements rather than outcomes. The goal is to prevent errors rather than repair them. For example, QA might investigate a patient's death by conducting a review of the patient's record to identify any gaps in care. QI would examine all the records of all mortality in a defined population and identify commonalities that could be the focus of improvement efforts.
- *Quality management* (QM) is an organization-wide philosophy that oversees activities that have an impact on ensuring the excellence of processes, policies, and practices. The focus is on the prevention of errors, the use of data-driven decision making, and continuous performance improvement. QM depends on quality planning, QC, QA, and QI to evaluate and achieve consistent quality standards, using a deliberate methodology to monitor and effect change. QM professionals need to understand organizational processes and statistical analytics.

Organizations Making an Impact on Quality and Safety Standards

Many agencies, both governmental and private, have had an impact on improving patient safety, especially since media attention has brought gaps in safety to the attention of the public. The organizations discussed next have driven changed practices and really forced health care organizations to better assess and improve their quality and safety.

Institute of Medicine

The IOM is a nonprofit, nongovernmental advisory agency that is part of the National Academy of Sciences. Although founded by Congress in 1970, it is an independent organization, comprised of volunteer experts and scientists, with the mission of advising policy makers, professionals, and health and science leaders about improving the nation's health.

Highly publicized incidents of patients dying in well respected health care institutions spurred the IOM to explore issues related to patient safety. The result was the 1999 report, *To Err Is Human: Building a Safer Health System* (edited by Kohn, Corrigan, and Donaldson). This report stated that not only is health care of poor quality but it is actually dangerous. As many as 98,000 people die in hospitals every year due to medical errors, a startling observation that brought patient safety to the forefront of national attention. That staggering number revealed to the public that something was seriously broken in our health care system. The IOM made these recommendations to respond to what was obviously a crisis in health care delivery:

1. Improve leaders and knowledge.
2. Identify and learn from errors.
3. Set performance standards and expectations for safety.
4. Implement safety systems in health care organizations.

In 2001, the Committee on Quality of Health Care in America of the IOM published another report, *Crossing the Quality Chasm: A New Health System for the 21st Century*, which recommended a redesign of the American health care system, offering performance expectations; direction for policy makers and health care leaders; guidance for improving the patient-physician relationship; suggestions as to how to align efficiency, cost savings, and quality; and other innovations to try to close the quality gap or, rather, the quality chasm. The report proposed six aims for improvement, saying health care should be: safe, efficient, effective, patient-centered, timely, and equitable. Although none of these concepts is new, the publicity surrounding these recommendations was a powerful motivator for health systems to examine their delivery systems. The IOM stressed that performance standards needed to be set to ensure improved safety.

Unfortunately, even with this spur to action, health care has not changed very much, and patient safety and efficiency of services are still poor. Improvements have been glacially slow in coming. In fact, a 2013 study in the *Journal of Patient Safety* estimates that as many as 440,000 patient deaths a year are caused by preventable medical errors (J. James 2013). It is not obvious why health care has resisted meaningful change. Whether due to a lack of professional oversight, unwillingness of leaders to invest resources in improving and sustaining safe practices, reluctance of clinicians to value **quality data**, or fear of malpractice suits, medical care remains fragmented, highly individualized, costly—and frequently unsafe.

In 2006, the IOM published yet another report, sponsored by the CMS, on the prevalence and cost of preventable medication errors, and outlined a national agenda to reduce and prevent them. The report, titled *Preventing Medication Errors*, found that medication errors are surprisingly common and costly, estimating that conservatively over 1.5 million preventable adverse drug events (ADEs) occur in the United States each year, with an annual cost of $887 million for treating ADEs in the Medicare population alone.

To improve this situation, the report recommends changing the way health care does business. Physicians, caregivers, pharmacists, and patients have to improve communication. The paternalistic tradition of "doctor knows best" and patient knows nothing has to be transformed so that physicians listen to patients and educate them about their medications, informing them "about the risks, contraindications, and possible side effects of the medications they are taking and what to do if they experience a side effect" (http://iom .nationalacademies.org/~/media/Files/Report%20Files/2006/Preventing-Medication-Errors-Quality-Chasm-Series/medicationerrorsnew.ashx).

The second step the report recommends is to make use of information technology (IT) in prescribing and dispensing medications and to put effective monitoring programs in place to track the incidence of ADEs and improvements. The third recommendation of the report is to improve packaging and labeling of medications to avoid look-alike, sound-alike medications that could be easily confused. These few reasonable changes do not seem difficult to implement or even technologically expensive and would increase the quality and safety of patient care; yet many organizations have not fully implemented these recommendations.

The Joint Commission

TJC is a nonprofit accrediting agency that has made a huge impact on improving patient safety by defining standards of care and surveying hospitals to assess whether they attain those standards. Over the years, TJC has articulated specific goals for patient safety and developed standards of care that need to be met for accreditation. Its mission is to continuously improve health care by evaluating and inspiring health care organizations to provide safe and effective care of high quality and value.

The organization has its roots in the work of Ernest Codman's concept of "end results" and his proposal that hospitals adhere to specific standards. As early as 1917, the American College of Surgeons (ACS) developed a one-page document called *Minimum Standard for Hospitals.* One year later, in 1918, when the ACS surveyed hospitals, only 89 of 692 hospitals met the minimum safety standards outlined in the document (http://www.employeescreen.com/wp-content/uploads/sites/6/joint_commission_history.pdf).

By 1951, the ACS was joined by other professional groups (the American College of Physicians, the American Hospital Association, the American Medical Association, and the Canadian Medical Association) to create the Joint Commission on Accreditation of Hospitals as an independent, not-for-profit accrediting organization. By the 1960s, accreditation by TJC was necessary in order to participate in Medicare and Medicaid programs. Few health care organizations could afford to ignore the Joint Commission on Accreditation of Hospitals' standards for accreditation, and efforts were made to comply. In 1987, the name of the organization was changed to the Joint Commission on Accreditation of Healthcare Organizations (JCAHO) to reflect its expanded scope, which included standards for home care agencies, managed care groups, ambulatory care, and laboratory certification, among others, and in 2007, the organization was renamed The Joint Commission (TJC).

Today TJC accredits over 20,000 health care organizations and publishes an annual report identifying hospitals that attain excellent standards. It also reports hospitals that use evidence-based standards that result in excellent patient outcomes based on performance measurements. TJC also rates top-performing hospitals on key quality measures for specified conditions, such as heart attack, heart failure, pneumonia, surgical care, children's asthma, inpatient psychiatric services, stroke and venous thromboembolism. Organizations and patient groups take these ratings very seriously.

In 2002, TJC established its National Patient Safety Goals (NPSGs) program, which targets specific areas of concern with regard to patient safety. The goals identify areas in which patient safety is vulnerable, such as the spread of infection due to multidrug-resistant organisms, catheter-related bloodstream infections, and surgical site infections. Solutions to these problems are recommended, based on evidence.

The NPSGs' focus on prevention efforts are fueled by the public's heightened awareness of medical errors. Because issues of safety are part of a national effort to improve health care, and organizations are required to measure improved outcomes and preventive efforts for accreditation, the goals have an impact. Both TJC and the CMS require that the NPSGs be met. Specific sets of NPSGs have been defined by these two organizations for different types of health care organizations: hospitals, long-term care facilities, behavioral health organizations, laboratories, networks, ambulatory centers, and office-based surgical centers.

Other TJC standards directly address the patient experience. For example, TJC has pain assessment and management standards to deal with chronic or acute pain. These standards apply to different kinds of health care organizations: ambulatory care facilities, behavioral health care organizations, critical access hospitals, home care providers, hospitals, office-based surgery practices, and long-term care providers. The standards require that patients be asked about their pain, and if appropriate, care and treatment should be provided. Patients should be screened initially and then on an ongoing basis for pain and should be educated about pain management.

In 2010, the CMS determined that it would oversee TJC's accreditation.

NATIONAL PATIENT SAFETY GOALS

The following list illustrates the kinds of problems the 2013 Hospital National Patient Safety Goals address and their suggested solutions:

Identify Patients Correctly

- Use at least two ways to identify patients. For example, patient name and date of birth.

Improve Staff Communication

- Get important test results to the right staff person on time.

Use Medicines Safely

- Label medicines that are not labeled (in syringes, cups, and basins).
- Take extra care with patients on blood thinning medications.
- Record and transfer information about patient medications.
- Make sure the patient knows which medicines to take at home.

Prevent Infection

- Follow hand hygiene guidelines from the Centers for Disease Control or World Health Organization.
- Use proven guidelines (evidence-based standards) to prevent infections after surgery, such as from catheters and from central lines.

Identify Patient Safety Risks

- Find out which patients are most likely to attempt suicide.

Prevent Mistakes in Surgery

- Make sure that the correct surgery is done on the correct patient at the correct place on the patient's body.
- Mark the correct place on the patients' body where the surgery is to be done.
- Pause before the surgery (time out) to ensure that a mistake is not being made.

Source: http://www.jointcommission.org/assets/1/6/2016_NPSG_HAP_ER.pdf

Centers for Medicare and Medicaid Services

The CMS is the government agency that reimburses hospitals for patients enrolled in the Medicare and Medicaid programs. Hoping to encourage health care organizations to participate in transparent quality and patient safety initiatives, the CMS is using its clout as the primary payer for health care services to offer financial incentives to hospitals that successfully report their compliance with specific quality measures. Quality measures can help health care organizations and consumers assess how well an organization provides care to its patients. These measures are based on scientific evidence and often reflect professional guidelines and established standards of care.

Organizations that do not report quality measures are penalized with reduced reimbursement. Oversight by the government agency that effectively holds the purse strings is among the most effective driving force for improved quality and changing practices that consumers have. Knowing that quality measures are being made available to the curious, increasingly educated, and cynical consumer of health care is helping to create accountability and further transparency of information.

Hospital Compare

The measures collected enable the CMS to track and trend patient safety issues over time and to publicly report quality of care indicators on their website. This resource for health care consumers is: www.hospitalcompare.hhs.gov. Hospital Compare, as this program is called, enables consumers to compare multiple hospitals on performance measures related to heart attack, heart failure, pneumonia, surgery, and other conditions.

It also displays information regarding 30-day mortality for heart attack and heart failure and mortality rates for pneumonia. Other additions include information on outpatient facilities, emergency departments, surgical process measures, as well as 30-day readmission measures for heart attack, heart failure, and pneumonia patients. Readmission rates serve as both a quality measure and a measure of organizational efficiency. Organizations are encouraged to investigate why patients return within 30 days. Was their discharge premature, was the care inadequate, or was the cause due to other factors?

Figure 1.4 shows a webpage from the Hospital Compare website that compares two hospitals for unplanned readmission for heart failure patients. Hospital A has more readmissions than the national average rate of 23 percent. Hospital B is just at the average. Neither hospital is below average, and it should be noted that the average is still quite high. If you or a member of your family were being treated for heart failure, you might want to find a hospital in the "green" zone—that is, one that performs better than the national average.

FIGURE 1.4. HOSPITAL COMPARE WEBPAGE FOR UNPLANNED READMISSIONS

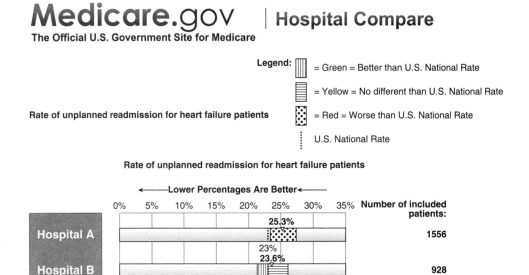

U.S. national rate of unplanned readmission for heart failure patients = 23.0%

Figure 1.5 shows another type of graphical information available to consumers, the "Average time patients spent in the emergency department before they were seen by a healthcare professional." The data show the number of minutes of three hospitals as well as the state average and the national average. If you live in an area with several hospitals, you might want to know this information. In an emergency, you would want to be seen quickly and the graph shows that hospital A has a shorter waiting time than hospital B or C.

Not only does the CMS publish information about process of care measures as part of Hospital Compare, but it has added a patient experience survey called Hospital Consumer Assessment of Healthcare Providers and Systems (HCAHPS). HCAHPS uses a standardized survey and collects and reports reliable data on the patient experience, such as noisiness, and perspective on hospital care, such as effective communication (see Chapter 4).

Patient Education

The CMS also promotes patient education by requiring hospitals to devise processes for clear communication about health status and care. For example, the CMS and TJC require documentation that patients who smoke and have

FIGURE 1.5. HOSPITAL COMPARE FOR WAITING TIMES

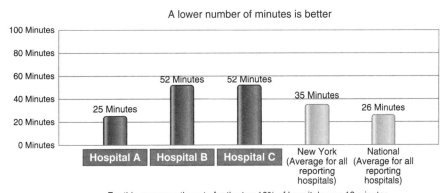

Medicare.gov | Hospital Compare
The Official U.S. Government Site for Medicare

Average time patient spent in the emergency department, before they were seen by a healthcare professional

A lower number of minutes is better

For this measure, the rate for the top 10% of hospitals was 13 minutes.

specific conditions (e.g., heart attack, pneumonia) are supposed to receive counseling about smoking cessation during their hospitalization. It would seem only common sense that patients who smoke receive cessation counseling because it is well known that smoking results in poor health outcomes. National guidelines also recommend inpatient education because research shows that educated patients are more likely than uneducated patients to stop smoking (Keating 2016). Yet, despite common sense, experience, and guidelines, few hospitals have complied with this recommendation. Therefore, the government decided to get involved and reward compliant hospitals with financial incentives to improve care.

Pay for Performance

In response to the IOM's reports (Committee on Quality of Health Care in America, IOM 2001; Kohn et al. 1999) on the poor quality and high cost of care, the CMS launched the pay-for-performance (P4P) initiative as part of its breakthrough initiatives to change the way care is delivered and improve the quality and efficiency of care. The CMS has defined the goal of P4P: to provide the right care for the right patient every time. "Right" care is based on the IOM definition of providing patients with care that is safe, efficient, effective, patient-centered, timely, and equitable.

P4P is a new model for financing health care, breaking with the traditional fee-for-service–based payment, which reimburses providers for what was done *to* the patient. P4P refocuses the payment model to reimburse providers based on what was done *for* the patient. Providers who provide their patients with better outcomes would be financially rewarded; providers would be penalized for poor performance and poor outcomes, such as preventable complications or medical errors. The P4P program attempts to use the payment structure for medical care to improve quality of care and reduce costs (see Chapter 2).

Never Events

In yet another effort to improve poor clinical performance, the CMS has attached a financial consequence to never events, which are defined as serious and preventable events (e.g., wrong-site surgery, retained foreign object) that should never occur. By making organizations effectively pay for poor-quality care, the CMS is hoping to force providers to develop methods to control preventable problems. The never event initiative has the further advantage of involving the chief financial officer in quality metrics for clinical care and improvement efforts. Money is a powerful incentive to improve. In addition to financial consequences, because never events are publicly reported, there are public relations and market share consequences as the public becomes aware of which organizations have not eliminated never events.

In collaboration with other organizations, such as the National Quality Forum (NQF), the Centers for Disease Control and Prevention, the Federal Drug Administration, the Agency for Healthcare Research and Quality (AHRQ), the CMS has defined a list of errors and mistakes that should never happen. The list of never events is divided into six categories: surgical, product or device, patient protection, care management, environment, and criminal. Examples include: medication errors, hospital-acquired pressure injuries, hospital-acquired infections, patient falls, postoperative complications, wrong-site surgery, foreign object retained after surgery, blood incompatibility, and many others. A complete list of never events can be found on the AHRQ website at http://psnet.ahrq.gov/primer.aspx?primerID=3.

Institute for Healthcare Improvement

The IHI is an independent, not-for-profit organization dedicated to optimizing health care delivery through accelerating improvements. It focuses on building a will for change, encouraging new ideas for improvements, and working with health systems to put new ideas into action. Its goal is to help to close the quality "chasm" identified by the IOM (Committee on Quality of Health Care in America, IOM 2001) through stressing the importance of quality improvement not only as an approach for ensuring good care but also as a business strategy. Good care is cost effective; poor care is expensive.

The IHI has initiated important projects that many health care organizations have adopted. Transforming Care at the Bedside is one such plan that focuses on improving the discharge process and the transition to home in order to reduce or avoid readmission. Another project measures patient harm through reviewing patient records for "triggers" (i.e., clues to identifying patients who have experienced adverse events). Many hospitals now call multidisciplinary Rapid Response Teams to the bedside when a patient's condition deteriorates, a practice that the IHI supports. The IHI also supports the widespread deployment of medication reconciliation plans at all transition points in care. These, and other commonsense ideas, have made an impact on the quality and safety of inpatient care.

The IHI developed a framework for optimizing health system performance called the Triple Aim initiative. The three aims, which remain a constant challenge, are to:

1. Improve the patient experience and satisfaction.
2. Improve the health of populations.
3. Reduce the cost of health care.

The IHI is working with volunteer organizations across the United States to implement these goals.

Sepsis, a serious, often deadly, medical condition characterized by an inflammatory state caused by severe infection, has been targeted by the IHI for improvements. Mortality rates for the approximately 750,000 new sepsis cases diagnosed each year is 25 percent, or 210,000 patients (Resar et al. 2012). The IHI is hoping to reduce this number by encouraging health care organizations to develop processes for early detection and to implement standardized evidence-based practices. To promote use of evidence-based practice guidelines, the IHI has developed the "Severe Sepsis Bundle," which is a series of treatments, based on evidence, that when implemented as a group (or bundle) will improve outcomes.

The **bundle** concept was developed in 2001 (Resar et al. 2012) to improve intensive care unit care through enhancing teamwork and communication for multidisciplinary teams. Improvements were significant, and the bundle concept was adapted to other high-volume areas of concern.

Agency for Health Research and Quality

The mission of the AHRQ, which is part of the U.S. Department of Health and Human Services, is to improve the quality and safety of health care and the efficiency and effectiveness of health care services. Its charge covers a wide range of expertise, including gathering data on the cost and use of health care services, acquiring information about the results of medical treatments, defining efforts to promote quality and safety, reducing medical errors, using information technology effectively, developing prevention initiatives, and educating patients about their health care options.

In 2004, the AHRQ began a series of reports called *Closing the Quality Gap: A Critical Analysis of Quality Improvement Strategies* (Shojania, K. G., et al. 2004); these reports evaluate quality strategies related to chronic conditions and practice areas. Examples of topics the reports include information about bundled payments, health disparities, effectiveness of medication adherence interventions, and improving palliative care, among many others. Quality measures are developed, based on these reports, as are educational materials and tools and guidelines for care. The CMS adopted the Patient Safety and Quality Indicators developed by the AHRQ that focus on preventable complications, such as unnecessary death and surgical wound infections, for inpatient hospitalizations for its report on hospital performance. The AHRQ is also concerned with prevention and has developed initiatives, such as the Patient-Centered Medical Home model of care (see Chapter 2), which focuses on coordinating primary care across the health care system and ensuring that the care is comprehensive and accessible to the population served.

The AHRQ supports various quality improvement and patient safety initiatives. Some of the safety initiatives sponsored by the AHRQ include the administration of the Patient Safety and Quality Improvement Act of 2005, which collects, analyzes, and provides feedback to providers about patient safety events. Quality indicators measure health care quality and track changes over time. The organization publishes an annual National Healthcare Quality Report that measures effectiveness, safety, timeliness and efficiency of care. Another initiative, **TeamSTEPPS** (Team Strategies and Tools to Enhance Performance and Patient Safety), is an evidenced-based system designed to improve communication and teamwork skills among health care providers. Another tool, a patient safety culture assessment tool, is used by hospitals, nursing homes, and medical offices to evaluate their patient safety culture and assess the impact of interventions to improve quality and safety.

The AHRQ also has a medical research component. By synthesizing scientific evidence for conditions that are high volume and important to the Medicare and Medicaid programs, this component provides evidence-based guidelines on treatments that have proven most effective. Patient-centered outcomes research compares drugs, surgeries, and different health care delivery options so that patients and their families can evaluate options and risks by going to the website: http://www.ahrq.gov/health-care-information/topics/topic-patientcentered-outcomes-research. Another program, the Centers for Education and Research on Therapeutics, conducts research about drugs and medical devices and provides education about them.

IT activities that improve decision making for health care providers and the quality and safety of medication management are also supported by the AHRQ. Other initiatives involve ensuring that there is value to health services. The Medical Expenditure Panel Survey (http://meps.ahrq.gov/mepsweb/) is the only national source of data about how Americans use services, how frequently, and at what cost.

National Quality Forum

In 1999, the President's Advisory Commission on Consumer Protection and Quality in the Health Care Industry recommended that a forum for quality measurement and reporting be established as a combined effort of public and private sectors. The National Quality Forum (NQF), a nonprofit public service coalition of purchasers, providers, hospitals, and quality improvement organizations, was established in response to that recommendation and charged with developing a plan for implementing quality measurements, including data collection and reporting standards. The NQF would also endorse measures and ensure that these quality measurements and performance data were accessible to the public.

The NQF reviews and recommends standardized health care performance measures; the measures are used to evaluate organizational structure, processes and outcomes of care as well as patient perceptions about their care. The NQF recommends preferred practices that can lead to improved outcomes and develops frameworks for organizing practices. Data from performance measures are used for public reporting, such as for the CMS Hospital Compare. The data also support P4P initiatives, where excellent performance receives financial rewards and poor performance receives less reimbursement for certain conditions acquired during a patient's hospital stay. The NQF was instrumental in defining for the CMS which preventable errors should be considered never events and not reimbursed. In the future, the NQF will recommend quality measures for payment and accountability programs.

The Leapfrog Group

Established in 2000, the Leapfrog Group was formed as a response to the 1999 report *To Err Is Human*, which not only focused attention on the high death rate from preventable medical errors but also recommended that large employers use their enormous purchasing power to try to influence the quality, safety, and value of health care. Employers who spend billions of dollars on providing their employees with health care wanted some control—a way to assess whether their investment was returning value. A group of large corporations, including General Motors, IBM, and Toyota, among others, joined forces to find a way to use their influence; they realized that "leaps" forward could be attained by rewarding hospitals that were able to implement significant safety and quality improvements. Today the Leapfrog Group is comprised of a coalition of 65 employers.

The group developed a survey to compare hospital performance on national standards of safety, quality, and efficiency. Through the transparent reporting of the results of the Leapfrog Hospital Quality and Safety Survey, vast numbers of employees—over 37 million—can evaluate the safety, quality, and efficiency of different hospitals and make informed choices about where to spend their health care dollars. Leapfrog recommends that employees choose hospitals that meet four criteria, proven to reduce error and promote quality and safety:

1. The use of computer physician order entry for medication orders to reduce prescribing errors
2. The use of evidence-based hospital referrals, which use scientific criteria, such as volume of procedures performed and outcome data
3. The use of intensivists, specially trained physicians, in intensive care units
4. A high Safe Practices Score reflecting adherence to procedures and practices recommended by the NQF and AHRQ

The Leapfrog Group believes that with these criteria, preventable medical mistakes will be significantly reduced.

The Leapfrog Group publicly reports Hospital Safety Scores based on CMS data and its own survey (http://www.hospitalsafetyscore.org/) that ranks hospitals on 26 measures of safety and uses incentives to reward hospitals that perform the best. The project, launched in 2012, assigns a letter grade to hospitals based on how well they protect patients from accidents, injuries, and errors. Over 2,600 hospitals across the country have been assigned a grade. The Hospital Safety Score is considered a standard measure of patient safety and has broad media approval, endorsed by the *Wall Street Journal*, *USA Today*, and the *AARP* magazine.

Data: The Foundation of Quality Management

The quality theorists, methodologies, and organizations reviewed in this chapter have all referred to data as the foundation of monitoring safety and quality of care. In this section, some of the fundamentals of quality data are introduced.

The quality theorist Edwards Deming is said to have quipped: "In God we trust. Everyone else has to use data." The reason data are critical to evaluating care is that with data, there is some objective standardization, a way to quantify and define the concept of "good" care or "quality" care. How else could an administrator or caregiver offer evidence that the delivery of care or the hospital services are excellent and responsive to patient expectations? Of course, a person could say "Trust me, I know my business," but today's health care customers are sophisticated enough to want more than paternalistic reassurance. By using data, the assessment of processes, services, outcomes and experience can be objective and effectively communicated.

Health care is awash in information, in numbers, and in data—about organizational processes, clinical processes, regulatory processes, financial information, patient information, staff information, organization-specific information, national information, and so on. But simply having data does not ensure a better understanding of processes or outcomes. The vast amount of data has to be organized and analyzed before it is meaningful and useful.

Case Example: Falls

Patient falls can be used as an example. Patient falls can result in fractures, surgery, or other problems; patients who fall often complain and sometimes institute lawsuits against the organization. Falls may also result in longer length of stay (LOS) which has financial implications to the health organization. Much information about falls is available. Professionals can retrieve data about prevalence of falls (how many people fall during a specified time period), outcomes of the falls (injuries), treatment that was required (surgery, medications), cost of the falls to the organization, and so on. Falls in one organization can be compared to falls in others. Information about the patients who fall, their ages, diagnoses, and risk factors, and about staffing ratios, times of day of falls, and medications associated with falls can be gathered and analyzed.

The issue is what to do with all this available information. When information is collected in a focused way with a question to answer (why are patients falling?) or a hypothesis to test (elderly patients on diuretics fall more than elderly patients not on diuretics), the data being gathered are quality data. The main reason to gather quality data is to evaluate whether improvements are necessary and what interventions might be effective to mitigate a problem. Those determinations cannot be made unless the causes, dimensions, and scope of the problem are known. There is a saying in quality circles: You can't manage until you measure. Information is key to performance improvement, which requires data specifically focused on specific improvement goals. If data collection efforts are not tailored to specific issues, the result may be a great deal of information that clouds the issue rather than sheds light on it.

Once the problem is defined, the data collection efforts can be focused and finely tuned. If data show that 10 patients fall during a month on a specific unit, how should this result be interpreted? Is 10 an acceptable number, or is it an indication of a flawed process? In order to decide whether this number is acceptable, compare it to the total number of patients on the unit. If the unit consists of 10 patients and 10 patients fall (100 percent), there is a serious problem. If the unit contains 100 patients and 10 fall (10 percent), that is less serious but perhaps still requires some investigation.

Quality Indicator

In other words, rather than a simple raw count of the number of falls, you need a percentage to better define the scope of the problem. Being a fraction, a percentage allows you to capture information about the incidence of the problem (how many people fall?) in the **numerator**, compared to the number of people who had the opportunity to fall (the number of [elderly] patients on the unit) in the **denominator**. This percentage is a quality indicator, indicating the scope of the problem. When you define, collect, and examine information with a specific purpose, you are developing a quality indicator.

The numerator and denominator of the quality indicator can be defined to examine or explore a problem very specifically. For example, if the improvement effort is focused on falls that resulted in hip fractures in patients who were 85 or older, that population would be the numerator. Or the number of patients over 85 who fell and had resulting hip fractures and who were on diuretics can be counted as the numerator. The specific population of interest defines the numerator; the general population from which the numerator comes is the denominator. In this case, the denominator represents those patients over 85 who had the opportunity to fall (see Figure 1.6).

Barriers to Using Quality Data to Assess Care

Although it sounds eminently sensible to collect information using quality measures, it is a relatively new conceptualization of how to assess care. The move toward using objective information for decision making has been slow. Numbers that reveal poor outcomes are interpreted as failures rather than opportunities for improvement, and few professionals want to admit to failure. When faced with data that reveal poor outcomes, physicians often question the accuracy of the data, the competency of the coders, the appropriateness of the risk adjustment, and so on, rather than accept the numbers and try to improve the process and outcomes.

In decades past, physicians evaluated the delivery of care, discussing problems in mortality and morbidity (M&M) conferences. If a patient died, or if the mortality rate or any other problem was at a certain level, the medical literature was reviewed to see if that level was appropriate for a specific condition. Sometimes issues of competency may have been addressed; sometimes the mortality was accepted as part of the natural progression of the disease.

M&M methods do not readily result in quality management or performance improvement initiatives because there is little interest in analyzing the population with the high mortality, understanding the patient characteristics,

FIGURE 1.6. QUALITY INDICATOR

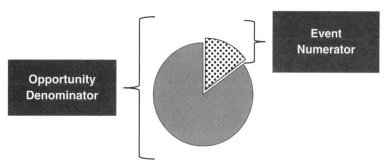

Numerator	The specific population that you are interested in; the Event (the number of patients over 85 who fell, had hip fracture, and were on diuretics)
Denominator	The entire population from which you are collecting information; the Opportunity (the number of patients over 85)
Quality Indicator	$\dfrac{\text{Event or Numerator}}{\text{Opportunity or Denominator}}$
Rate	$\dfrac{\text{Numerator}}{\text{Denominator}} \times 100$

reviewing the processes of care that might have led to the mortality, or developing measures in order to review the mortality rates over time. In terms of indicators, physicians may have discussed the numerator, but rarely would the denominator be discussed. Little effort was made to introduce, develop, and implement improvement processes. Patients were individuals who were cared for by individual physicians. Aggregating information about patient populations in order to improve patient safety is a recent development, an outgrowth of the 1999 IOM report on preventable medical errors.

Case Example: Cardiac Surgery Mortality

Often an organization is comfortable continuing its care practices and is not looking to change. However, if an external agency reviews the care provided and ranks it as poor, that shakes things up. For example, New York State was among the first to publish data about mortality rates for cardiac surgery. One of the flagship hospitals in the health care system in which we work was reported to have a higher mortality rate than comparable hospitals. Needless to say, such publicity is not good for business, and the governing board of trustees and the chief executive wanted to understand what was going on and then take steps to remediate the situation.

When questioned about the high mortality rates, the medical staff gave the kinds of responses that they had been giving for years: Their patients were sicker than patients at other hospitals and therefore at higher risk for dying. The chief executive and the governing board weren't satisfied with that explanation and charged the quality management department with analyzing the situation.

The New York State mortality data introduced new ways of understanding data. The data were **risk-adjusted**, a very important concept. *Risk adjustment* refers to a complex statistical process that adjusts for variation among patients in order to account for differences in the patient population. Risk adjusting allows for fair and accurate comparisons of patient outcomes across organizations. By risk adjusting the cardiac mortality via a statewide cardiac advisory group, physicians could no longer assert that their patients were sicker than others as a reason for a higher mortality rate. By normalizing the population, new explanations for unexpected mortality could be formulated. As physicians became more comfortable looking at published data and learned to respect and trust the quality management department, performance improvement efforts could be undertaken to try to lower the high mortality rate.

Investigating the cause of the high mortality rate in the hospital and coupling the New York State data with available administrative data, the fact that many cardiac mortalities were associated with a secondary diagnosis of sternal wound infection or sepsis was uncovered. Patients who had had emergency surgery, had bleeding (when patients have planned surgery, often they stop taking blood thinners, but emergency patients had no warning and so remained on their blood-thinning medication), had prolonged hospital stays, and were often readmitted. Once the source of the problem was understood, solutions could be implemented to alleviate the problem: Clotting medication was administered to emergency surgery patients. Two years later the Department of Health reported that the hospital mortality rate was the lowest in the state. Administrators and physicians saw the tremendous value of using data to analyze patient outcomes.

Risk-adjusted data has made a difference in promoting changed practices. The government and private agencies dedicated to improving health care and patient safety have made a difference in spurring organizations to change. Quality management, quality metrics, and quality methodologies have become the foundation of performance improvements.

Summary

Quality management has evolved over time, with prominent health care and quality theorists contributing to improving patient safety and performance. Familiarity with the foundations of quality offers perspective on the changes being implemented in the reform environment. This chapter introduces:

- the contributions of quality theorists to quality management
- the basics of quality management methodologies
- the governmental, regulatory, and private organizations that are changing the way health care organizations monitor safety and improve care
- several examples of how quality data can be used to improve performance and encourage changed practices

Key Terms

bundle, control chart, denominator, end results, evidence-based medicine, numerator, outcomes measurements, Pareto principle, Plan-Do-Study-Act, quality data, risk-adjusted, Six Sigma, statistical quality control, TeamSTEPPS, transparency, zero defects

Quality Concepts in Action

The occurrence of never events in a hospital setting is a marker of poor care and poor processes and will have negative financial repercussions for the organization. As a hospital administrator or nurse manager, how would you react to reports of never events? Would you:

- challenge the data and defend the care as appropriate?
- implement new programs in the hope of improvement?
- focus on prevention to avoid the occurrence of never events?
- punish the offending staff members?
- hire new staff to combat never events?

Defend your position and explain what specific steps you would take and why.

References

Batalden, P. B., and J. J. Mohr. 1999. "An Invitation from Florence Nightingale: Come Learn about Improving Health Care." In Joint Commission on Accreditation of Healthcare Organizations, *Florence Nightingale: Measuring Hospital Care Outcomes.* Oakbrook Terrace, IL: 11–16.

Best, M., and D. Neuhauser. 2005. "W. Edwards Deming: Father of Quality Management, Patient and Composer." *Quality and Safety in Health Care* 14: 310–312.

Best, M., and D. Neuhauser. 2006. "Joseph Juran: Overcoming Resistance to Organisational Change." *Quality and Safety in Health Care* 15 (5): 380–382.

Codman, E. A. 1934. *The Shoulder: Rupture of the Supraspinatus Tendon and Other Lesions in or about the Subacromial Bursa.* Boston: Thomas Todd.

Committee on Quality of Health Care in America, Institute of Medicine. 2001. *Crossing the Quality Chasm: A New Health System for the 21st Century.* Washington, DC: National Academy Press.

Creech, B. 1994. *The Five Pillars of TQM: How to Make Total Quality Management Work for You.* New York: Truman Talley Books.

Crosby, P. 1979. *Quality Is Free.* New York: McGraw-Hill.

Donabedian, A. 2005. "Evaluating the Quality of Medical Care." *Milbank Quarterly* 83 (4): 691–729.

Health Policy Brief. 2012, December 13. "Reducing Waste in Health Care." *Health Affairs.*

Holusha, John. 1993, December 21. "W. Edwards Deming, Expert on Business Management, Dies at 93." *New York Times.*

Institute of Medicine of the National Academies. 2006. *Preventing Medication Errors: Quality Chasm Series.* http://www.nationalacademies.org/hmd/Reports/2006/Preventing-Medication-Errors-Quality-Chasm-Series.aspx

James, B. C. 1989. *Quality Management for Health Care Delivery.* Chicago: Hospital Research and Educational Trust of the American Hospital Association.

James, J. 2013. "A New, Evidence-based Estimate of Patient Harms Associated with Hospital Care." *Journal of Patient Safety* 9 (3): 122–128.

Joint Commission on Accreditation of Healthcare Organizations. 1999. *Florence Nightingale: Measuring Hospital Care Outcomes.* Oakbrook Terrace, IL: Author.

Keating, S. 2016 . "Presurgical Tobacco Cessation Counseling." *American Journal of Nursing* 116 (3): 11.

Kohn, K. T., J. M. Corrigan, and M. S. Donaldson, eds. 1999. *To Err Is Human: Building a Safer Health System.* Washington, DC: National Academies Press.

Lohr, K. N., ed. 1990. *Medicare: A Strategy for Quality Assurance*, Vol. 1. Washington, DC: National Academies Press.

Mead, M. 1955. *Cultural Patterns and Technical Change.* Geneva: UNESCO.

Mullan, F. 2001. "A Founder of Quality Assessment Encounters a Troubled System Firsthand. *Health Affairs* 20: 137–141.

Resar, R., F. A. Griffin, C. Haraden, and T. W. Nolan. 2012. *Using Care Bundles to Improve Health Care Quality.* IHI Innovation Series White Paper. Cambridge, MA: Institute for Healthcare Improvement.

Shojania, K. G., K. M. McDonald, R. M. Wachter, and D. K. Owens. 2004. *Closing the Quality Gap: A Critical Analysis of Quality Improvement Strategies Vol. 1. Series Overview and Methodology.* Rockville, MD: Agency for Healthcare Research and Quality.

Suggestions for Further Reading

Berwick, D. M. 1991. "Controlling Variation in Health Care: A Consultation from Walter Shewhart." *Medical Care* 29 (12): 1212–1225 [abstract].

Campbell, S. M., M. O. Roland, and S. A. Buetow. 2000. "Defining Quality of Care." *Social Science & Medicine* 51 (11): 1611–1625.

Codman, E. A. (1918) 2013. "A Study in Hospital Efficiency: As Demonstrated by the Case Report of the First Five Years of a Private Hospital." *Clinical Orthopaedics and Related Research* 471 (6): 1778–1783.

Deming, W. E. 1967. "Walter A. Shewhart, 1891–1967." *American Statistician* 21: 39–40.

Deming, W. E. (1993) 2000. *The New Economics for Industry, Government, Education*, 2nd ed. Cambridge, MA: MIT Press.

Deming, W. E. 1986. *Out of the Crisis*. Cambridge, MA: MIT Press.

Dlugacz, Y. D., A. Restifo, and A. Greenwood. 2004, *The Quality Handbook for Health Care Organizations: A Manager's Guide to Tools and Programs*. San Francisco: Jossey-Bass.

Dlugacz, Y. D. 2006. *Measuring Health Care: Using Quality Data for Operational, Financial, and Clinical Improvement*. San Francisco: Jossey-Bass.

Donabedian, A. 1980. *Explorations in Quality Assessment and Monitoring: The Definition of Quality and Approaches to Its Assessment*. Ann Arbor, MI: Health Administration Press.

Donabedian A. 1989. "The End Results of Health Care: Ernest Codman's Contribution to Quality Assessment and Beyond." *Milbank Quarterly* 67 (2): 233–256.

Fenter, T. C., and S. L. Lewis. 2008. "Pay-for-Performance Initiatives." *Journal of Managed Care Pharmacy* 14 (6): S12–S15.

Jha, A. K., E. J. Orav, A. B. Ridgway, J. Zheng, and A. M. Epstein. 2008. "Does the Leapfrog Program Help Identify High-Quality Hospitals?" *Joint Commission Journal on Quality and Patient Safety* 34 (6): 318–325.

Juran, J. 1988. *Quality Control Handbook*, 4th ed. N.P.: McGraw-Hill.

Juran, J. 2004. *Architect of Quality: The Autobiography of Dr. Joseph M. Juran*. New York: McGraw-Hill.

Mallon, W. J. E. 2007. "Amory Codman Considered Father of Evidence-Based Medicine." 9 (3). http://www.aaos.org/news/bulletin/janfeb07/research1.asp

Mallon, W. 2000. *Ernest Amory Codman: The End Result of a Life in Medicine*. Philadelphia: WB Saunders.

"Medical Errors in the USA: Human or Systemic?" 2011. *Lancet* 377 (9774): 1289.

Pelletier, L. R., and C. Beaudin. 2008. *Q Solutions: Essential Resources for the Healthcare Quality Professional*, 2nd ed. Glenview, IL: National Association for Healthcare Quality.

Roberts, J. S., J. G. Coale, and R. R. Redman. 1987. "A History of the Joint Commission on Accreditation of Hospitals." *JAMA* 258 (7): 936–940.

Useful Websites

http://www.ahrq.gov/

http://www.ahrq.gov/health-care-information/topics/topic-patientcentered-outcomes-research.html

http://www.ahrq.gov/legacy/qual/patientsafetyculture/hospdim.htm

http://www.ahrq.gov/qual/patientsafetyculture/

http://www.ahrq.gov/research/findings/final-reports/pscongrpt/psini2.html

http://www.ahrq.gov/professionals/education/curriculum-tools/teamstepps/index.html

http://www.certs.hhs.gov/

http://www.employeescreen.com/wp-content/uploads/sites/6/joint_commission_history.pdf

http://iom.nationalacademies.org/~/media/Files/Report%20Files/2006/Preventing-Medication-Errors-Quality-Chasm-Series/medicationerrorsnew.ashx

http://www.jointcommission.org/about_us/history.aspx

http://www.jointcommission.org/assets/1/6/Joint_Commission_History.pdf

http://www.jointcommission.org/assets/1/6/2016_NPSG_HAP_ER.pdf

http://www.hospitalsafetyscore.org

http://www.medicaid.gov/Federal-Policy-Guidance/downloads/SMD073108.pdf

http://www.medicare.gov/hospitalcompare/search.html

http://www.nytimes.com/1993/12/21/obituaries/w-edwards-deming-expert-on-business-management-dies-at-93.html

http://www.who.int/patientsafety/education/curriculum/who_mc_topic-7.pdf

http://meps.ahrq.gov/mepsweb/

http://psnet.ahrq.gov/primer.aspx?primerID=3

CHAPTER TWO

UNDERSTANDING THE IMPACT OF HEALTH CARE REFORM

Chapter Outline

The Affordable Care Act
New Models of Payment
New Models of Providing Care
New Models for Collecting Data
Improving Interpersonal Communication
Summary
Key Terms
Quality Concepts in Action
References
Suggestions for Further Reading
Useful Websites

Key Concepts

- Understand the goals of health care reform.
- Highlight important aspects of the Affordable Care Act.
- Define the challenges to health care professionals working in the reform environment.
- Outline new models of providing care and financing care.
- Discuss the advantages and challenges involved in health information technology.
- Explain new techniques for improving communication in the health care setting.

Health care reform is more than government policy about changing the way we finance medical care. It is a full-scale paradigm shift, involving new ways of thinking about, understanding, managing, implementing, and documenting the delivery of health care. The reforms are an attempt to make health care services available to more of the population than in the past and to increase consumers' choices for health care providers and specialists.

Generally, the goals of reform are to increase the quality of care, decrease the cost of care, better understand the relationship between process and outcome, and improve communication between providers and patients. The impetus for reforming health care is the result of well-documented evidence that although the United States spends more on health care than other developed countries, the quality ranks among the last on many variables (http://www.commonwealthfund.org/publications/fund-reports/2014/jun/mirror-mirror).

Health care professionals need some familiarity with the reform environment since they are working within it. Regardless of the specifics, there are commonalities: The focus of reform is on the process of care and which processes can be associated with improved outcomes and lowered costs. In the new model of care, the hospital is no longer the center of care delivery; care should reside primarily in the community.

New challenges for health care professionals, especially those involved with the "business" of health care, include developing the skills necessary to transform the organization by emphasizing new structures and behaviors. Leaders must evaluate whether sufficient intellectual resources exist within the health care system to make the required changes. Financial management is changing, and developing methods to remain financially viable during the process of transformation is challenging. Risk is now be associated with population management, and insurers financially reward or punish organizations and individual physicians.

The Affordable Care Act

Although the financial details are complicated and dependent on income levels, the Patient Protection and Affordable Care Act (ACA), which was signed into law on March 23, 2010, attempts to improve access and quality of care by:

- expanding Medicaid eligibility;
- subsidizing insurance premiums;
- providing incentives for businesses to offer health care benefits;
- prohibiting denial of insurance coverage for preexisting conditions; and
- supporting medical research.

It also empowers the Centers for Medicare and Medicaid Services (CMS) to test different models of payment and care delivery, examples of which are discussed next.

Accountable Care Organizations

The ACA encourages the establishment of Accountable Care Organizations (ACOs), which is a model of care that ties provider reimbursement to quality metrics and reduced costs for a defined patient population. According to the CMS an ACO is comprised of groups of doctors, hospitals, and other providers who agree to be accountable for providing Medicare patients with high-quality, low-cost coordinated care (https://www.cms.gov/Medicare/Medicare-Fee-for-Service-Payment/ACO/index.html?redirect=/Aco/). ACOs are not based on altruism. ACOs have financial incentives; if they succeed in delivering high-quality, low-cost care to their patients, they will share in the savings of Medicare spending (ACO Shared Savings Program).

The guidelines for ACOs were established by the Department of Health and Human Services (HHS) in 2011, which explained the steps that must be completed to participate in the Medicare Shared Savings Program. ACOs accept responsibility—that is, are accountable for—the overall quality and cost of at least 5,000 Medicare beneficiaries for a three-year period. Specifically, the ACO must:

- provide a sufficient number of primary care physicians to serve their population;
- promote evidence-based medicine in the practice;
- encourage **patient engagement**;
- monitor and evaluate quality and cost measures;
- be patient centered; and
- coordinate care across the continuum.

For ACOs to succeed and for care to be coordinated across the continuum, communication and information transfer have to be seamless and complete. And with the new payment models, such as bundled care and **pay for performance** (P4P), providers receive financial rewards for eliminating unnecessary tests and services and proactively maintaining wellness. To focus on populations, quality management must exist beyond the walls of the hospital, with community physicians complying with quality standards.

DEFINING TERMS FOR ACOS

Some of the terms involved in ACOs may be unfamiliar.

Evidence-based medicine refers to "integrating individual clinical expertise with the best available external clinical evidence from systematic research" (Sackett et al. 1996, 71)—that is, making use of high-quality research to inform clinical decisions for individual patients.

Patient engagement refers to the way patients interact with increasingly complex health care services. Patients are expected to decide when to seek care, how to choose providers and insurers that meet their needs, how to manage

their health, and how to determine the best course of treatment among conflicting advice from providers in a climate of advanced communication and
information technology.

   Patient-centered care refers to the active involvement of patients in their
health care services, including making decisions about treatment options. In
Crossing the Quality Chasm (2001), the Committee on Quality of Health Care
in America and the Institute of Medicine (IOM) defined patient-centered care
as "care that is respectful of and responsive to individual patient preferences,
needs, and values, and ensuring that patient values guide all clinical decisions"
(p. 3). Patient-centered care cannot be achieved without patient engagement.
Perhaps patients also will become involved in quality management; if so, it
remains to be seen how and to what degree.

ACOs are committed to improving and maintaining the health of a population, such as patients with diabetes or heart failure, not simply reducing
expenses and costs. They value prevention and wellness as well as proactive
rather than reactive care. The focus is on good outcomes, not volume of services. This paradigm shift has an impact on **quality measurements.** Although
quality measurements exist for hospital care, where rules, norms, and mores
are defined, measures now have to be developed for the community, where
behavior is much more fluid.

Financial rewards are linked to documenting standards of performance.
The five areas to be measured include:

1. patient/caregiver experience of care,
2. care coordination,
3. patient safety,
4. preventive health, and
5. at-risk/elderly health.

Specifics of the performance measures can be found at: https://www.cms.gov/
Medicare/Medicare-Fee-for-Service-Payment/sharedsavingsprogram/
Downloads/ACO-Shared-Savings-Program-Quality-Measures.pdf.

Accompanying all the changes is the need for new measures to assess
whether care delivery is improving while costs are being contained. Developing measures to evaluate good outcomes and success is a time-consuming
challenge. Measures and performance improvement strategies that have
been used in hospitals must be adapted to outpatient services. It is not
enough for **electronic health records** (EHRs) to be introduced into the health
care delivery system; it has to be used productively for data collection and

analysis as well. The greater availability of data is creating an important shift in the responsibilities of quality management departments, moving away from regulatory compliance to a more analytic and statistics-based model of evaluating care processes and patient safety.

Health Insurance Exchanges

According to the ACA (Section 1311), for a health insurance plan to be qualified to participate in the Health Insurance Exchange programs that have expanded insurance coverage to millions of Americans, the plan must be accredited, meet specific quality requirements, and collect and report quality data. HHS selected the National Committee for Quality Assurance (NCQA) to be the accrediting organization for the health exchanges, web portals which provide consumers with competitive information about insurance plans. The NCQA uses the clinical quality measures of the Health Effectiveness Data Information Set (**HEDIS**). These performance measures are used by more than 90 percent of health plans across the country, which enables a fair comparison among them. HEDIS data also include a patient experience survey, the Consumer Assessment of Healthcare Providers and Systems (**CAHPS**), which measures patient satisfaction in such areas as customer service, timely care, and processing claims.

To maintain NCQA accreditation, which is considered the gold standard of accreditation, health plans must allow the results of clinical quality and patient experience measures to be publicly reported.

The ACA requires all health plans, group, private, and those in the health exchanges to submit annual reports on:

- improving health outcomes,
- preventing hospital readmissions,
- ensuring patient safety and reducing medical errors, and
- implementing wellness and health promotion activities.

The NCQA evaluates plans by comparing the HEDIS data of over 80 performance measures across five domains of care to regional and national benchmarks. Among the measures HEDIS reports are:

- measures of wellness and prevention, such as preventive screenings, medical assistance with smoking cessation;
- chronic disease management measures, such as those associated with diabetes, cholesterol, high blood pressure and asthma;
- behavioral health measures, such as antidepressant medical management; and
- safety measures, such as limiting imaging studies for low back pain.

The measures are designed to address overuse, waste, and appropriateness of care and are regularly updated.

Using quality indicators to evaluate resource utilization reveals that some plans deliver higher-quality care than others for the same condition in a more efficient way, avoiding hospitalizations and unnecessary surgeries and treating patients with medications in outpatient care. Because the measures are so specific, performance of different plans can be fairly compared, and consumers will have information on which to base their choice of health plans. In this way, HEDIS data are used to improve quality of care and service.

The CAHPS satisfaction or experience survey focuses on measures that reveal how well plans are meeting member expectations, the areas that most affect satisfaction, and the areas that need improvement. Measures evaluate: access to care, including specialists, tests, and treatments; timeliness of care; physician communication effectiveness; customer service; coordination of care; and other plan information.

New Models of Payment

New models of reimbursement are being developed and encouraged in order to redo the way providers are currently paid, which is on a fee-for-service basis. The hope is that new models might avoid the potential drawbacks of the fee-for-service model. Being paid for volume and complexity of provided services may lead to increased costs and not necessarily higher-quality care.

Bundled Payment

Under the Bundled Payments for Care Improvement Initiative, a provision of the ACA, the CMS is exploring new payment relationships with hospitals that volunteer to participate in the program. The payment arrangements are expected to lead to higher-quality, coordinated care that will result in lower costs to Medicare. Traditional models reward quantity of services rather than quality; the more services provided, the greater the reimbursement; the more acute the care, the more financial payment.

The bundled payment model is a new way to finance health care services, replacing the conventional method of paying various physicians for the various services they provide during an episode of care. Under the bundled payment model, one fee will be set for a defined episode (such as a stroke or hip replacement), and payment will be divided among the hospital and caregivers for all medical services. The episode involves the entire continuum of care and is not defined solely by the hospitalization.

The CMS is testing four different models of bundled payment: acute care, post acute, combined acute and post acute, retrospective, and prospective payment. All models require that care be redesigned using defined treatment plans grounded in evidence-based medicine, standardizing protocols for surgery, and improving information transfer. Although the four different prongs of the model differ, the goal remains constant: improved care, greater efficiency, lower cost, and improved accountability and communication across the entire continuum of care. In short, the new model of payment rewards physicians for quality and coordination of care rather than for volume of services provided.

All models rely for success on reducing variation in care and eliminating waste along with providing a positive patient experience and good outcomes. Required evaluative measures will monitor quality improvements, process improvements, health outcomes, expenses/costs, and detect unintended consequences, such as stinting on care or manipulating patient selection or shifting costs.

Pioneer and Advance Payment Accountable Care Organization

Another model of payment launched by the CMS Innovation Center is the Pioneer and Advance Payment Accountable Care Organization. It is designed to show how payment arrangements of ACOs improve care and generate Medicare savings. Those ACOs that have successfully shared in the Medicare Savings program will have the opportunity to move to population-based payment after two years.

Comprehensive Primary Care Improvement

Still another payment model being tested is the Comprehensive Primary Care Improvement initiative which has the goal of strengthening primary care. Those practices that participate in the initiative will be given resources to improve the care coordination for their Medicare patients and be offered financial incentives, such as bonus payments, if they better coordinate care for their patients.

Value-Based Purchasing

Another weapon in the arsenal of the ACA is to improve the quality of care and reduce costs through Value-Based Purchasing (VBP). In 2012, the CMS began rewarding hospitals that provide high-quality care for their Medicare patients through the Hospital VBP Program. VBP is quite different from traditional fee-for-service payments, which reward health care practitioners for how much they do and often leads to costly, complex, and unnecessary services. Like other reforms, VBP focuses on the *quality* of care rather than the amount of care and requires that communication about patient outcomes be transparent. With the introduction of VBP, hospitals and health care systems will be paid for quality, not quantity.

Hospitals receive financial rewards based on specific quality measures that are associated with improved processes and patient satisfaction. For example, a quality process measure is: how often heart failure patients receive effective discharge instructions. The idea behind the measure is the assumption that effective discharge instructions may reduce the readmission rates for heart failure patients by better educating them on how to manage their medications and other treatment responsibilities. From a quality management point of view, measures should connect process and outcomes. Many organizations send questionnaires to patients about their posthospital care and use those for quality indicators. More sophisticated quality tools need to be formulated to meet the new environment.

Since 2012, hospitals have received financial incentive rewards for how well they perform on a set of quality measures and also on how much they improve in performance as measured against a baseline. The better a hospital does on its quality measures, the greater the reward it receives. Incentive payments are based on hospital performance as compared to other hospitals and improvement over time. Therefore, the incentives offered under the VBP program award the continual improvement of care.

The CMS plans to update the measures as needed to continue to improve quality and add measures on improved patient outcomes and prevention of hospital-acquired conditions such as pressure ulcers. The measures of the VBP program are publicly reported on the government's Hospital Compare website. Not only hospitals, but the law requires the CMS to develop value-based purchasing programs for home health agencies, nursing facilities, ambulatory surgical centers, specialty hospitals, long-term care facilities and hospice programs. Such an approach will require quality management programs to take a proactive approach to define end results of a quality intervention—a provocative and exciting challenge.

Pay for Performance

In 2006, the IOM published *Preventing Medication Errors*, which recommended that profits be tied to quality and patient safety. In another report published that same year, *Rewarding Provider Performance: Aligning Incentives in Medicare*, the IOM recommended P4P programs as an "immediate opportunity" to offer financial incentives for improved performance.

P4P is a general term for initiatives that improve quality, efficiency, and value of health care. It links payment to value and improves on the reimbursement practice that allows physicians and hospitals to bill for services related to patient harm, such as falls.

P4P programs financially reward hospitals, physician practices, and other providers if they meet expectations of selected performance measures. The measures cover clinical quality and safety, efficiency, patient experience/satisfaction, and adoption of **health information technology** (**HIT**).

Government agencies, such as the CMS, health insurance plans, employers, and others can sponsor P4P programs. The ACA encourages P4P approaches, especially for the Medicare population, and suggests that new effective programs be identified.

In an attempt to improve the way health care does business, the CMS introduced the P4P model in a three-year demonstration project that involves more than 200,000 Medicare beneficiaries. Practices involved in this project are expected to meet quality standards for prevention and management of chronic disease, such as diabetes. If a practice meets the standards, it will be eligible for rewards for improved patient management. Hospitals will also be compensated if they meet specific quality measures. Physicians who make use of HIT to manage their chronically ill Medicare patients and who show improved outcomes will be financially rewarded as well. The CMS also offers disincentives. If the quality measures are not met, the hospital will receive a reduction in payment. Never events will not receive reimbursement.

Case Example: Communicating with Clinicians through P4P Data

Linking payment to quality care is not as straightforward as it may seem. There is a great deal of diversity among health care organizations, between community and tertiary hospitals, among physician practices, and among surgical centers. There is also variation among the patient populations of different health centers. Therefore, ranking hospitals on the instances of infection they have, for example, might be unfair.

Under P4P and value-based performance, hospitals with a high infection rate, for example, are penalized, and those with lower rates are financially rewarded. The government tries to make comparisons legitimate by calculating a standardized infection ratio (SIR) for different types of health centers. For example, a tertiary hospital with a large burn unit can be expected to have a higher infection rate than a small community hospital without such a unit. The government says if the SIR is greater than expected, the organization is penalized; if the SIR is less than expected, the organization is rewarded.

The SIR is calculated as the observed number of infections (the actual raw number) divided by the expected number (what the government anticipates and risk-adjusts for). The challenge for many organizations, especially smaller ones, is to realize that even a single instance of infection could cause them to be in the red and thus penalized financially.

Figure 2.1 is an example of a dashboard report that shows different types of infections that occurred in a small community hospital for a year. The figure shows that a single occurrence of the infection methicillin-resistant *Staphylococcus aureus* (MRSA) and a single occurrence of a colon surgical site infection (SSI) caused the hospital to be higher than the number of infections expected and therefore in the red. The organization was penalized financially.

FIGURE 2.1. VALUE-BASED PERFORMANCE AT A COMMUNITY HOSPITAL

	Observed Infection Count	Expected Infection Count	Standardized Infection Ratio	Threshold Value	% −/+ Threshold
ICU CLABSI	0	0.44	0.000	0.457	−100.00
ICU CAUTI	0	0.81	0.000	0.845	−100.00
C-DIFF	12	8.79	1.365	0.750	82.00
MRSA	1	0.54	1.845	0.799	132.08
CMS Ab Hyst SSI	0	0.01	0.000	0.698	−100.00
CMS Colon SSI	1	0.53	1.883	0.751	150.76

Green =   Red =

FIGURE 2.2. VALUE-BASED PERFORMANCE AT A TERTIARY HOSPITAL

	Observed Infection Count	Expected Infection Count	Standardized Infection Ratio	Threshold Value	% −/+ Threshold
ICU CLABSI	4	16.20	0.247	0.457	−45.97
ICU CAUTI	17	26.20	0.649	0.845	−23.20
C-DIFF	117	173.01	0.676	0.750	−9.83
MRSA	16	19.70	0.812	0.799	1.67
CMS Ab Hyst SSI	4	3.55	1.127	0.698	61.43
CMS Colon SSI	17	12.86	1.344	0.751	78.90

Green =   Red =

Figure 2.2 shows infection information for a large tertiary hospital. Even with 117 instances of *Clostridium difficile* (*C. difficile* or *C. diff.*), the hospital is still in the green, below 1, because the expected infection count is higher than the observed. However, four instances of abdominal hysterectomy SSIs puts the hospital in the red, because the expected rate was just a bit lower, at 3.55.

The difference between being in the red and the green for this infection at this hospital was one instance of the infection.

These examples of infection dashboards are designed to focus clinicians on the importance of every single instance of infection. Busy clinicians are often impatient with looking at raw numbers, especially a single instance of infection, which they may well consider acceptable. However, the government thinks one instance is unacceptable in many cases. P4P helps improve safety and quality by educating clinicians, through quality tables, in the importance of individual issues and problems and forces them to focus on the raw numbers. The financial incentive is effective pressure.

The preceding examples are about infection, but the same type of reports can be produced for mortality, readmission, safety, and others. Performance improvement initiatives can and should be developed to bring each variable into the expected rate. Every complication, morbidity, and mortality should be investigated with the goal of improvement. Ideally, hospitals want zero instances of issues for which they will not be reimbursed.

New Models of Providing Care

The ACA enables more people access to care than previously and improves that care through innovative approaches for the way care is delivered.

Patient-Centered Medical Homes

Although the concept of patient-centered medical homes (PCMHs) predates the ACA, the principles of PCMHs are entirely congruent with the ACA and the two models work in concert. According to the Agency for Healthcare Research and Quality (AHRQ), PCMHs provide coordination of services and ACOs provide the infrastructure and incentives to facilitate collaboration across different types of providers and organizations.

In 2002, several family medicine groups created the Future of Family Medicine project with the purpose of transforming family medicine. The project recommended that every American should have a "personal medical home" through which to receive his or her acute, chronic and preventive care. The care should be "accessible, accountable, comprehensive, integrated, patient-centered, safe, scientifically valid, and satisfying to both patients and their physicians" (Martin et al. 2004). PCMHs are patient-centered care based on improving quality and safety, financial and clinical outcomes, and physician and staff satisfaction as well as patient engagement while also lowering costs. Like ACOs, PCMHs are based on improved outcomes rather than volume of services.

By 2005, the American College of Physicians had developed an Advanced Medical Home model that supported the use of evidence-based medicine, clinical decision support tools, and improved access to care. It encouraged quantitative indicators of quality and HIT and recognized the importance of payment reform.

The PCMH is a model of care that transforms thinking about and managing primary care. It is a philosophy, not a place, that encompasses care that is patient centered, comprehensive, team based, coordinated, accessible, and focused on quality and safety. It is called a "home" because it values the patient experience and should provide an environment where patients can expect to be treated with respect, dignity, and compassion. In the PCMH model, care is facilitated by information technology (EHR, registries, decision support tools) to ensure that patients get the care they need when and where they need it in a culturally and linguistically appropriate manner.

FIVE CORE ATTRIBUTES OF PCMHs

1. *Comprehensive care.* PCMHs provide prevention and wellness services, addressing mental and physical health needs, and managing acute care and chronic care health issues. Comprehensive care requires a team of providers, which may include physicians, physician assistants, nurses, pharmacists, social workers, nutritionists, and others. In order to provide care, the team has to share information and communicate effectively.
2. *Coordinated care.* Care has to be coordinated not only among providers but across different care venues, such as hospitals, long-term care facilities, home health care, and community support. Care coordination is especially critical at points of transfer between sites.
3. *Patient centered.* PCMHs are committed to addressing the whole person, partnering with patient and family and respecting their values, culture, wishes, preferences, and needs. Patients are considered a crucial part of the medical team and partners in their medical management.
4. *Accessible care.* PCMHs transform traditional office hours and office visits and makes care accessible 24/7 via e-mail, telephone, shorter waiting times, and longer office hours.
5. *Quality and safety.* PCMHs use evidence-based medicine for clinical decision making. Physicians share information about treatment decisions with the patient and family. Performance measurements about outcomes and satisfaction are collected, reviewed, and acted upon. Data are transparently reported and shared throughout the health system and community. Population health management is expected.

Source: https://pcmh.ahrq.gov/page/defining-pcmh

Community Health Centers

The need for community health centers (CHCs) is not a new concept. In fact, in 1965, President Lyndon Johnson, in an effort to overcome known health disparities, especially their impact on racial and ethnic minorities, as well as on the poor and uninsured, launched CHCs to improve health care for these vulnerable populations. CHCs provide patients with low incomes or who are uninsured comprehensive primary care health services, including dental and mental health services. To improve and ensure access, they also provide transportation and translation services. CHCs are not only for the uninsured but also provide care for Medicaid and Medicare beneficiaries and others.

The ACA health care reform legislation dedicated $11 billion for new health centers and to expand existing health centers and another $1.5 billion to fund the National Health Service Corps, a program that rewards physicians for working in underserved areas. It is anticipated that CHCs will grow as the number of insured people grow, due to the reform bill and the health insurance exchange program. By 2015, CHCs served over 40 million patients. The legislation also provides $2 billion every year after 2015 for prevention screenings and immunization programs and grants for employers who establish "wellness" programs for their employees. In addition to providing a real safety net for people who previously were medically disenfranchised, the health care reform law has dedicated $230 million over a five-year period for community-based teaching programs and development of primary care residency programs in CHCs.

With more and more people expected to use CHCs for their primary care, it is important that the care be up to standard. A 2012 study by Goldman et al. concluded that CHCs provide better care than private practices. Based on records from the National Ambulatory Medical Care Survey gathered by the National Center for Health Statistics, the researchers evaluated how well physicians complied with guidelines for 18 measures, including treatments for specific diseases and screenings. For 13 of the measures, CHC physicians performed as well as those in private practice, but in five measures, such as administering ACE (Angiotensin Converting Enzyme) inhibitors for congestive heart failure, using beta blockers, using appropriate medication for asthma, conducting blood pressure screening, and avoiding electrocardiograms in low-risk patients, a higher percentage of CHC physicians followed recommendations, despite the fact that CHCs often deal with patients who have chronic conditions and complex socioeconomic challenges.

Prevention and Wellness

The ACA provides unprecedented support for prevention and wellness services by reducing costs and expanding services, such as increased prevention services for Medicare patients and offering grants to employers for wellness programs. The National Prevention Council, composed of various federal agencies, coordinates wellness, prevention, and health promotion strategies at the federal level. The council has developed a National Prevention Strategy that attempts to shift the focus of health from sickness to wellness.

To strengthen and support prevention efforts, the strategy identifies four goals and seven priorities to reach those goals. The goals are to:

1. promote healthy and safe community environments to increase the number of Americans who are healthy;
2. support clinical and community preventive services by recognizing those communities that promote health and wellness through prevention;
3. empower people to make healthy choices; and
4. eliminate health disparities.
    (http://www.surgeongeneral.gov/priorities/prevention/strategy/ national-prevention-strategy-fact-sheet.pdf)

According to the surgeon general, priorities of the strategy are based on recommendations that come from evidence-based medicine about factors that can cause preventable death and major illness and can have an impact on the greatest number of people. The priorities are:

1. tobacco-free living,
2. preventing drug abuse and excessive alcohol use,
3. healthy eating,
4. active living,
5. injury- and violence-free living,
6. reproductive and sexual health, and
7. mental and emotional well-being.

The Centers for Disease Control and Prevention (CDC) estimates that reducing smoking and improving activity levels and healthy eating would reduce the incidence of heart disease and stroke, of Type 2 diabetes, and of cancer (http://www.cdc.gov/chronicdisease/pdf/2009-Power-of-Prevention .pdf).

Local Prevention Efforts

Another aspect of the ACA is a program that offers support via Community Transformation Grants to states and communities that attempt to repair poor health and reduce chronic disease through promoting healthy lifestyles. The ACA also created a Prevention and Public Health Fund to prevent disease through early detection and focusing on the causes of chronic disease through worksite wellness and other programs. This fund highlights the national commitment to wellness and prevention. Cost sharing is waived for preventive services and new funding is provided for community prevention services and workplace wellness programs. The CDC evaluates these programs to define best practices.

These prevention and wellness efforts require commitment from states and local communities. Prevention efforts, such as screening tests, immunizations, and early detection programs, are cost effective as well as clinically sound. Research conducted by the Urban Institute and the New York Academy of Medicine showed that community-based programs helped to reduce Type 2 diabetes and high blood pressure by 5 percent in two years and reduced heart and kidney disease and stroke within five years. Some forms of cancer, arthritis, and chronic obstructive pulmonary disease could be reduced by 2.5 percent within 10 years (Trust for America's Health 2008).

In July 2008, a report conducted by the Trust for America's Health, called *Prevention for a Healthier America: Investments in Disease Prevention Yield Significant Savings, Stronger Communities,* concluded that a small investment returns great results. The report said that investing $10 per person per year in community-based programs to improve eating habits, increase exercise, and prevent smoking could save more than $16 billion annually.

Prevention efforts help people become better educated about what constitutes good health habits. Community, schools, and religious organizations can offer information about preventive services that are available and help to educate about the benefits of prevention. Community centers and other public spaces can offer preventive services, such as screenings and immunizations, as can retail outlets. Health care providers should offer recommended preventive services routinely as part of wellness visits and remind patients about preventive health screenings and immunizations. Worksites can offer employees access to preventive services and offer them on site if possible.

Local communities can invest in education campaigns. The New York Academy of Medicine summarized many efforts that have resulted in success. Included among the success stories was a coronary health improvement project (CHIP) community intervention that targeted coronary risk in a high-risk group. With a monthlong 40-hour educational curriculum and with nutritional assessments, participants were told to improve their diet, stop smoking, and exercise daily. After the monthlong intervention, cholesterol levels, glucose levels, blood pressure, and weight showed significant reductions (Englert et al. 2007).

An intervention in California looked at the impact of increasing the price of cigarettes by 25 cents and using 5 of those cents for an anti-tobacco educational campaign. After three years, mortality from coronary heart disease had decreased by 2.93 deaths yearly per 100,000 people. Smoking decreased by 2.72 packs per person per year (Fichtenberg and Glantz 2000).

Falls are the leading cause of injury in people over 65, and more than half of falls occur at home. Falls are also the leading cause of traumatic brain injury in the elderly. According to the National Center for Injury Prevention and Control (2006), fall-related death rates and hip fracture hospitalizations are on the rise for this population. Clearly it would be an advantage to prevent seniors from falling. Community interventions have proven successful in doing this.

A program developed in New South Wales, The Stay On Your Feet program, addressed factors that contribute to falls, such as footwear, vision, balance, medications, chronic health issues, and home hazards. The program worked with health professionals and local government and used education, raising awareness, and media campaigns. After four years, there was a decrease of a statistically significant 20 percent in fall-related hospitalizations. Increased awareness, safer footwear, and improved balance were reported (Kempton et al. 2000).

Case Example: Influenza Vaccination

As a response to the 2009 H1N1 influenza epidemic, health care providers worked with local government agencies, especially regional Departments of Health, to ensure outreach to identified high-risk groups, the underserved, and groups with poor access to health care services as well as to the general population. Communication was critical because the guidelines from the government and state were updated and changed daily, and people were understandably confused.

Personnel in schools, hospitals, community and faith-based organizations, town officials, members of emergency medical services, and others in the community were kept informed via media coverage, county executive public messages, and legislative forums. An ongoing dialogue with state Departments of Health and the CDC was established to gather the most up-to-date information to release to the public. Statistical analysis and mapping conducted by quality analysts helped to evaluate the efficacy of the program and identify potential areas of improvement for vaccinating at-risk population groups in the region. Robust communication strategies and partnering with community groups and regional health care facilities enabled local public health officials to quickly, efficiently, and responsibly distribute the H1N1 vaccine to the community.

Working collaboratively with so many groups enabled quality and clinical professionals to study why many pregnant women, one of the high-risk groups recommended to receive the vaccine, did not choose to be immunized. The results showed that providers needed to be more supportive of immunization; increased education and awareness of providers should help increase immunizations of pregnant women in the event of future influenza outbreaks (Dlugacz et al. 2012).

New Models for Collecting Data

HOW DOES HIT DIFFER FROM EHR?

Health information technology (HIT) provides the infrastructure for technologies that design, develop, store, share, and analyze information for health information. Electronic health records (EHRs) are subset tools of the many tools available through HIT.

EHRs are digital versions of a patient's paper medical chart. One of the advantages of the digital version is that it enables the sharing of information among providers as well as with laboratories, specialists, pharmacies, and others. EHRs can also contain medical histories, treatment plans, medications, allergies, and other pertinent patient information.

Background

The changing health care landscape relies on increasingly sophisticated information technology (IT), including the EHR, which the government has encouraged health care organizations to adopt. In fact, the ACA requires health plans to use EHRs to retrieve data that will promote efficiency and communication, reduce medical errors, and improve the quality of care.

As early as 2004, President George W. Bush issued an executive order that required implementation of an interoperable electronic patient system by 2013. He established the Office of the National Coordinator for Health Information Technology to lead efforts in transforming the traditional paper-based records system into an electronic system using HIT. In 2009, Congress passed the Health Information Technology for Economic and Clinical Health (HITECH) Act as part of the American Recovery and Reinvestment Act. HITECH called for the voluntary adoption of HIT for health care systems and established incentive payments as of 2011 for using EHRs. After 2015, those health systems that fail to use EHRs will be penalized.

The goal of the HITECH Act is to enable coordination of information across the country to significantly improve care delivery through the **meaningful use** of interoperable EHR, such as electronic prescribing and submitting clinical quality and other measures electronically. The government defines the term *meaningful use* as:

- improving care coordination,
- reducing health disparities,
- engaging and involving patients and families in their health care,
- improving population and public health, and
- ensuring privacy.

Meaningful use also refers to using EHR technology for exchanging health information to improve the quality and efficiency of care.

Advantages of Electronic Health Records

EHRs convert the traditional paper, handwritten patient charts into computerized versions. Advocates claim that EHRs are improvements over paper because the information is complete, up to date, and accurate; they can easily identify patients for preventive visits, immunizations, and screenings. With a comprehensive patient record, providers can diagnose problems more quickly and reliably. In addition, in case of a crisis, in emergency settings, care providers have instant access to medical history, allergies, conditions, and medications. EHRs can alert providers to potentially dangerous drug interactions and help to reduce medication errors by verifying medications and dosages and eliminating mistakes due to handwriting. Clinical alerts, and interfaces with lab reports and registries, part of EHRs, can enhance clinical decision making.

Because EHRs move with patients, information can be shared across providers and across organizations. Sharing information through effective communication is crucial in an environment where health care is a team effort; multiple providers have easy access to the same information. EHRs are useful when patients have to make transitions between care settings. EHRs can also benefit specific populations of patients, such as those who suffer from a specific condition, because physicians can be alerted to preventive measures; and risk factors for specific conditions may be more easily identified as well.

EHRs are faits accompli of the new health care environment. Students and professionals working in health care need to find a way to use EHRs as sources of data and, based on the records, to establish registries by disease. In this way, patients can be followed more easily, preventive visits can be kept track of, readmission to hospitals can be reduced, and the community can be better educated. As measures are developed to define improved patient care, new variables may be required to be entered into EHRs. EHRs make data mining relatively easy, and certainly easier than trying to find variables in multiple handwritten pages of a patient's medical record.

Another real advantage to EHRs for health professionals is that they contain primary data: data observed, collected, and documented directly by the investigator. Previously, data analysis on aggregated patient issues and health phenomena was based on secondary data, such as billing data. Billing data are entirely dependent on the accuracy and education of the coders. When using EHRs, health professionals can analyze several variables for potential correlation and even causation. For example, in an attempt to better understand mortality rates, an analyst can collect information about age and other demographics, secondary diagnoses, treatments and procedures, and other variables, which can lead to informed database development and better understanding of disease-specific populations and outcomes.

Due to EHRs and other HIT, health professionals require a relationship with highly trained analytic teams. In today's health care environment, in order to understand how to develop performance improvement initiatives and understand the philosophy and tools involved in quality management, students and professionals need to expand their education to include an increased familiarity with information that is entered into medical records, an understanding of the pros and cons of the new technology, and an ability to communicate effectively with IT departments. EHRs and other HIT can make available many opportunities for analysis, including efficiency in the operating room, turnaround time for procedures, even procedures by specific physicians.

And managing these new frontiers is not sufficient to work in today's health environment. Administrative and policy leaders also need to establish effective communication with clinicians. Because EHRs are primary data, administrators and leaders need to understand restrictions of **HIPAA** (the Health Insurance Portability and Accountability Act), which is designed to protect patient privacy. They also must recognize and become familiar with institutional review board requirements, which also are involved in protecting patient privacy. These new models of care as well as population-based care management, integrated delivery systems, and report cards require a quality management program that includes aggregated data and relies heavily on sophisticated IT infrastructure.

Challenges to Effective Use of Electronic Health Records

Although theoretically EHRs have the potential to promote improved quality and efficiency, not all health care professionals and policy leaders are entirely comfortable with making the change. Many see ethical and social problems inherent in the use of EHRs, especially since research has not demonstrated that they are consistently accurate or accessible to disadvantaged patients. Privacy issues are of concern, especially when data are shared without specific patient consent or even knowledge. Security of data may also be a problem, and patients who fear that their records may be insecure may not divulge important health information.

Physicians complain that EHRs are difficult to use and time-consuming. *The New York Times* reported a survey of physicians across the country who said that they received tens of thousands of alerts, most of them false alarms, from EHRs and so they tended to ignore them (Wachter 2015). Physicians also say that since electronic records are highly structured and constrained environments (check yes/no), they are difficult to work with, and they may even include less information than written notes where there is no limit on the amount and kind of information entered.

Other issues are that insurers believe that EHRs may make fraudulent billing easy. The interoperability of EHRs—that is, getting various electronic systems to "talk" to each other—is very challenging technically; often different systems don't speak the same language even within the same health care organization.

Aware of these concerns, HHS requested that the IOM study the effectiveness of the EHR. In 2011, the IOM reported that there was risk associated with IT problems and called on the Food and Drug Administration to regulate HIT and to investigate adverse events related to HIT (http://www.nationalacademies.org/hmd/Reports/2011/Health-IT-and-Patient-Safety-Building-Safer-Systems-for-Better-Care.aspx). EHRs are works in progress, with a steep learning curve.

International Classification of Diseases Codes

The term *International Classification of Diseases* (**ICD**) refers to the codes developed by the World Health Organization and used by physicians and health care professionals to report diagnoses and procedures. The codes are the basis on which payers pay for procedures and services and are updated periodically. As of October 1, 2014, as part of the reform initiative to incorporate HIT to improve care and efficiency, the CMS required that health providers replace the 30-year old ICD-9 codes with the revised ICD-10 codes. The CMS considers this transfer crucial to health care reform because the updated codes fulfill the reform goals of better care, better access to care, and lower costs through meaningful use of HIT. Since 2015, the ICD-10 has been required under the meaningful use reform incentives, and there are penalties for noncompliance. It is also thought that use of ICD-10 codes will help to reduce fraudulent claims for Medicare and Medicaid payments and eliminate redundant procedures.

The ICD-10 codes enable providers to record more specific details and therefore to code the diagnosis or procedure more precisely. These codes incorporate innovations and improvements in medical procedures that the ICD-9 did not include. Another advantage to the ICD-10 is that it uses standardized terminology that crosses the entire continuum of care and will be a critical element in EHRs. The improved codes should enable easier data sharing and better-quality management because many quality measures are based on ICD codes. It is also thought that the greater specificity of the ICD-10 codes will improve public health because the new codes will be able to capture information on diseases for research, reporting, and surveillance.

Improving Interpersonal Communication

Using HIT is only one way to improve communication. It is particularly effective in promoting better coordination and standardization of information for providers and insurers. In addition to establishing criteria for HIT, the health care environment encourages prioritizing patient-centeredness, including an understanding of their experience, over practices that stress efficiency and productivity alone. Patient-centered care is an approach that focuses on more than the patient's illness; it includes the patient's concerns, the social context in which the patient functions, personal preferences, and other psychosocial aspects of the patient experience. The movement is away from treating only an illness or a disease toward treating the entire person as an active partner in care. Effective communication and collaboration between the care provider and the patient is crucial to establishing patient-centered care. Communication is critical because often there is a disconnect between what patients want from their providers and what providers imagine or think their patients want.

Understanding new communication strategies and being familiar with new ways to manage patients and clinical care is important for administrative and quality professionals as well as for clinicians, if they are to provide a patient-centered environment of care and a standard endorsed by regulatory agencies, to improve patient satisfaction, and to satisfy CMS expectations. Meeting these responsibilities requires some knowledge of how patients think and feel about their care, of what their expectations are about the patient-physician relationship, and of how to meet those expectations.

Narrative Medicine

Prioritizing patient-centeredness, including an understanding of their experience, over practices that stress efficiency and productivity alone requires physicians to adopt new strategies for communicating with their patients. Narrative medicine techniques genuinely treat patients as active partners in the relationship of care and break through the rigid boundaries and barriers that have characterized traditional medical practice.

Some medical school programs have introduced narrative medicine. The goals are to improve communication between provider and patient, promote a better therapeutic relationship between the clinician and patient, understand and validate the patient's experience, and encourage reflection from physicians about their own and their patients' feelings about illness. Training in narrative medicine teaches physicians to actively listen and to ask the right questions to elicit information in a compassionate and creative way. Ideally, together, the physician and the patient develop a narrative—a story—that leads the patient away from "sick" to health through the creation of shared meanings, life history, and feelings. It is thought that "narrative provides meaning, context, perspective for the patient's predicament. It defines how, why, and what way he or she is ill. It offers, in short, a possibility of understanding which cannot be arrived at by any other means" (Greenhalgh and Hurwitz 1999, 48).

Since clinical care is dependent on various kinds of written and spoken texts—a patient recounts symptoms to a care provider, the listening clinician writes an account or report of what the patient relates, and other providers may add reports or comments—understanding these different accounts as a multivoiced narrative of illness might lead to improved understanding and better outcomes. However, many physicians, already hard-pressed for time, find the idea of actively listening to a patient's story of illness impractical. But this resistance may be based more on physician perception than reality. One study of patients with complex medical histories showed that two minutes of listening was enough for 80 percent of patients in a general practice to explain their concerns. Physicians in this practice had been trained in active listening (Langewitz et al. 2002).

Narratives can serve as a bridge between large-scale clinical trials (the basis of evidence-based medicine) and the art of applying an individual practitioner's knowledge to a particular patient. In other words, evidence-based medicine and narrative medicine work in a complementary way and should be integrated as "narrative evidence-based medicine" (Charon, Wyer, and NEBM Working Group 2008). Narratives are developed not only to explore the patient's experience. They are also useful for physicians to describe their own experience with treating illness. This type of self-reflection leads to greater empathy on the part of physicians for their patients' situations.

Absorbing the techniques of narrative medicine takes time and a willingness to revise old routines with self-reflection, active listening skills, empathy, and attention. The patient-provider relationship is enhanced by reducing boundaries and promoting transparency. For example, knowing how to manage mortality in a patient-centered environment is among the new challenges faced by health care professionals. It is expensive to die in a hospital. Administrators as well as clinicians need to be able to understand the clinical, financial, and ethical issues involved in placing patients in hospice care, palliative care, or the intensive care unit.

Administrators also need effective tools to manage improved communication. Informed consent includes clinical information but also has ramifications that may be legal and financial. Do patients understand what they are signing? Who has explained it to them, and with what skill? Communication between physicians and patients and their families about appropriate levels of care is critical.

Physicians recognize and acknowledge that they need more skills to help their patients understand end-of-life issues and also for themselves to feel more comfortable with the discussion and the inevitable death of their patients. Narrative medicine, self-reflection, active listening, and shared communication help everyone. In today's health care environment it is important that patients feel satisfied with their care and with the communication between them and their care providers.

Improving Documentation

In the new world of health care reform, another challenge for organization's management is to effectively make use of EHRs and to translate entries into usable data, measurements, and databases to provide information to leaders about the best ways to keep people out of the hospitals. Quality management professionals will need to develop new models for analysis in order to meet this challenge. To understand how to improve processes in the community and improve compliance with certain indicators in specific population groups, new ideas and methodologies have to center on improving care, reducing costs, and increasing satisfaction in the community ambulatory setting in order to reduce hospitalizations and focus on prevention.

With the shared risk paradigm of health care reform, insurers want proof—that is, documentation—that patients are being managed effectively; that populations with specific diseases, even high-risk patients, are understood and treated in the community; that waste is reduced; that utilization of medical resources appropriate; and that patients are placed in appropriate levels of care. Quality managers have to identify what kind of data best serve this new paradigm. The denominator of measures—that is, the population being examined—needs to be defined to best answer the new questions being asked.

In addition to compliance, quality managers have to:

- define which variables contribute to certain problems and conditions and need to be monitored;
- identify the clinical requirements for preventive care;
- describe the appropriate treatments, interventions, and levels of care for certain diseases; and
- monitor health across the continuum of care.

Looking Ahead

These innovative models of care and payment require care delivery to be rethought and restructured. They are upending traditional modes of practice. Providing more coordinated care may involve more staff and IT resources and certainly leadership commitment. Hospital infrastructure may have to be redesigned to accommodate the demands of these new models and to manage the continuum of care. The community is crucial to new health care models; urgent care centers are being located in local pharmacies and stores. The CMS is encouraging all participants in these programs to collect performance data and make use of that data to improve health outcomes. The CMS also is collecting and evaluating qualitative data to better understand the strengths and weaknesses of each model from participants' points of view.

For professionals involved in health care administration and policy as well as for clinicians, the paradigm shift means looking away from the hospital and episodes of care to merged health care systems that provide various levels of care, from outpatient centers through long-term care facilities. Patients/consumers are expected to be fully involved in care. Chronic disease management will be centered in the home. End-of-life care will have to be managed differently from how it currently is managed.

The data that are becoming available for quality assessment provide richer opportunities to explain improvements, processes of care, values, and expectations through new analytics. As more measurements are used by regulatory agencies, the media, peer review organizations, and others, clinicians and hospitals are beginning to assess care via data and to create new variables that reflect processes of care. Some measures are already integrated into EHRs. New concepts, such as predictive modeling, human engineering, data mining, defining populations, and a focus on the continuum of care rather than the hospital episode, challenge quality professionals to develop new skills. Graduate training and continuing education must respond to these demands.

Summary

Health care professionals and quality managers need to understand the impact of health care reform since they are working within its framework. Health care reform changes the financial and clinical aspects of health care. To be better informed, professionals should be familiar with the:

- highlights of the Affordable Care Act;
- specifics of Accountable Care Organizations;
- new payment models, such as bundled payments, value-based purchasing, and pay for performance;
- pros and cons of heath information technology;
- innovations in prevention and improving community health; and
- new communication strategies.

Key Terms

CAHPS, electronic health record, evidence-based medicine, health information technology, HEDIS, HIPAA, ICD, meaningful use, patient-centered care, patient engagement, pay for performance, quality measurements

Quality Concepts in Action

Under the bundled payment model, the health care organization is responsible for an entire episode of care. Imagine that a physician refers a patient to be evaluated for cardiac surgery. As an administrator, how would you:

- evaluate how to allocate health care resources and for what elements of the episode?
- determine the variables you need to analyze in order to ensure a profit for the organization?
- document that the patient was treated efficiently and was satisfied with the care delivered?

Discuss each of these points with specific reference to the Affordable Care Act.

References

Charon, R., P. Wyer, and NEBM Working Group. 2008. "Narrative Evidence-Based Medicine." *Lancet* 371 (9609): 396–397.

Committee on Quality of Health Care in America, Institute of Medicine. 2001. *Crossing the Quality Chasm: A New Health System for the 21st Century.* Washington, DC: National Academies Press.

Dlugacz, Y., A. Fleischer, M. T. Carney, N. Copperman, I. Ahmed, Z. Ross, et al. 2012. "2009 H1N1 Vaccination by Pregnant Women during the 2009–2010 H1N1 Influenza Pandemic." *American Journal of Obstetrics and Gynecology* 206 (4): 339.e1–339.e8.

Englert, H. S., H. A. Diehl, R. L. Greenlaw, S. N. Willich, and S. Aldana. 2007. "The Effect of a Community-Based Coronary Risk Reduction: The Rockford CHIP." *Preventive Medicine* 44 (6): 513–519.

Fichtenberg, C. M., and S. A. Glantz. 2000. "Association of the California Tobacco Control Program with Declines in Cigarette Consumption and Mortality from Heart Disease." *New England Journal of Medicine* 343 (24): 1772–1777.

Goldman, L. E., P. W. Chu, H. Tran, M. J. Romano, and R. S. Stafford. 2012. "Federally Qualified Health Centers and Private Practice Performance on Ambulatory Care Measures." *American Journal of Preventive Medicine* 43 (2): 142–149.

Greenhalgh, T., and B. Hurwitz. 1999. "Narrative-Based Medicine: Why Study Narrative?" *BMJ* 318: 48–50.

Institute of Medicine of the National Academies. 2006a. *Preventing Medication Errors.* Washington, DC: National Academies Press.

Institute of Medicine of the National Academies. 2006b. *Rewarding Provider Performance: Aligning Incentives in Medicare.* Washington, DC: National Academies Press.

Kempton, A., E. Van Beurden, T. Sladden, E. Garner, and J. Beard. 2000. "Older People Can Stay on Their Feet: Final Results of a Community-Based Falls Prevention Programme." *Health Promotion International* 15 (1): 27–33.

Langewitz, W., M. Denz, A. Keller, A. Kiss, S. Rütimann, and B. Wössmer. 2002. "Spontaneous Talking Time at Start of Consultation in Outpatient Clinic: Cohort Study." *BMJ* 325 (7366): 682–683.

Martin, J. C., R. F. Avant, M. A. Bowman, et al. 2004. "The Future of Family Medicine: A Collaborative Project of the Family Medicine Community." *Annals of Family Medicine* 2, Suppl. 1 : S3–32

National Center for Injury Prevention and Control. 2006, September 7. "Falls among Older Adults: Summary of Research Findings." http://bexar.tx.networkofcare .org/aging/library/article.aspx?id=1465

Sackett, D. L., W. M. Rosenberg, J. A. Gray, R. B. Haynes, and W. S. Richardson. 1996. "Evidence-Based Medicine: What It Is and What It Isn't." *BMJ* 312 (7023): 71–72.

Trust for America's Health. 2008, July. *Prevention for a Healthier America: Investments in Disease Prevention Yield Significant Savings, Stronger Communities.* http:// healthyamericans.org/reports/prevention08/

Wachter, R. M. 2015, March 21. "Why Health Care Is Still So Bad." *New York Times.*

Suggestions for Further Reading

Adashi, E. Y., H. J. Geiger, and M. D. Fine. 2010 "Health Care Reform and Primary Care: The Growing Importance of the Community Health Center." *New England Journal of Medicine* 362: 2047–2050.

Agency for Healthcare Research and Quality, U.S. Department of Health and Human Services. 2010. *The Roles of Patient-Centered Medical Homes and Accountable Care Organizations in Coordinating Patient Care.* AHRQ Publication, Rockville, MD.

American College of Physicians. 2005. *The Advanced Medical Home: A Patient-Centered, Physician-Guided Model of Health Care.* Philadelphia: American College of Physicians Position Paper.

Anderko, L., J. S. Roffenbender, R. Z. Goetzel, F. Millard, K. Wildenhaus, C. DeSantis, and W. Novelli. 2012. "Promoting Prevention Through the Affordable Care Act: Workplace Wellness." *Preventing Chronic Disease* 9: 120092.

Anderson, G. F., U. E., Reinhardt, P. S. Hussey, and V. Petrosyan. 2003. "It's the Prices, Stupid: Why the United States Is So Different from Other Countries." *Health Affairs* 22 (3): 89–105.

Bechtel, C., and D. L. Ness. 2010. "If You Build It, Will They Come? Designing Truly Patient-Centered Health Care." *Health Affairs* 29 (5): 914–920.

Blumenthal, D. 2010. "Launching HITECH." *New England Journal of Medicine* 362 (5): 382–385.

Centers for Medicare and Medicaid Services. 2011. "CMS EHR Meaningful Use Overview." *EHR Incentive Programs*. Washington, DC: Author.

Charon, R. 2001. "Narrative Medicine: A Model for Empathy, Reflection, Profession, and Trust". *JAMA* 286 (15): 1897–1902.

Dasgupta, S., and R. Charon. 2004 "Personal Illness Narratives: Using Reflective Writing to Teach Empathy." *Academic Medicine* 79 (4): 351–356.

Hicks, L. S., A. J. O'Malley, T. A. Lieu, T. Keegan, N. L. Cook, B. J. McNeil, B. E. Landon et al. 2006. "The Quality of Chronic Disease Care in U.S. Community Health Centers." *Health Affairs* 25: 1712–1723.

Hoo, E., D. Lansky, J. Roski, and L. Simpson. 2012, April. *Health Plan Quality Improvement Strategy Reporting Under the Affordable Care Act: Implementation Considerations*. The Commonwealth Fund.

Institute of Medicine of the National Academies. 1997. *The Computer-Based Patient Record: An Essential Technology for Health Care*. Washington, DC: National Academies Press.

Kalitzkus, V., and P. F. Matthiessen. 2009. "Narrative-Based Medicine: Potential, Pitfalls, and Practice." *Permanente Journal* 13 (1): 80–86.

Layman, E. J. 2008. "Ethical Issues and the Electronic Health Record." *Health Care Management (Frederick)* 27 (2): 165–176.

McClellan, M., A. N. McKethan, J. L. Lewis, J. Roski, and E. S. Fisher. 2010. "A National Strategy to Put Accountable Care into Practice." *Health Affairs* 29 (5): 982–990.

Sepucha, K., C. A. Levin, E. E. Uzogara, M. J. Barry, A. M. O'Connor, and A. G. Mulley. 2008. "Developing Instruments to Measure the Quality of Decisions: Early Results for a Set of Symptom-Driven Decisions." *Patient Education and Counseling* 73 (3): 504–510.

Shrank, W. 2013. "The Center for Medicare and Medicaid Innovation's Blueprint for Rapid-Cycle Evaluation of New Care and Payment Models." *Health Affairs* 32 (4): 1–6.

U.S. Department of Health and Human Services. 2012. *Annual Progress Report to Congress: National Strategy for Quality Improvement in Health Care*. http://www.ahrq.gov/workingforquality/nqs/nqs2012annlrpt.pdf

Zlabek, J. A., J. W. Wickus, and M. A. Mathiason. 2011. "Early Cost and Safety Benefits of an Inpatient Electronic Health Record." *Journal of the American Medical Informatics Association* 18 (2): 169–172.

Useful Websites

http://www.cdc.gov/chronicdisease/pdf/2009-Power-of-Prevention.pdf

http://www.cms.gov/eHealth/ListServ_ICD10_AHealthCarePriority.html

http://www.cms.gov/Medicare/Medicare-Fee-for-Service-Payment/ACO/index.html?redirect=/aco/

http://www.cms.gov/Medicare/Medicare-Fee-for-Service-Payment/sharedsavings program/Quality_Measures_Standards.html

https://www.cms.gov/Medicare/Medicare-Fee-for-Service-Payment/sharedsavings program/Downloads/ACO-Shared-Savings-Program-Quality-Measures.pdf

http://www.commonwealthfund.org/publications/fund-reports/2014/jun/mirror-mirrorhttp://www.healthaffairs.org/healthpolicybriefs/brief.php?brief_id=78 oct 12, 2012

http://www.healthcare.gov/news/factsheets/2011/03/accountablecare03312011a.html

http://healthyamericans.org/assets/files/NYAM_Compendium.pdf

http://www.hhs.gov/hipaa/for-professionals/privacy/laws-regulations/index.html

http://www.hhs.gov/secretary/about/priorities/promote_prevention.htmlTop of Form

https://www.hnfs.com/content/hnfs/home/tn/prov/clin_quality_initiatives/hedis.html

http://www.iom.edu/Reports/2011/Health-IT-and-Patient-Safety-Building-Safer-Systems-for-Better-Care.aspx

http://www.nationalacademies.org/hmd/Reports/2011/Health-IT-and-Patient-Safety-Building-Safer-Systems-for-Better-Care.aspx

http://www.ncqa.org/HEDISQualityMeasurement

http://www.ncqa.org/Portals/0/Public%20Policy/2012%20Updates/NCQA_Accreditation_Alignment_with_Exchange_Accreditation_Requirements_11.13.12.pdf

http://www.surgeongeneral.gov/priorities/prevention/strategy/national-prevention-strategy-fact-sheet.pdf

https://innovation.cms.gov/initiatives/Pioneer-ACO-Model/Pioneer-ACO-FAQs.html

http://kff.org/health-reform/issue-brief/community-health-centers-in-an-era-of-health-reform-overview/

https://pcmh.ahrq.gov/page/defining-pcmh

CHAPTER THREE

MAKING THE CASE FOR CHANGE

Chapter Outline

Key Concepts

- Understand the rationale for changing traditional processes of care delivery.
- Define the role of quality metrics and analytics in improving care.
- Describe the role of leaders in creating an environment for change.
- Explain the relationship between effective communication and culture change.

The new paradigms associated with the health care reform environment have quality management strategies, tools, and techniques as their foundation. The next generation of leaders, both administrative and clinical, and policy makers will help to change and improve the present system, which is acknowledged to be inefficient, expensive and even harmful. Many theorists are attempting to define "cures" for the ailing health care system of the United States. Most policy thinkers agree that until there is a profound transformation in the way care is delivered and the way profits are made and costs are reimbursed, changes will simply be temporary and superficial (Commonwealth Fund, 2008).

The demand for change and for improved quality and safety is a response to the increasing awareness of how unsafe and inefficient hospital care has been. Concern began in 1999, when the Institute of Medicine (IOM) released a scathing report, *To Err Is Human: Building a Safer Health System,* alerting the public that medical errors accounted for 98,000 unnecessary deaths per year (Kohn et al. 1999). The public took note; the government took action; and the delivery of health care began to change.

What Is Involved in Change?

To accomplish these changes, and to improve quality and safety, old traditions and former modes of behavior need to be reconsidered.

New Models of Care

In the past, health care delivery and financial success involved patients being hospitalized for episodes of acute care. Health care leaders, professionals, and policy makers knew and understood the way hospitals worked and how care was organized—and paid for. The more services and interventions a patient required, the greater the remuneration to the hospital. Hospitals and physicians worked on a fee-for-service basis.

This model led to a focus on quantity of services rather than quality of care. Hospitals became inefficient; care was costly, patients were harmed. Today, with new models of health care delivery moving toward a focus on wellness, good outcomes, prevention, and payment-for-performance (P4P) models, and with physicians and hospitals ranked for quality, safety, and the patient experience, health care professionals need to develop new methods to work effectively and efficiently within these new models.

Therefore, administrative and executive leaders need to eliminate unnecessary duplications of services, departments, and programs. They need to pare down and streamline the supply chain. They need to understand their community and offer appropriate services that stimulate and reinforce activities in specific patient populations, such as encouraging ongoing physician visits in order to reduce hospital (re)admissions. Concepts, such as appropriate end-of-life care and intensive care, have to be reinterpreted, reconceived, and reevaluated. Databases have to be developed to monitor efficiency and effectiveness of services, and those data need to be presented across levels of the organization to provide objective information about care delivery.

Case Example: Advanced Illness Screening

To better meet the needs of end-of-life patients and their families, and to provide the appropriate level of care for patients with advanced illness, whether hospice, palliative, or other, information is required about these patients and their condition. One community hospital developed a screening tool to assess whether patients met one or more of a dozen potential triggers that would alert caregivers to provide palliative care consultations (see Figure 3.1).

Most of the patients were readmitted to the hospital, many with end-stage disease and/or dementia. The goal of screening these patients is to ensure that they have advanced directives, understand end-of-life options for care, have considered providing a "Do Not Resuscitate" form, and have accepted comfort care rather than more medically aggressive options. About half

FIGURE 3.1. SCREENING TOOL TO IDENTIFY ADVANCED ILLNESS

- ❑ Severe/Advanced Dementia with urinary and/or bowel incontinence
- ❑ Congestive Heart Failure limiting ambulation
- ❑ Oxygen-dependent COPD, pulmonary hypertension, pulmonary fibrosis
- ❑ Severe CNS compromise (e.g., major stroke, tumors, hypoxic encephalopathy)
- ❑ Neuromuscular/Autoimmune Diseases that compromise ADLs (e.g., ALS, MS)
- ❑ Cirrhosis with change in mental status
- ❑ End-Stage Diseases (including but not limiting kidney, cancer, liver, dementia)
- ❑ Patients with multiple comorbidities or life-altering symptoms/conditions (e.g., poor nutritional status with weight loss, presence of pressure ulcers, inability to ambulate)
- ❑ Recent significant decline in ADLs
- ❑ Repeated unplanned hospitalizations or ED visits for any reason in past 6 months
- ❑ Repeated unplanned hospitalizations or ED visits for any reason in past 30 days
- ❑ Hospice

If one or more are checked, a patient is appropriate for a palliative care consult.

of these patients met more than one trigger—that is, a predetermined identifier—alerting caregivers about the conditions of patients most debilitated by advanced illness. Screening tools such as this one ensure that seriously ill end-of-life patients and their families have opportunities to best prepare themselves for death and that providers provide appropriate care.

Improving Quality

The U.S. government supports improved quality and safety efforts and is now requiring such efforts for reimbursement. Accordingly, regulatory, government, and professional agencies that oversee hospital care have developed various tools and procedures to improve safety. For example, wrong-site surgery should never occur. To improve patient safety, these agencies recommend marking the surgical site and having a "time out" in the operating room—that is, a pause before surgery to ensure that everyone involved knows who the patient is and what the correct procedure is. However, even with these innovative protocols, wrong-site surgery still occurs today. Another example: There are policies and procedures in place to count sponges and other surgical equipment involved in surgery, and yet we still have incidents of so-called foreign bodies left inside patients.

Surgical safety is not solely an American problem but a worldwide one. The statistics on patient harm reveal how many errors are made that are preventable. In fact, the World Health Organization (WHO) has promoted a global program, "Safe Surgery Saves Lives" which encourages checklists and other simple safety procedures. The WHO reports that complications of surgery occur in 25 percent of surgery and that at least half the cases where surgery led to harm were preventable (http://www.who.int/patientsafety/safesurgery/en/).

According to the IOM (2006), medication errors are also common, both for inpatient and ambulatory patients. Patients acquire hospital infections. The Centers for Disease Control and Prevention (CDC) reports that almost three quarters of a million acute care patients acquire hospital infections yearly in the United States (http://www.cdc.gov/hai/surveillance/). Patients continue to get pressure ulcers and to fall.

Quality and safety have to be monitored with measures, not with opinions or instincts. Measures of quality are more than complying with regulatory requirements, which was their focus in the past. Today **quality metrics** have to actually measure quality of care—that is, provide an objective measure as to whether patients are doing better, feeling better, and using health services more effectively than otherwise. Quality metrics will determine whether and how successfully care is being provided and resources are being used effectively and efficiently. Financial rewards will be tied to meeting these measures.

Managing and Measuring Quality in the Reform Environment

With the center of gravity shifting from a hospital episode to the community and ambulatory care and with the new payment paradigms (such as bundled payment and P4P), health care administrators and providers have to change the way they think about treatments, interventions, and the provision of patient-centered, customer-friendly care. In this new environment, the source of revenue will shift away from the hospital to the physician's office or outpatient centers; the resulting decentralization will require that new methods be adopted to collect and analyze information. The challenge will be how to provide and document efficient and effective care in a complex and competitive marketplace across multiple levels of care and across the continuum.

Measuring Quality Performance

For health care organizations to make a profit, they will need to document quality performance in new ways. For example, the Centers for Medicare and Medicaid Services (CMS) requires that organizations track pneumonia. However, it is not sufficient to simply count the number (volume) of hospitalized pneumonia patients. For leaders to understand their pneumonia patient population and to better manage that disease process, which is especially important in a bundled payment model, they require information about immunizations, the effectiveness and appropriateness of hospital discharge instructions, and the availability and use of rehabilitation services. They also need to track follow-up visits, readmission rates, mortality, and morbidities associated with hospitalizations. Data **dashboards** just for this one measure are expected to be revised and enlarged to encompass the entire spectrum of care.

In such a complex care environment, new ways to conduct performance improvement activities also have to be devised, with new methods, new measurements, and new reporting mechanisms. Partnerships will have to be forged among clinicians, administrators, and analysts to develop meaningful databases and to interpret the results. The new generation of health care leaders will have to be more analytically sophisticated than in the past in order to understand the **scope of care**, the environment of care, the regulatory requirements, and how to prioritize resources for improvements. Therefore, in addition to monitoring financial variables, leaders will have to correlate quality variables and service variables with financial and clinical ones. Quality variables, such as the Healthcare Effectiveness Data and Information Set (HEDIS), the CMS measures, The Joint Commission (TJC) measures, and so on, underline and support the goals of reform because they measure clinical effectiveness, quality, efficiency, utilization, and satisfaction.

Measuring Care in the Community

In this new environment, quality management professionals will have to monitor more than compliance with regulations and standards; they will have to develop new methodologies to respond to care focused in the community. What previously had been distinct measures, such as sepsis or pressure injuries, now will move out of the hospital walls into the nursing facilities, rehabilitations centers, home care, and private physician offices. Data about these measures will be transparent and public so that consumers will know which organizations have better or worse measures of quality.

FROM PATIENT TO COMMUNITY

Measurements are regarded differently today from in the past. The evolution of the language surrounding quality measures is instructive. In the past, the "patient"—that is, a sick person in a hospital—received treatment that resulted in specific outcomes, which were measured for accreditation. Then, with the competitive marketplace emerging as a response to the **transparency** (information that is available and accessible) and public reporting of measures, health care organizations wanted to serve their "customers," to attract the biggest share of the market for their services. As patient satisfaction became one of the measures ranking health organizations, there was competition for "clients," developing long-term relationships between providers and individuals. The competition was based on documentation of being ranked the best on many quality variables. And finally, in today's environment, with sharing risk for care, health care organizations have to serve the "community" and its citizens. Serving the community entails prevention efforts, effective management of chronic diseases, understanding the demographics and psychosocial needs of the population being served, and providing services that satisfy the expectations of the community.

Measures change as thinking about health care quality evolves. With Accountable Care Organizations providing care in the ambulatory and community settings and value-based purchasing strategies targeting quality outcomes, measurements need to be redefined. For example, in the past, pressure injuries were expected to be monitored and controlled for the hospitalized "patient," with the goal of reducing severity and volume of skin injuries. Therefore, quality measures tracked volume and severity. As patients became "customers," however, not only were pressure injuries considered preventable (never events), but the patient's communication, pain management, and other needs were incorporated into databases so that leaders could monitor whether patient satisfaction was high and pressure injuries were low.

Serving their "clients" required health care organizations to understand which patients were especially vulnerable to pressure injuries, such as elderly diabetic bedridden patients, and to take action to reduce that vulnerability and manage their pain and suffering all while satisfying their expectations. For the "community" citizen, the issue is whether the variables that make a patient vulnerable to pressure injuries can be prevented. Perhaps better fall prevention programs would reduce hip fractures and thus reduce the number of bedridden patients. Or better management of diabetes, including nutritional counseling and improved education regarding self-management, might eliminate hospitalizations.

In the future, quality management will develop new paradigms and models to conduct performance improvement activities outside of the hospital and to design new methodologies to reach new goals. Today we look to see whether we are fulfilling criteria of indicators and complying with regulations and standards. The issue is not fuzzy: yes or no. But when dealing with the community, it is more difficult to define how to improve compliance when there is so little control outside a hospital setting. Providing care that is patient-centered is easier when the patient is within the four walls of the hospital, a kind of captive audience; doing so in the community requires different thinking and methods.

What steps need to be taken to change lifestyle habits, such as exercise and diet, and to improve an understanding of and compliance with medication regimes? Health care organizations may have to go into the community and set up markets with healthy food and locate screening activities in community centers or pharmacies. Clinical, administrative, and quality management leaders will have to forge collaborations with community leaders to help develop wellness and prevention programs that will get population buy-in, collaborations that, in turn, will require an understanding of the characteristics of that population. To develop citizen-centered preventive care in the community might require physicians to go to centers to offer immunizations, screenings, and education. Medicine may have to be readily available.

Who Is Involved in Change?

Change should be coupled with intelligent planning and strategies for implementation. It is not effective to distribute a memo saying a culture change is needed. If a hospital is not working efficiently, if it is losing money and, more important, delivering inadequate patient care or care below the quality benchmark established by the government, then leaders have to make change. Meaningful change must address underlying causes, among them poor communication between silos, poor **information transfer**, and poor accountability for patient experience and safety.

Leaders

Leaders have to lead the charge for change. A survey of diverse industries and organizations, reported by Srinivasan and Kury in the *Harvard Business Review* (2014), found that when leaders took seriously their commitment to quality, with every manager committed to integrating quality into the delivery of care, quality improved. The first place to focus improvement efforts is with leaders, whether a health care organization has poor accreditation scores and hopes to raise them, an incident occurred that alerted the state Department of Health to a problem that requires correction or if an organization hopes to compete more effectively for market share, or an organization has serious financial trouble.

Leaders have to be clear about their mission and vision, their goals, their priorities, and the importance of quality within their organization. If the leadership goal is to promote quality and safety, then integrating quality management into every level of a health care organization may involve reassessing the existing quality infrastructure and making improvements, developing new and improved processes of care and tracking their success with data and measurements, and providing quality education to staff, especially about how to use measurements effectively to enhance communication and accountability.

Most organizations that are not as successful as they would like to be need to prioritize improvement efforts. To prioritize, leaders must have clearly defined goals: Is it financial success, excellent customer service experience, recognized clinical excellence, passing regulatory surveys, or something else? New strategies focus on providing **value**—that is, aligning best outcomes and lowest cost with organizational goals. However, notions of value are quite slippery. What is valuable to one organization may not be to another. If financial concerns are primary, cost-effective care would be a goal. However, if the care is cost effective but quality suffers, that is not a good solution. Quality can be stressed, but if it is at tremendous resource allocation, change may not be practical or sustainable. Patient satisfaction can be a yardstick for value, but that may not ensure either superior outcomes or cost effectiveness. Whatever the organization values, measures are required to ensure improved processes and outcomes.

Managers

Once the organization's leaders define their top priorities, they need to evaluate whether there is an existing infrastructure to realize their goals. If not, then new and improved structures need to be developed, using quality management tools and techniques to improve clinical and financial outcomes. Managers need to be educated in tenets of quality management and performance improvement. Since accountability and communication are critical to change, managers have to make responsible data-driven decisions. Even with an infrastructure in place, leaders often have to choose among competing priorities and concentrate improvements on only a few key areas because it is impractical to attempt to fix everything simultaneously. Identifying the areas for improvement efforts requires managers to collect information to assess the current state of care, develop accurate measurements, and track improvement efforts with data. Managers are also responsible for educating all staff on proposed changes, devoting time and training to new processes, and explicitly defining roles, responsibilities, and accountability for improvements.

THE ROLE OF LEADERS IN MAKING CHANGE

Effective change requires leaders to:

- assess the current state of care to target improvement efforts;
- develop accurate measurements and databases to track changes;
- educate staff on changes;
- prioritize training for deployment of changed processes;
- define accountability and lines of communication; and
- evaluate sustainability of improvements.

To move away from old patterns requires education, takes time, and involves objective data. Senior leaders, middle management, clinicians, and staff need to be educated about using quality methodologies to improve patient care and safety. The links between quality care and financial success need to be recognized and explained (Dlugacz 2010). A patient-centered environment should be defined, as should the value of transparency, how to use measurements and analyze data to monitor and improve care, and how to improve lines of communication and really work in teams. The existing information technology structure should be evaluated for adequacy. The level of decision support available should be assessed, and suggestions should be gathered from experts on how to elevate analytics. The value of databases and dashboards to monitor improvements, identify best practices, and locate gaps in the delivery of care needs to be recognized. These strategies, and others, can bring floundering hospitals into financial viability and successful accreditation. Patient satisfaction surveys can reflect these improvements. Hospital rankings can improve.

Governance

Good-quality programs are not only useful for failing hospitals; often the senior leaders or governing board wants to excel and achieve superior rankings. Board presidents or chief executive officers may not feel that the care and safety of their health care organization is at the level of excellence that they would like it to be, even though their TJC scores are acceptable and the organization is financially sound. If the quality management program is rudimentary, most likely the organization would not be able to compete with more sophisticated ones. Investing in quality management, in database development, in dashboards, and in quality education for the staff makes good business sense and improves an organization's competitive edge.

Case Example: Developing a Quality Structure for Change

When a local health care organization wanted to establish an infrastructure that would promote superior quality outcomes, it incorporated several strategies for success. The organization had the necessary leadership commitment to incorporate quality into a focused strategic plan that would grow its clinical reputation. It was willing to commit resources to develop sophisticated quality analytics, database reports, and a communication structure that would monitor the delivery of care, locate gaps in care, and target improvement efforts.

The organization identified a physician champion of quality and change who would drive the improved quality campaign and encourage physician buy-in. Administrative and clinical leaders met to explicitly articulate their most pressing short-term goals and then to develop a longer, multiyear plan based on an analysis of what could realistically be improved quickly and what would require resources of personnel, time, and money for longer-range performance improvement. With improved information and communication, the organization was able to make the cultural change it had hoped for and the one that it felt was crucial to its success.

Administrators and Clinicians

For change to happen, for patient safety to be central to the delivery of care, for processes to be efficient, for data and measurements to be used to monitor improvements, new roles and responsibilities for quality and safety have to be defined, with clinical and administrative leaders understanding that their previous roles are inadequate in today's health care environment. What was once the sole responsibility of the medical staff is now becoming important to the administration and vice versa. Roles are merging; responsibilities are changing.

In the past, it was the administrator's job to manage the business—that is, the financial aspect of the organization—and to encourage physicians to bring in patients. The relationship was based on money. Physicians who brought in patients with a high case mix, who needed surgery and other expensive interventions, made money for the health care organization (fee for service) and were highly valued and largely independent.

However, today, because reimbursement is tied to such quality indicators as mortality, readmission, and disease management, administrators require knowledge of and familiarity with issues involved in providing care; they need to understand cause of death, reasons for readmission, and the specifics of disease management. Today's administrators need to supervise the entire scope of care (the different levels of care, such as acute, hospice, palliative, ambulatory) as well as maintain their traditional responsibility of developing strategies to maximize payments and monitoring the budget. Decisions about where patients should be placed, on which level of care, were once completely in the medical realm; administrative leaders were not involved and did not expect to be. But today administrators are encouraged to understand clinical care because of the link between establishing proof—through data—of quality care and financial rewards or penalties.

Administrators are not alone in enlarging their responsibilities. Today clinicians are being held accountable for meeting set expectations regarding good outcomes and improved performance, as shown through quality metrics. If those expectations are not met, the organization will not be reimbursed for expensive services rendered. Physicians are encouraged to take on administrative responsibilities, leading performance improvement efforts and developing, providing, and monitoring strategies for greater efficiencies. Peers are beginning to hold one other accountable for the quality of their product, like members of a sports' team who share a common goal.

MAGNET HOSPITALS

A hospital that is awarded Magnet status by the American Nurses Credential Center has met a set of criteria for outstanding nursing quality. Not only are the nurses expected to deliver excellent patient outcomes, but they are expected to be involved in quality data analysis and clinical research. Other criteria include high job-satisfaction scores and low job turnover rates. A 2013 study reported that Magnet hospitals had a 14 percent lower mortality rate than non-Magnet hospitals (http://www.nursing.upenn.edu/chopr/Documents/Lower%20Mortality%20in%20Magnet%20Hospitals.pdf). Health care organizations are promoting the Magnet designation as a badge of superior care.

Private physician practices are also undergoing change. Independent physicians are finding it impractical and difficult to manage in today's environment and are joining forces into larger group practices and affiliating with health care organizations in order to succeed financially and have support for the extensive documentation necessary for ensuring that quality standards are being met. Relationships are changing because as reimbursement moves away from volume (fee for service) to quality, prevention, and efficiency (pay for performance), new demands are being placed on clinicians to prove they are meeting standards. Therefore, clinicians have to understand quality standards, quality metrics, quality reports, and their role in improving the financial aspect of the organization.

Monitoring Quality

It is important for both administrators and clinicians to monitor whether patients have been appropriately placed and treated efficiently, without unnecessary costs to the organization. Both groups are concerned with patient care and want patients to be treated effectively because otherwise they might require hospital readmission, for which the organization will not be paid. Quality measures should go across the entire continuum of care and keep track of how the patient fares from the initial office visit to after medical discharge. One effective way to do this is to focus on **service lines** (groupings of patients with similar clinical conditions, such as orthopedics, cardiac) so that, for example, diabetic patients are monitored for everything, not only their glucose levels, but also their vision and their feet, their medication management and compliance. Focusing on service lines is a different mind-set and thus a different set of measurements for quality.

Likewise with tracking costs; costs for a service should be tracked. This is the thinking behind the movement toward bundled payments, where a health organization will get a lump sum for managing a condition, let's say, again, diabetes. The entire treatment, care, services rendered, and so on, for the diabetic patient will then be tracked for cost effectiveness. Again, this is a new way of thinking about the finances of health services.

Today's administrators and clinicians need to take the patient experience more seriously than ever before because the economic model of care is shifting to a customer-based or patient-centered model rather than a hospital-centered one. This change in perspective forces the health care organization to develop long-term relationships with customer/patients and with the community, making seamless transitions between home and hospital, acute care and prevention services.

Quality Managers

Quality management is changing along with every other aspect of health care. Traditionally quality professionals provided information about regulatory requirements and prepared hospitals for regulatory surveys. When incidents occurred, quality management staff helped with documentation required by the state agencies. But today, since reimbursement is based on quality and clinicians and administrators need to be educated and familiar with quality standards and to report quality metrics, quality management is becoming part of the leadership team. Again, traditional walls are collapsing. New quality data requirements are central to this reform environment.

Changing Communication

Both administrators and clinicians have to improve the effectiveness of communication and information transfer, with a focus on moving accurate information across the continuum of care. Information has to be consistent and provide the same detail and accuracy across providers and into different levels of care, moving smoothly from the emergency departments to the floors, from the intensive care units through to the discharge process and into the community.

Improved methods of communication are now a part of the administrators' and leaders' responsibilities. Administrators have begun to attend multidisciplinary team meetings, so-called huddles, which are frequent, short meetings, and to support and encourage various communication transfer strategies such as TeamSTEPPS (see Chapter 4). Simply put, in order for patient care to be successful, everyone involved in health services has to standardize and improve the way they communicate with each other and standardize what is said and how it is said in order to have the best outcomes.

Breaking Down Silos

Communications about quality care should be consistent, accessible, and effective. Improving communication requires a culture change, which means implementing new processes and procedures that internalize those new modes of thought. Traditionally health care services have been individualized and specialized, with each department, discipline, and service line having its own hierarchy, leadership styles, communication methods, and particular functions. Often these functions are not integrated so that one specialist is responsible for a specific aspect of care (perhaps pulmonary function) while another specialist is called in for a different issue (perhaps skin care). Often no specialist is responsible for the coordination of care. Communication suffers. Unless these specialists carefully record their findings in the patient record for everyone to read or they all speak to each other about the patient, care remains fragmented, and important information can be lost.

Health care organizations are so big and unwieldy that it is not surprising that islands or silos within the system are created. Silos are extremely difficult to penetrate, especially since they have been working relatively well for many years. Silos are especially powerful in disciplines or units where turnover is low and the environment is stable. Why change what seems to be successful? Since independent silos are inherent to hospital culture, leaders face a challenge to try to change the system to increase communication and establish a multidisciplinary approach to patient-centered care. Even with serious attempts, barriers to effective multidisciplinary communication exist.

Educating Patients

The role and responsibility of the patient is also changing. With today's focus on transparency, patient-centered care, and the patient experience, the patient and family are now expected to become involved in—that is, to partner in—their own care. In order to do so, patients and families have to be made privy to the kind of information and given the kinds of choices that would have been unthinkable generations ago when the physician provided information and patients received it without comment. In the past, responsibilities for treatment decisions were exclusively the purview of the medical staff. However, today the patient is considered part of the team.

Case Example: Confronting Choices

Although theoretically patient participation is a good thing, in practice it may be very difficult, both for the health care provider to manage and for the patient as well. My personal experience is a case in point. When I was diagnosed with cancer, I consulted three specialists, each one highly regarded and recommended by prominent physicians of my acquaintance. Because my cancer is very rare, there is little science about it: no studies, no data, no information. Even so, each of the three specialists offered me different and even contradictory advice about how to proceed with treatment. How was I to decide what would be the best option for me? On what basis? And yet a decision had to be made.

This experience brought home to me the importance of patient education, teaching physicians how to communicate effectively and patients how to listen well and ask questions. With education, patients understand their treatment options and can determine a plan; with education, compliance is improved. For example, when a physical therapist explained to me the value of exercise and the importance of movement after surgery, I was eager to start exercising and moving, even with some pain. When the consequences of different treatment options were explained to me, and I was able to ask questions and get responsive and coherent answers, I felt confident that I could make a decision.

Different physician communication styles made a difference as well. One physician was extremely authoritative, another most reasonable, the third had very poor communication skills. I determined that I was most comfortable with the reasonable one, the one with whom I felt I could communicate. Because my experience is not unique, medical training is beginning to include programs in effective communication, narrative medicine, listening, mindfulness, and empathy skills.

Health Literacy

Issues of health literacy for patients are crucial to understand and manage if care is to be successful. Technology may work well to consolidate information for organizations, but unless patients understand their treatment plan and the expectations physicians have of them, care will not be effective. The cost of low health literacy has been estimated to be $200 billion a year in the United States (Vernon et al. 2007). For these reasons, improving health literacy has become a national priority.

Health literacy refers to a person's ability to obtain, process, and understand basic health information and the services needed to make appropriate health decisions. Poor health literacy has been associated with poor understanding of medical information, limited knowledge of chronic disease management, and poor clinical outcomes. According to the National Assessment of Adult Literacy (2003), sponsored by the U.S. Department of Education (http://files.eric.ed.gov/fulltext/ED493284.pdf), over 77 million people have basic or below-basic health literacy skills, which means they would have difficulty following instructions on a prescription drug label; and only 12 percent of adults have enough proficiency to be able to use a table and calculate insurance costs. Addressing and improving health literacy can improve these behaviors and outcomes for both adults and pediatric patients. Medical professionals need to be sensitized to this important issue.

The problem of health literacy is the most acute for the most vulnerable patients: those with limited education, who are of lower socioeconomic status, the uninsured or undocumented, people with physical and mental disabilities, those with low English proficiency, nonnative speakers of English, and the elderly. Patients with low health literacy have difficulty managing their chronic conditions and complying with their treatment requirements. For example, diabetics with low health literacy have poor glycemic control; studies have revealed that diabetics with low literacy did not recognize their symptoms or know how to treat hypoglycemia and did not know what the normal glycemic range should be, even though they had participated in educational programs for diabetes (Rothman et al. 2004).

Low-literate patients may be misdiagnosed because of poor verbal communication between themselves and their providers, which may result in more hospital readmissions and unnecessary emergency department visits. Low literacy is also associated with higher mortality (Berkman et al. 2004).

Since patients may be embarrassed or uncomfortable telling their health professionals that they do not understand or cannot interpret written material, it is up to the professionals to ensure that information is effectively communicated and comprehended.

Medication management poses an enormous challenge for those with low health literacy. This is a most serious problem because 70 percent of preventable adverse drug events are due to errors in medication administration (Zandieh et al. 2008). Patients with low literacy have trouble interpreting prescription drug labels, such as: *Do not take dairy products, antacids, or iron preparations within 1 hour of this medication* (Davis et al. 2006). In addition, the written materials that accompany medication often are targeted to a tenth-grade reading level, which is too high for most of the U.S. population who read at an average of a fifth-grade level, and certainly too difficult for those with low literacy.

The situation is further exacerbated because many elderly patients have multiple chronic diseases and are given prescriptions for multiple medications. It is not rocket science to realize that providing simplified and appropriate levels of health information to the majority of patients (written at the fifth-grade level) and doing other techniques such as "teach back" (a method to ensure patient understanding by asking them to articulate in their own words what they need to do) would be effective for improving comprehension and management, would reduce unwanted complications, and would reduce cost.

The importance of health literacy and medication management has been a focus of the Agency for Healthcare Research and Quality, The Joint Commission, and the IOM, which have issued statements calling for health literacy awareness and improvements. The American College of Physicians has recommended to the IOM that drug labeling and medication instructions, both oral and written, be reviewed to accommodate a low-literate patient population (https://www.nationalacademies.org/hmd/~/media/Files/Activity%20Files/ PublicHealth/HealthLiteracy/Commissioned-Papers/Improving%20Prescrip tion%20Drug%20Container%20Labeling%20in%20the%20United%20States .pdf). The Accountable Care Act recognizes this problem as well and calls for more efficient and effective models of care, especially for the management of chronic illness, which requires health professionals to address cultural, social, and linguistic barriers to self-management.

In 2012, the IOM published "Ten Attributes of Health Literate Care Organizations" (Brach et al.), which highlights how important it is for health care organizations to recognize that not only is literacy an issue that negatively affects outcomes but that even people with normal literacy skills might have limited skills when they are sick and frightened.

HEALTH-LITERATE ORGANIZATIONS

A health-literate organization should incorporate the following 10 attributes into daily management. A health-literate organization:

1. Has leaders who make health literacy integral to its mission, structure, and operations.
2. Integrates health literacy into planning, evaluation measures, patient safety, and quality improvement.
3. Prepares the workforce to be health literate and monitors progress.
4. Includes populations served in the design, implementation, and evaluation of health information and services.
5. Meets the needs of populations with a range of health literacy skills while avoiding stigmatization.
6. Uses health literacy strategies in interpersonal communications and confirms understanding at all points of contact.
7. Provides easy access to health information and services and navigation assistance.
8. Designs and distributes print, audiovisual, and social media content that is easy to understand and act on.
9. Addresses health literacy in high-risk situations, including care transitions and communications about medicines.
10. Communicates clearly what health plans cover and what individuals will have to pay for services.

Source: Brach et al. 2012.

Interventions designed to deal with health literacy issues should be rigorously evaluated. Organizations should develop metrics to measure success in comprehension and management with an awareness of literacy issues and should identify areas for improvement. The idea is to promote qualitative and quantitative methods to promote safety and improve quality for all patients. High-risk areas of communication, such as informed consent for surgery, end-of-life directives, discharge instructions, and other transitions, should be highly monitored with safeguards internalized to avoid miscommunication.

For example, videos can be used to explain end-of-life decisions and promote understanding of palliative care. In the health system in which we work, we developed a video for caregivers for raising awareness about fall prevention. This educational video is part of new employee orientation in keeping with the commitment to sensitize everyone involved in hospital care about the dangers of falls and prevention strategies, from environmental risks, such as poor lighting or obstructions in the rooms, to quick response to call bells.

Communicating across Institutions and Organizations

Effective communication needs to improve not only among providers and between provider and patient but throughout the organization. In any large multihospital system, each hospital, whether it is community, tertiary, children's, behavioral health, long-term care, or others, has its unique history, culture, style, and goals. Because system leadership required the same standard of care to be provided regardless of specific institution, the basics of effective communication have to be explicitly defined, monitored, and supported. Information has to be moved throughout the organization in efficient and effective ways, which requires a defined accountability structure so that a specific person or entity takes responsibility for collecting and transferring information appropriately.

The best way to initiate and maintain change and to improve communication is through data and measurements. Objective information is more effective in changing behavior than memos and meetings. If a physician is confronted with accurate and valid data that show that his or her cardiac mortality rate or infection rate is higher than that of comparable doctors in comparable settings, that information makes an impact. Since so much information is now available, because every aspect of the delivery of care is expected to be monitored, measured, analyzed, and presented, the issue for quality managers is to determine how to analyze and present useful information from the vast morass of data.

Organizing Information

When leaders charged the quality management department of our large health care system with the responsibility of communicating information, it seemed that a reasonable method of confronting the challenge would be to focus information reports according to dimensions of care (see Figure 3.2).

Considering the complexity of data from all the individual hospitals in the system and aggregating that data for analysis, bucketing information into large categories in order to better organize and interpret the available data provides a coherent structure. Information is collected and analyzed according to various dimensions of care that are important to leaders: system initiatives for performance improvement, regulatory expectations, informatics, utilization management, and applied research. Therefore, when leaders require information about the health system's performance improvement initiatives, that information and no other is communicated. If leaders want a report on regulatory or accreditation compliance, information about TJC or the Department of Health is available. If sentinel events (unexpected occurrences that cause harm or death to patients) are of particular interest, because they are reported to the Department of Health, information can be reported about those events. Because too much irrelevant information can easily be overwhelming and therefore useless, categorizing information along

FIGURE 3.2. DIMENSIONS OF CARE

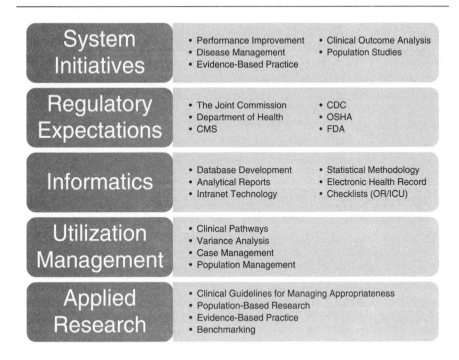

System Initiatives	• Performance Improvement • Disease Management • Evidence-Based Practice	• Clinical Outcome Analysis • Population Studies
Regulatory Expectations	• The Joint Commission • Department of Health • CMS	• CDC • OSHA • FDA
Informatics	• Database Development • Analytical Reports • Intranet Technology	• Statistical Methodology • Electronic Health Record • Checklists (OR/ICU)
Utilization Management	• Clinical Pathways • Variance Analysis • Case Management • Population Management	
Applied Research	• Clinical Guidelines for Managing Appropriateness • Population-Based Research • Evidence-Based Practice • Benchmarking	

these dimensions ensures that leaders receive the data on exactly the topic they want to understand. As priorities change, the reporting structure is sufficiently robust to accommodate new categories.

Communicating Information

However, to report even on these defined categories, a method had to be devised to transfer information effectively and efficiently. In order to improve communication and define accountability, high-level committees were developed, which we call Joint Conference Professional Affairs Committees (JCPACs). These committees are chaired by members of the board of trustees who have the final responsibility for providing oversight (see Figure 3.3).

Board members, senior clinical leaders, senior quality leaders, and administrative leaders formed committees for different aspects of care: acute care, long-term rehabilitation, ambulatory, behavioral health, safety and environment of care, and service quality. The role of these committees is to give direction and set prioritization goals.

The board and senior leaders identified goals for improving clinical quality, service quality, and operational performance. Each of the individual Joint Conference committees reports to the quality committee. Information from

FIGURE 3.3. LINES OF COMMUNICATION

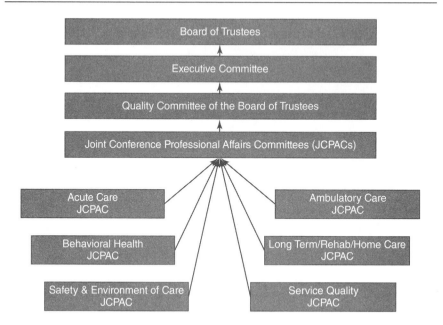

the quality committee is transferred to the executive committee of the board and then to the full board of trustees. The JCPACs are responsible for reviewing the scope of care for all facilities. This structure enables communication to funnel to executive leaders and creates a platform for culturally diverse institutions to work together.

The JCPAC committees receive information from the system performance improvement coordinating groups (PICGs), which in turn receive information from site-specific PICGs (see Figure 3.4). As the name suggests, these committees are responsible for identifying, prioritizing, and assessing improvement activities as well as for sharing best practices and warnings about vulnerabilities in the delivery of care. The JCPACs also receive information from the medical boards from across the system, which report on matters associated with the clinical staff, such as credentialing and termination, and from the nurse executive and administration. This structure gives individual hospitals from across the system access to the board. Quality managers from across the system can communicate about regulatory changes and performance improvement initiatives, best practices, gaps in care, plans, and priorities using standard reports developed by quality management leaders. This structure has evolved

FIGURE 3.4. JCPAC COMMUNICATION

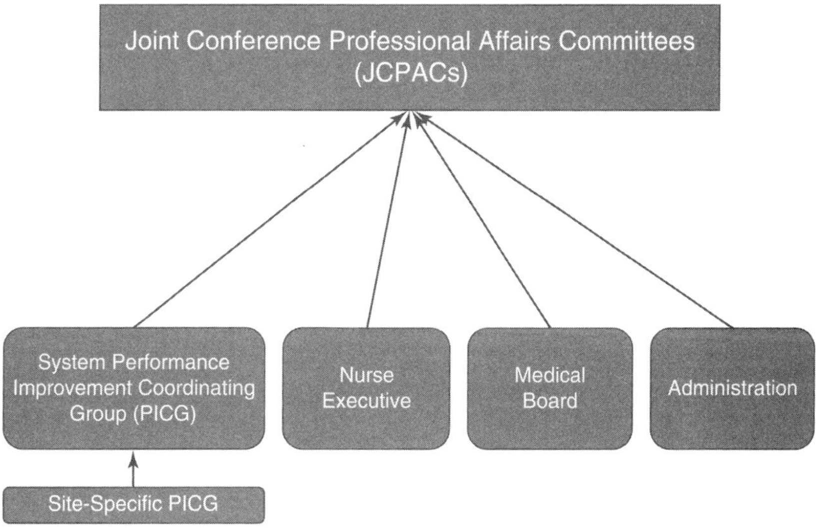

to a single oversight quality committee of the board that receives quarterly reports from specialized subcommittees.

The information does not have to move just from the senior clinical, quality, and administrative leaders to the board of trustees; information also has to be shared "down" the lines to the bedside caregiver and to everyone in between. Even when change can be seen in the upper levels of the organization, it may not filter down to the frontline workers. If there are collaborations, such as between health organizations and the Institute for Healthcare Improvement, for example, the bedside worker may not even be aware of it. All staff members in the hospital or health care setting need to be aware of the implications of their work to the patient.

For example, the people responsible for maintaining the cleanliness of the patient rooms should understand something about infection and their role in preventing it. The workers who deliver food, and sometimes leave it beyond a bedridden patient's reach, need to be educated about the role of nutrition in managing disease and recovery. Using data to educate and define accountability has to be part of every level of the orientation and training of staff.

This communication structure, endorsed by the board of trustees, enabled the system quality management department to transform the culture of the organization, moving it from reliance on investigating individual patient safety issues in a random and subjective way to a formal, objective process that defines, standardizes, and integrates the quality of care across the system and throughout the entire continuum of care.

The Role of Data in Promoting Change

An additional benefit of establishing a defined committee structure to transfer information is that it educates and informs via data. Reports to these committees are based on data. Quality management develops the measurements, "cleans" the gathered data to ensure validity and accuracy, analyzes the data for information, and then creates reports based on the data. Familiarity and comfort with data are important because health care organizations are using quality data combined with financial data to understand their organizational successes and deficits. Also, data are reported to government agencies for reimbursement and for transparency, and are publicly reported; therefore, the more confident health care professionals are in understanding and using data, the better they can function in today's data-driven health care environment.

For clinical and administrative staff, missing information, incomplete information, inappropriate information, or incorrect information may cause problems in understanding patients' health status or the success or failure of treatment and procedures. The medical record is the source of data, which is increasingly moving away from physician subjectivity to the more objective electronic health record. Organizations are moving to dashboards of quality indicators, which are graphic presentations of information, similar to car dashboards, and tables of measures to define what to improve and to understand what population would best benefit from the improvements.

Tables of Measures

Organizations struggle with how to integrate the data required by different regulatory bodies, different measurement systems, different information technology systems, and incompatible electronic health records. Health care leaders have to resolve these issues in order to be successful.

Leaders receive information about inpatient quality indicators that are of concern to them, measured across time so that at a glance they can assess issues related to the delivery of care and identify whether trends are moving in an improved direction. Table 3.1 shows a subset of inpatient quality indicators, compared over time. Leaders can see that unplanned readmissions within 30 days, for example, can be reflective of both organizational efficiencies and clinical care. If the rate is increasing, leaders may want an investigation into the cause. Are patients being discharged prematurely? Are discharge instructions ineffective? Are clinicians at fault? Was the care less than optimal? Evaluating

TABLE 3.1. INPATIENT QUALITY INDICATORS

Indicator	Prior 12-Month Average	Prior 3-Month Average	Current Month
Volume (Discharges)			
Discharges ALOS (Average Length of Stay)			
Unplanned Readmissions within 30 Days			
Admissions with Preexisting Pressure Injuries (%)			
Nosocomial Pressure Injury Rate (%)			
Nosocomial Infection Rate (%)			
Suspected Drug Reactions			
Medication Incidents Relative to Discharges (%)			
PCD (Patient Care Days) Fall Index (1,000 patient care days less newborns)			

these measures allows the board to assess what concerns require improvement efforts and resources. If the rate of hospital-acquired infections is rising or medication incidents are not decreasing, leaders may require explanations and improvements from the appropriate clinician or unit manager.

Data about ambulatory services are also monitored, measured, and reported, including both operational and clinical indicators. At a glance, Table 3.2 reveals a great deal of information about organizational efficiency, such as the number of new patients, missed appointments, and clinical prevention services, such as immunizations. These kinds of data reports are of great use to both clinicians and administrators in summarizing the success of care delivery.

Quality Measures

Performance improvement is data driven. If professionals do not understand how to measure the quality of a particular process or outcome, a program to improve cannot be developed. The basic goal of quality management is to quantify good care and safe care, which is why the government and not-for-profit patient safety organizations require that health care organizations measure their care and report out quality measures. The government does not leave it up to health care organizations to monitor and oversee themselves, and since the government is the largest payer of health care in the country, it can exercise control and force compliance with measures.

TABLE 3.2. TABLE OF MEASURES FOR AMBULATORY SERVICES

Operational Indicators	Prior 12-Month Average	Prior 3-Month Average	Current Month
Total Visits			
Total Appointments Scheduled			
Appointment Compliance (Rate)			
New Patients			
Revisits			
No-Show Rate			
Rescheduling Rate (for High-Risk Patients)			
Immunization of 2-Year Olds			
Compliance Rate for PAP Smear			
Compliance Rate for Mammography			
Adult Immunization (over 65 years old)			
Pneumonia Vaccination (every 5 years if indicated)			

Government and regulatory agencies require health care organizations to report on over 60 indicators, from patient satisfaction to measures related to the treatment of specific diseases, the so-called bundles rewarded by the CMS, and organizations collect information, via quality indicators, to understand their delivery of care. They describe what to measure and what kind of data to use, as well as how often to report and in what manner to report in order to comply with regulations. TJC insists that a structure be established within health care organizations to collect and communicate data. When organizations are surveyed for accreditation, they have to show compliance with collecting data for the measures.

Health care organizations also collect measures to assess the delivery of care. Nursing measures, such as falls and pressure injuries, are collected; measures related to length of stay (LOS) are collected. Many of these indicators or measures (the terms are used interchangeably) are reported to administrative and clinical leaders on a regular basis so trends in the delivery of care and patient outcomes can be tracked. Quality measures have evolved from operational (volume, LOS) and outcomes (mortality, infection) to encompass psychosocial and cognitive patient characteristics (e.g., did the patient understand the discharge instructions?) to prevention strategies in the community (e.g., vaccination rates).

Quality indicators are used to explain certain phenomena in addition to encompassing a broader range of the health care experience. For example, if the surgical site infection rate is higher than leaders consider appropriate, data can be collected to better understand the elements in the process to attempt to locate the source of the infection. Information about sterilization procedures, staff education and competence, and proper pre- and postoperative treatments can be collected and analyzed. If data reveal the source of the problem, improvement efforts can be made. Numerators and denominators have also evolved (see Chapter 1), and today health care administrators look to measurements and databases to monitor the delivery of care.

Performance Improvement

As quality has evolved, from quality assurance to quality improvement to quality management, the use of quality measures has evolved as well. From simple numerical counts to note volume and mortality, for example, to indicators with numerator and denominators to evaluate processes and outcomes, to the introduction by the CMS of evidence-based measures (based on scientific data), to publicly reporting data and comparing organizations to national or internal benchmarks, measures are now used for performance improvement. Measures are analyzed and communicated, and today, those who work in health care as nursing professionals or administrators use data to ask and answer complex questions about organizational and clinical processes.

For example, if data reveal that elderly people in the hospital die of sepsis, a life-threatening complication of infection, and demographic data link these elderly patients to nursing homes, as more and more data accumulate, intelligent assumptions can be developed. If analysis reveals that elderly people who live in nursing homes contract pneumonia, come to the hospital in crisis, develop sepsis and die, then improvements can be instituted. The nursing home staff can be educated about the importance of compliance with vaccinations, or the environment can be improved so as to avoid contagion. Data enable targeted improvements.

Summary

Among the goals of this book is to help health care professionals and students become familiar with issues involved in assessing and implementing improved quality care. These issues involve:

- new models of care based on quality data;
- new responsibilities for clinical and administrative leaders;
- new approaches to inpatient, ambulatory, and community services;
- new structures to communicate information; and
- new sophistication and commitment to using and interpreting quality data.

Key Terms

dashboards, information transfer, quality metrics, scope of care, service lines, transparency, value

Quality Concepts in Action

Consider the following conflict:

The board of trustees receives information/data that the hospital has a higher-than-expected cardiac surgery mortality rate and has been ranked near the bottom of comparable hospitals in the region. A board member asks the medical director for an explanation, and the director in turn asks the appropriate surgeons. The surgeons say that their patient population is complicated, their patients have many comorbid conditions, and no other institution is willing to operate on such high-risk patients. Since some of these surgeries are successful, shouldn't they take a chance on prolonging the lives of these patients? This emotional plea is impossible for board members to answer since it is not their role to determine medical suitability for surgery. Although this ethical dilemma is difficult to resolve, the board wants to resolve the difference between what the surgeons say and what the data show.

Consider the pros and cons of the following actions:

1. Since the surgeons are highly respected and well qualified and bring in many patients and therefore much revenue to the hospital, the board agrees to ignore the data and leave things alone.
2. The board asks quality management to find a way to frame the data so that the community is reassured that the hospital is delivering good care.
3. Quality management analyzes the mortality data and tries to ascertain the difference between those patients who have successful outcomes and those who do not, hoping to target improvements and develop processes for better outcomes.
4. The board and senior leaders decide to fire the surgeon with the worst outcome under the assumption that the rankings will then improve.
5. The board and senior leaders determine that hiring a consultant to review the data and make changes in the department will lead to improvements.

If you were the director of quality management, consider each of these options, and discuss pros and cons. What would be your recommendation, and why?

References

Berkman, N. D., D. A. DeWalt, M. P. Pignone, S. L. Sheridan, K. N. Lohr, L. Lux, S. F. Sutton, et al. 2004. *Literacy and Health Outcomes* Evidence Report/Technology Assessment No. 87 (Prepared by RTI International–University of North Carolina Evidence-based Practice Center under Contract No. 290-02-0016). AHRQ Publication No. 04-E007-2. Rockville, MD: Agency for Healthcare Research and Quality.

Brach, C., D. Keller, L. M. Hernandez, C. Baur, R. Parker, B. Dreyer, P. Schyve, et al. 2012. "Ten Attributes of Health Literate Health Care Organizations." Washington, DC: Institute of Medicine of the National Academy of Sciences.

Commonwealth Fund. 2008, April 21. "Fundamental Change Needed to Improve Health Care in the U.S.: Delivery System Requires Major Fix, Say Health Care Leaders."

Davis, T. C., M. S. Wolf, P. F. Bass III, M. Middlebrooks., E. Kennen, D. W. Baker, C. L. Bennett, et al. 2006 "Low Literacy Impairs Comprehension of Prescription Drug Warning Labels." *Journal of General Internal Medicine,* 21 (8): 847–851.

Dlugacz, Y. D. 2010. *Value-Based Health Care: Linking Finance and Quality.* San Francisco: Jossey-Bass.

Institute of Medicine of the National Academies. 2006. *Preventing Medication Errors: Quality Chasm Series.* Washington, DC: National Academies Press.

Kohn, K. T., J. M. Corrigan, and M. S. Donaldson. 1999. *To Err Is Human: Building a Safer Health System.* Washington, DC: National Academies Press.

Rothman, R. L., D. A. DeWalt, R. Malone, B. Bryant, A. Shintani, B. Crigler, M. Weinberger, et al. 2004. "Influence of Patient Literacy on the Effectiveness of a Primary Care-Based Diabetes Disease Management Program." *JAMA: The Journal of the American Medical Association,* 292 (14): 1711–1716.

Srinivasan, A., and B. Kury. 2014, April. "Creating a Culture of Quality: Financial Incentives Don't Reduce Errors. Employees Must Be Passionate about Eliminating Mistakes." *Harvard Business Review*: 22–25.

Vernon, J., A. Trujillo, S. Rosenbaum, and B. DeBuono. 2007. "Low Health Literacy: Implications for National Health Policy." University of Connecticut. http://publichealth.gwu.edu/departments/healthpolicy/CHPR/downloads/LowHealthLiteracyReport10_4_07.pdf

Zandieh, S. O., D. A. Goldmann, C. A. Keohane, C. Yoon, D. W. Bates, and R. Kaushal. 2008. "Risk Factors in Preventable Adverse Drug Events in Pediatric Outpatients." *Journal of Pediatrics* 152 (2): 225–231.

Suggestion for Further Reading

Committee on Quality of Health Care in America, Institute of Medicine. 2001. *Crossing the Quality Chasm: A New Health System for the 21st Century.* Washington, DC: National Academies Press.

Nielsen-Bohlman, L., A. M. Panzer, and D. A. Kindig, eds. 2004. *Health Literacy: A Prescription to End Confusion.* Washington, DC: National Academies Press.

Useful Websites

http://www.ahrq.gov/professionals/quality-patient-safety/quality-resources/tools/literacy-toolkit/healthlittoolkit2.html

http://www.cdc.gov/hai/eip/antibiotic-use.html

http://www.cdc.gov/hai/surveillance/

http://www.jointcommission.org/assets/1/18/improving_health_literacy.pdf

https://www.nationalacademies.org/hmd/~/media/Files/Activity%20Files/PublicHealth/HealthLiteracy/Commissioned-Papers/Improving%20Prescription%20Drug%20Container%20Labeling%20in%20the%20United%20States.pdf

http://www.nursing.upenn.edu/chopr/Documents/Lower%20Mortality%20in%20Magnet%20Hospitals.pdf

http://www.who.int/patientsafety/safesurgery/en/

http://files.eric.ed.gov/fulltext/ED493284.pdf

CHAPTER FOUR

NEW CHALLENGES FOR HEALTH CARE PROFESSIONALS

Chapter Outline

Meeting Statistical Expectations for Standards of Care
Meeting Patient Expectations
Role of Dashboards
Role of Data Analysis
Understanding Different Kinds of Data
Managing Care for Chronic Illness across the Continuum
Managing Aggregated Patient Care Issues
Improving Communication
Summary
Key Terms
Quality Concepts in Action
References
Suggestions for Further Reading
Useful Websites

Key Concepts

- Highlight the impact of public reporting of quality measures.
- Describe the importance of assessing the patient experience.
- Illustrate how dashboards can be used for objective decision making.
- Compare the analytic value of different kinds of data.

- Outline innovations in care for managing chronic illness across the continuum.
- Define techniques and processes developed to improve communication in the health care setting.

The definition of quality has undergone an evolution in the last several decades. In the past, accreditations scores from survey organizations, such as The Joint Commission (TJC), would signal whether a health care organization was in compliance with defined standards or not. If so, the organization was considered good; if not, improvements were implemented. But accreditation scores are static. Either the organization is in compliance or not, and the better the compliance, the higher the score. These surveys were episodic, occurring every few years, and the entire health care organization would gear up and put on its best face for the survey. After the surveyors departed, it was generally back to business as usual until the next survey. Although senior leaders wanted to achieve the highest score, they relegated compliance issues to quality management departments.

Meeting Statistical Expectations for Standards of Care

Today, however, with the publication of risk-adjusted data about quality variables and the use of that data to compare one organization to another (as the New York State cardiac mortality data do), leaders are more committed to an examination of quality care (https://www.health.ny.gov/statistics/chac/indicators/). If one organization ranks below another, or if one organization has a higher mortality or infection or readmission rate than expected and compares unfavorably with others in the region, leaders want the situation analyzed and improved. Improving quality variables requires a more sophisticated analysis of processes than just improving compliance with standards. Quality management has evolved to meet the challenge of evaluating and improving processes for better outcomes.

For example, the cardiac mortality data published by the New York State Department of Health has helped to educate consumers by explaining the health risks that adversely affect patient outcomes in coronary bypass surgery. The data also provide patients with information that enables them to make comparative decisions about where they want their surgery to take place. Due to this public exposure, health care organizations have begun to focus on developing methodologies to study the effects of treatments on outcomes.

The Evolution of Quality

Quality analysts have started to focus on **patient populations**, analyzing those characteristics that make one patient a higher risk for mortality (or other quality variable) than another. Individual hospital and physician performance are assessed over time and compared against statistical national benchmarks. The continuum of care is also examined, which includes preoperative assessment, case selection, intra-operative management, postoperative clinical decision making, and provider communication. All of these analyses have moved quality management from concentrating on compliance with regulatory standards to using data and statistics to help understand the relationship between process and outcomes and to develop accurate measurements to assess the delivery of care.

Publishing mortality rates was only the beginning of the transformation of the role of quality management in health care organizations. Today there is pressure from the Centers for Medicare and Medicaid (CMS) to monitor and report over 70 quality and **performance measures** of clinical care and efficiency. The measures are based on evidence and represent best practice standards. They are highly specific and broad ranging. For example, quality measures on heart attack care that are reported on the CMS website, Hospital Compare (https://www.medicare.gov/hospitalcompare/compare.html), include: the average number of minutes before an outpatient with chest pain is transferred to an appropriate hospital for specialized care, the number of patients who received clot-busting drugs within 30 minutes of arrival at a hospital, and the number of patients given aspirin at discharge.

CMS measures are updated regularly as evidence increases, and they are displayed on the CMS website (https://www.cms.gov/) quarterly or annually. Achieving compliance with so many clearly defined clinical quality and performance measures requires not only excellent and efficient processes of care but also effective data collecting and reporting strategies. These data reports are more complicated than in the past and contain more detail about the processes involved in the delivery of care. Managing data is more complicated than ever before. Data come from various places, are stored differently, and pose challenges to combine and aggregate for meaningful interpretation and reporting to users.

Nonetheless, if leaders want to capture market share, they need to carefully monitor how the organization functions compared to others; therefore, they have to be familiar with and understand the data being reported. Customers of health care services can choose where to go for health services based on highly specific available information about facilities. When data are less than optimal, leaders who are newly invested in monitoring quality encourage changed processes to improve. Improved outcomes have a financial analog in that financial incentives are based on good performance.

Measures of Quality

Another change in the way quality is evolving is that measurements are replacing accreditation standards as benchmarks for performance. For example, in the past, to maintain compliance, organizations were simply required to have a process to review blood utilization. Quality management would create a database of blood usage, cataloging which patients, what processes, and so on were involved. Even if the results of blood utilization were poor, simply having a process to do the review met the standard of yes or no. There was no interpretation of the data, no statistical analysis of good or bad outcomes. Today, new questions are being asked about blood products and utilization. In 2011, TJC recommended seven standardized measures to evaluate the blood utilization process. These measures are publicly available on the TJC website: http://www.jointcommission.org/patient_blood_management_performance_measures_project/.

Today, measurements are collected to show that blood was utilized appropriately and efficiently. Quality management and clinicians review the numbers of transfusions and work with the blood bank to better understand not only volume of usage but diagnosis, procedures, even individual clinicians' use of blood. Translating guidelines into numbers helps to evaluate whether there is overuse, underuse, or appropriate use of resources.

Regulatory agencies are setting numerical expectations: **deciles** (a ranked order of 10 equal groups), observed rates, expected rates. A specified number has to be achieved rather than a yes or no about a process; and the process has to be shown to be successful. Deciles are creating new benchmarks for organizations to evaluate themselves against, and those benchmarks are moving targets. As one organization improves, the rankings of all others are affected. Trying to close the gap between the actual and the desired performance (both of which can be objectively quantified) has become a new goal for administrative and clinical leaders. Leaders are asking new questions, moving away from asking whether care delivery complies with the regulatory standard to more complex questions: What does it take to be a top performer (i.e., in the top decile), and what processes result in improved outcomes?

In the past, regulatory agencies required the use of multidisciplinary teams to evaluate care, but the agencies did not evaluate the efficacy of team efforts. Today, as measurements become more complex, multidisciplinary teams are essential to understand those and relate the process to the outcome. Measurements today lead to efforts to improve the numbers, to take action.

For example, if the pressure injury rate (a never event) is higher than expected and higher than the rate in comparable organizations, leaders want to improve. To improve, the multidisciplinary team has to understand the root causes of the problem and evaluate which interventions work most successfully. In this example, perhaps teams would involve internists, nutritionists, physical therapists, nurses, geriatricians, nursing home personnel, and social workers. They have to determine what is absent in the process, what the gaps in care are that result in a poor outcome, and then determine what processes need to be implemented to improve (i.e., lower) the pressure injury rate. Examining processes in light of numbers goes beyond any individual physician and any individual patient. Such activity forces proactive team building, and working in teams has become routine for analyzing processes and improving outcomes.

Case Example: Heart Failure Readmission

Today, if hospital readmission rates are high, the organization is penalized financially. Leaders of a local organization wanted to reduce their higher-than-anticipated readmission rate for heart failure (HF) patients. HF is a progressive disease; if not managed well, patients can have episodic crises and be readmitted to the hospital for intervention. To assess the cause of the high readmission rate, a multidisciplinary team was formed that included members from the hospital quality management, nutrition, and psychiatry departments; clinicians; and social workers. When the team analyzed the rates of unplanned readmission for HF patients, the volume numbers by themselves offered no explanation. After careful review, however, the team was surprised to discover that psychosocial issues were a major contributor to readmissions.

HF patients are often elderly, depressed, living alone, and easily confused about their medication regime and health management. Many of the patients who were readmitted were not managing their condition appropriately; as a result, their condition deteriorated and they often required hospital services. After identifying the problem, the team was able to develop interventions to specifically address the problem, such as improving the clarity of discharge instructions, simplifying medication instructions, making home visits to assess patient health, and making follow-up phone calls to check patient weight, swelling, and other specific indications of HF. Due to this analysis and the solutions put in place, readmissions for this population were reduced.

Meeting Patient Expectations

Improving **patient satisfaction** is another new challenge for health care organizations. Data are being collected not only to assess care processes but also for patient satisfaction scores, which reflect the consumers' "voice." If the data collected result in scores that are not in the top decile, administrative leadership might well pressure employees to improve their communication skills with patients and institute other nonclinical services that increase satisfaction, such as reduced noise and improved cleanliness.

HCAHPS

In 2008, the CMS began publishing comparative data on patient satisfaction scores, and it announced that in 2013 it would link Medicare payments to performance. The Hospital Consumer Assessment of Healthcare Providers and Systems (HCAHPS) survey is a national survey of patient experiences of hospital care that is publicly reported as part of the CMS Hospital Compare website. The survey enables comparison across health care organizations on topics that are important to patients, such as about effective communication, cleanliness and quietness of the environment, staff responsiveness, pain management, and so on. By publicly reporting survey results, the CMS hopes to generate incentives for improved quality of care and increased accountability.

HCAHPS SURVEY

The HCAHPS survey asks discharged hospital patients to evaluate their experience on the following topics:

1. Nursing communication
2. Physician communication
3. Responsiveness of hospital staff
4. Pain management
5. Communication about medications
6. Discharge information
7. Cleanliness of hospital environment
8. Quietness of hospital environment
9. Overall rating
10. Willingness to recommend
    (http://www.medicare.gov/hospitalcompare/Data/Overview.html)

Questions are highly specific. For example, a question about nursing care is: "During this hospital stay, after you pressed the call button, how often did you get help as soon as you wanted it?" Patients are asked to rank the answer as: never, sometimes, usually, always, not applicable. Effective communication would be assessed with questions such as: "Before giving you any new medicine, how often did hospital staff describe possible side effects in a way you could understand?"

The survey questions can be found at: http://www.hcahpsonline.org/files/HCAHPS%20V9.0%20Appendix%20A%20-%20Mail%20Survey%20Materials%20(English)%20March%202014.pdf.

Leaders take the patient experience very seriously, especially now that results are publicly reported, and use the survey results to monitor success

FIGURE 4.1. INPATIENT LIKELIHOOD TO RECOMMEND

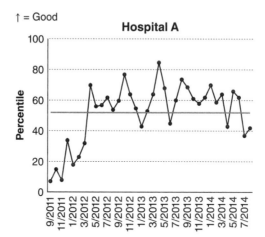

in implementing new programs. For example, after one of the hospitals in the health care system in which we work announced a serious commitment to improving the patient experience, the survey scores significantly increased, moving from below the 50th percentile to above. By graphing the results of the survey, leaders can easily view progress. Figure 4.1 shows that over a three-year period, the likelihood to recommend the hospital increased from about 10 percent to an average of above 50 percent.

In the 1980s, our health care system made an effort to increase the satisfaction of patients who had noncomplicated birth deliveries. There was competition for these patients in our area because leaders believed that satisfying young mothers and their babies would encourage them to be future customers of health care services. The patient satisfaction surveys were analyzed, and the results were taken seriously. Improvements were introduced based on survey results. Today we have instituted private rooms, with a pleasant environment, and improved communication between new parents and caregivers.

Case Example: Cleveland Clinic

The highly respected Cleveland Clinic also reacted to survey results with an improvement initiative. The clinic's satisfaction scores were very poor, and the chief executive officer (CEO) realized that a complete change of mind-set was required to change the way the organization functioned. Like most prestigious medical centers in the United States, the clinic stressed medical outcomes and did not prioritize the patient experience.

However, the CEO, Toby Cosgrove, realized that unless its patient satis- faction scores improved, the health care organization would lose patients to competitors. Therefore, he made the patient experience a strategic priority, appointed a leader for the initiative, devoted resources to the project, and insisted that everyone involved in the patient experience, from the top sur- geons to the janitors, become involved in the improvement effort, attending multidisciplinary meetings and training sessions—no exceptions. During a three-year period, the scores moved from below average to the top 8 percent of the 4,600 hospitals included in the CMS survey.

Cosgrove determined to do more than a superficial prettying up of the patient experience (such as introducing new gowns and better food) and con- ducted in-depth surveys and studies to elicit patients' input and to understand their needs. The surveys and studies revealed that patients wanted not sim- ply superficial changes but cultural ones. They wanted reassurance that their caregivers understood their concerns; they wanted improved communication about their plan of care and better coordination of care.

To overcome physician reluctance to take patient satisfaction scores seri- ously as a priority, Cosgrove assigned a prominent surgeon to lead the newly formed Office of Patient Experience. When the results of the CMS survey for the clinic and for individual units were published, employees were shocked at the low scores. Metrics were developed to track and analyze complaints and to determine root causes of problems. **Best practices** were identified.

Improvements in processes were instituted, such as same-day appoint- ments for new patients. That campaign resulted in a 20 percent increase in new patients in one year. Weekly huddles were mandated on each unit, consisting of nurses, physicians, housekeepers, social workers, case managers, and others, to increase communication and identify and correct problems. Hourly nursing rounds were established where patients were asked whether they needed anything. The leadership commitment to these programs moved the clinic to top scores. Hospital executives from all over the country now come to the clinic to learn how to institute improvements in their own organizations.

Role of Dashboards

Today's health care challenges involve data—collection, reporting, and analysis—which are used for monitoring specifics of patient care and of the patient experience. Displays of multiple variables, or dashboards of key per- formance indicators, are among the most effective ways to assess and monitor care in real time. CEOs and other leaders use these dashboard displays for visualizing the delivery of care and services. Similar to the way car dashboards display crucial information about your car (gas level, overheating), health care dashboards reveal information about, for example, composite score on CMS measures, risk-adjusted readmission rates, HF, central line infections, among many other variables.

Leadership Reports

If the CEO wants the organization to rank in the top decile—that is, to be better than 90 percent of comparable organizations—he or she requires continuous feedback about performance indicators. Through dashboards and other database analytic reports, leaders know at a glance whether their organization is ranked among the best in the region. Not only leaders, but the general public knows as well. Therefore, there is tremendous pressure to comply with the CMS measures so that the organization is valued by the public and is competitive in the health care marketplace. In order to change the numbers—that is, to show improvement—constant vigilance by leadership is required, and that vigilance means tracking and improving the numbers through feedback and efforts to identify and close gaps in care.

In the health care system in which we work, leaders receive a monthly executive dashboard based on a focused review of aggregated data and statistical analysis. The variables that are reported have been prioritized by system leaders who have targeted mortality, readmission, and infection.

Figure 4.2 shows that the dashboard displays the actual index associated with each variable and also the threshold, reasonable goal, and stretch goal. The dashboard is color-coded and easily interpreted so that leaders can see at a glance whether goals have been met or not met.

WHAT IS AN INDEX?

Analysts often display data results as an index rather than a rate because an index enables a fair comparison. In Figure 4.2 the data have been risk adjusted; thus, factors such as comorbidities, age, and others have been taken into account. If the observed rate is worse than the risk-adjusted predicted or expected rate (compared to similar organizations), then the index is above 1. An index of 1.06 means that on that variable, the organization is performing 6 percent worse than expected. If the index is 0.99, then on that variable, the organization is doing better than expected.

The data have to be accurate, valid, and reliable. The exclusion and inclusion criteria for specific measures have to be carefully defined and communicated. For example, it was determined that the measure of HF readmission within 30 days should exclude from the denominator patients who were transferred from nursing homes. Carefully defining the

FIGURE 4.2. QUALITY AND SAFETY VECTOR OF MEASURES DASHBOARD

YTD as of	Indicator Name	YTD	Threshold	Goal	Stretch Goal	Desired Direction
Oct 2015	Risk Adjusted AMI, HF, PNE Mortality Index	0.99	1.29	1.17	1.05	⇗
Aug 2015	Risk Adjusted Readmission Index	1.03	1.17	1.06	0.95	⇗
Dec 2015	All CLABSI Count (excludes NICU)	94.00	82.50	75.00	67.50	⇗
Dec 2015	ICU CAUTI Count	87.00	192.50	175.00	157.50	⇗
Dec 2015	Employee Influenza Participation Rate	99.21	95.00	100.00	100.00	⇗
Dec 2015	Employee Influenza Vaccination Rate	88.34	85.00	90.00	95.00	⇗
Dec 2015	Fluid Bolus Initiated Within 30 Minutes of Severe Sepsis	55.45	44.70	49.70	54.70	⇗
Nov 2015	HCAHPS Inpatient Likelihood to Recommend-Percentile	40.00	51.00	59.00	64.00	⇗

● = MET   ● = NOT MET

FIGURE 4.3. HOSPITAL COMPARISON DASHBOARD

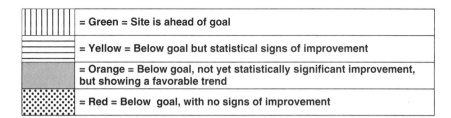

Indicator	Hospital A	Hospital B	Hospital C	Hospital D	Hospital E
Raw Mortality Rate					
Raw Readmission Rate					
Antibiotic within 180 min of Sepsis Identification					

	= Green = Site is ahead of goal
	= Yellow = Below goal but statistical signs of improvement
	= Orange = Below goal, not yet statistically significant improvement, but showing a favorable trend
	= Red = Below goal, with no signs of improvement

denominator—that is, identifying the appropriate patient population for the measure—demands statistical and analytic know-how.

Leaders also are supplied with dashboard data that enable comparison across several hospitals in the multihospital health system (see Figure 4.3). Comparing various institutions on one graphical display reveals information about which institution needs improvement and which hospital is ahead of or below the goal. Leaders can assess improvements or the lack thereof at a glance. Figure 4.3 shows three variables across five hospitals. Data reveal that mortality for hospitals A, B, D, and E are below the goal but improving, while hospital C is below the goal with no signs of improvement. Readmission rates are also poor, with all hospitals below the goal; three hospitals are showing improvement, although they remain below the goal. The data displayed show that improvements have been made in antibiotic delivery for sepsis patients and that three hospitals (A, D, and E) are ahead of the goal while two (B and C) are still below the goal but improving.

By reviewing the data, leaders can determine where resources might be most useful. Without such a graphical comparison of prioritized variables, this determination would be less objective.

Clinicians are also changing their attitude toward data and beginning to rely on data and dashboard reports to assess, monitor, and improve their delivery of care. Since the measurements are aggregated—that is, they reveal care for many patients—clinicians have begun to consider general as well as specific outcomes to processes. It is no longer sufficient for a physician to be concerned solely with the treatment and outcome of one patient at a time. In order to rate in the top decile, the population of patients must have good measurements. Therefore, clinicians have to be educated about data, measurements, and what is required and involved in changing processes for improvements.

Role of Data Analysis

In order to ensure valid and reliable data and to produce databases and dashboards that can be used for decision making, quality management departments are promoting more sophisticated analytics and incorporating research analysts and statisticians to maintain accurate measurements and develop meaningful dashboards. To analyze the processes of care, the interaction between the physician (treatment, interventions) and the patient (outcomes, complications) has to be recorded. The patient's medical record stores details of the patient's care. As data are now recorded in the electronic health record (EHR), analysts will be able to understand the process of care more objectively and perhaps generate improvements.

As more and more data become available through the EHR, quality management and other professionals are developing and analyzing bigger databases and defining which variables in these big datasets have an impact on the care environment and best expose the relationship between process and outcome. Quality professionals have begun to develop algorithms to transform entries from the EHR into useful analytics that can be used to assess and improve the delivery of care, first extracting the relevant data and validating the data and then analyzing the data for decision making.

Case Example: Assessing High-Risk Pregnancy

Understanding the issues involved in managing specific patient populations effectively and developing improved processes will improve care and be more efficient financially. Therefore, data analysis increasingly involves population studies. For example, the health care system in which we work participated in a Health Care Efficiency and Affordability Law (HEAL) 10 grant program, where New York State offered rewards to those programs that showed improved care coordination and management through the effective use of interoperable health information technology (HIT) in a patient-centered medical home model (see Chapter 2).

Quality management analysts assessed the effectiveness of information transfer, using HIT, and reported out results by defining and analyzing measures for high-risk obstetrical patients who were at risk for three clinically important conditions:

1. Preterm labor
2. Hypertension, chronic or gestational
3. Diabetes in pregnancy, pregestational or gestational

These three risk factors were selected because they have the greatest impact on maternal and fetal morbidity and mortality. The hypothesis was that information sharing across high-risk patients' continuum of care improves multidisciplinary communication to enhance care. The goal for evaluation was to discover whether communication is enhanced with utilization of EHRs and to assess whether information is transferred efficiently from the physician office to the labor and delivery room. Through evaluation of the effective use of EHRs, aggregate data and information for descriptive analysis relative to these three conditions was provided to obstetrician/gynecologists, thereby closing the feedback loop for evaluating the delivery of care for this high-risk population.

Data for Performance Improvement

Health care workers have to be educated about the value of quality metrics, the use the government is making of reported data, and the importance of monitoring populations with data in order for meaningful change to occur (Dlugacz 2006). Physicians also have to be educated about their role in these metrics. If the data reveal less-than-optimal care, often individual physicians ignore it because the data do not seem to be about *their* process of care, which they know to be good. Leaders have to drive the desire to change, or nothing will improve.

The organization has to embrace the evaluation of services based on data analytics that track information about care. Every hospital has a performance improvement structure where innovations can be discussed. Data and statistical information can and should be presented to clinicians to allow them to see aggregated care results. When problems are revealed, solutions are required. The old way of management actively discouraged employees from participating in organizational change; this outmoded point of view is being replaced by the requirements for the new health care environment, which demands active engagement of clinicians and administrators in monitoring the delivery of care.

A new culture is being established, based on numbers, evidence, risk adjustment, new goals and objectives, benchmarks, sophisticated information systems, e-learning (electronic learning) programs, and new curricula. As organizations transition from the fee-for-service payment system to the newer bundled payments and pay-for-performance models, employees need education and training. Measurements and data analyses drive continuous improvement and close the quality gap.

Understanding Different Kinds of Data

The 21st century is awash in data. We live in an age of information overload. However, simply having data is not the same as having useful information. For data to be useful, they have to be analyzed and interpreted. In health care, there are many different sources of data and many different kinds of data are being collected, and the data are used for different purposes.

A small sample of the kinds of data being collected includes: clinical data, demographic and census data, data on resource use, clinical outcomes data, health status data, financial data, and quality data. Types of data include administrative and claims data; data from regulatory studies, population studies, and registries; performance data; and patient satisfaction data. There are longitudinal data, retrospective data, and data collected at the point of care. And this is not an exhaustive list. The abundance and specialization of the data have to be addressed before the data can be applied meaningfully to improving clinical care or to achieve the 2001 goals of the Committee on Quality of Health Care in America and the Institute of Medicine of providing safe, effective, patient-centered, timely, efficient, and equitable quality care.

SOME TYPES OF DATA

Many kinds of data are collected and analyzed to better understand health care services and to suggest research activities and improved interventions. A very partial list follows.

Aggregated data collects information about a population of patients with a certain condition (e.g., pneumonia or malaria) or variable (administered blood thinners). Aggregated data are used for decision making and strategic planning because the data reveal statistical information about a multitude of patients.

Concurrent data are data collected within one to three months of treatment or intervention and are useful to alert clinicians to issues of importance. For example, if concurrent data reveal a high rate of infections of patients who had surgery, action should be taken to assess the cause.

Cross-sectional data are collected about different groups of people or populations at a single point in time. For example, cholesterol levels could be collected across age groups, exercise levels, ethnic groups, gender, and so on, to determine which variables, if any, seem most salient.

Longitudinal data are collected over time, tracking the same variables in the same group of patients at different points of time. For example, orthopedic patients who undergo hip replacement surgery can be tracked for mobility before surgery, directly after surgery, three months' postsurgery, and one year postsurgery. Since the same population is tracked for the same variable over time, physicians can assess the efficacy of the intervention.

Point-of-care data are collected where the care occurs, whether at the bedside, in the emergency department, in the ambulance, or elsewhere. The data are used for decision making for treatment, interventions, or improvements. For example, if infection occurs postoperatively, the status of sterilization procedures in the operating room (OR) might be examined.

> **Prevalence data** are collected at one point in time to discover the number or population of patients who have a specific condition. For example, to discover the prevalence of pressure injuries in a hospital, each person who has such an injury would be counted.
>
> **Retrospective data** examines conditions and events that have occurred in the past, often relating those events to a current condition. For example, a study could be conducted on the impact of a specific medication intervention given to high-risk cardiac patients over a number of years to analyze whether the intervention has been effective.

To cope with the broad range of data sources and applications, in 2010 the Institute of Medicine called for the development of a national strategy to use data to provide objective evidence for scientific guidelines to improve care. National initiatives, especially about the use of electronic data and HIT, are wrestling with the problems associated with the new technologies and potential usefulness of data sources. Electronic health data are expected to improve care coordination among providers, improve efficiency, reduce the burdens of reporting quality measurement, and improve safety by providing alerts for drug interactions and complications. Public health surveillance can also be increased.

Challenges with Health Information Technology

However, there are serious challenges to be overcome in using electronic data, basically because there is so much variation and so few standards that all systems adhere to. Even in the same health care system, data from different departments can be incomplete and fragmented. Often different data systems "speak" different languages and can't "talk" to each other. The systems are heterogeneous in quality and completeness.

Some data are highly coded, such as administrative and financial data, and others are somewhat complete, such as laboratory data. However, much clinical information is not computerized yet. Research shows that most American clinicians do not even use computers to document care, and when they do, they use free text, which is difficult to analyze (Jha et al. 2006, Ajami & Bagheri-Tadi 2013). Often data systems are not connected or even connectable so that a patient's medical history, risk factors, and treatment interventions are not always encoded in the same way in the same place. Improvement in the delivery of care is one of the primary goals of data collection. To improve care, best practices have to be identified, codified, and communicated to clinicians. Lack of standardization and fragmentation are barriers to this goal.

To come to grips with the world of electronic data, several national initiatives have been analyzing how best to move forward. For example, the Massachusetts Health Quality Partners, formed in 1995, is a coalition of physicians, hospitals, health plans, government, consumer organizations, academic institutions, and employers. Their charge is to promote valid, comparable measures for quality improvement. They publish a statewide quality report that compares physician networks to each other, the medical groups within the networks to each other, practice sites within the groups, and how individual physicians within the sites perform (www.mhqp.org). A dashboard reveals to consumers how well groups provide preventive care and manage chronic diseases. Public reports such as these strongly motivate physicians and physicians groups to improve performance.

But these dashboards have to overcome various technical challenges. Physicians may not enter information in a standardized or complete way. Therefore, capturing accurate quality metrics from the electronic record is a challenge. Also, there is often little standardization of data definitions among different EHR vendors, hospitals, laboratories, or radiology centers, again making consistent mapping of information for quality measures difficult. Even within the same network, different sites can use different codes, which forces computer analysts to link these incompatible systems. Finally, the continuum of care is difficult to capture. Clinical information about a patient who is seen in a physician office and then has an episode of care in a hospital may be difficult to track and standardize.

Different Data Sources and Clinical Research

Data are frequently collected and stored in various ways and places; data are collected by health care providers, payers, and government agencies for public health and planning. Professional societies and pharmaceutical companies generate large registries of data. Clinical trials are sources of data as well. Combining data can lead to important clinical research results. Even administrative data collected by health systems and insurance companies for billing and quality purposes, which are thought to be inappropriate for the study of clinical care, can generate useful and important clinical information.

One example is a study based on administrative data that showed that high-risk patients who took beta blockers had improved outcomes (Lindenauer et al. 2005). Studies using census data have revealed inequities of health services based on demographics, even having an impact on life expectancy (Ezzati et al. 2008). State registries, such as the New York State Cardiac Surgery Database, have produced scorecards comparing the care of different providers and hospitals. Pharmaceutical companies fund data collection and registries about common problems.

The federal government supports population-based databases for public health research, such as about smoking and diabetes. Among the best known is the Framingham Heart Study, which began in 1948 and has identified common characteristics that contribute to cardiovascular disease for several generations of patients (www.framinghamheartstudy.org). Both the Centers for Disease Control and Prevention and the National Institutes of Health support nutrition surveys to assess the connection between risk factors and disease. Combined with other large databases, such as national death registries, researchers were able to link diabetes, gender, and outcomes (Gregg et al. 2007).

Yet these extremely robust data sources have limitations when it comes to providing information for analyzing clinical care practices. Many large databases are based on observational data, not on randomized trials. This distinction is important because often randomized trials do not validate observational findings; this occurred when observational data encouraged hormone replacement therapy for women to protect against heart disease but a rigorous clinical trial found that to be incorrect (Rossouw et al. 2002).

Variation in timeliness of data also makes it difficult to merge databases from different data sources. Clinical data can be available to caregivers immediately; administrative data, which has to be coded, can take weeks or months to access; government databases used for research or planning often have a lag of several years. Another issue of concern is that with the increase in the availability of HIT, privacy issues and discrimination may be risks to patients.

Data and Quality

But on the local level, members of the medical community, including both clinical and administrative professionals, in individual hospitals and health systems are increasingly accepting of using data for quality assessment, performance improvement, understanding processes of care and expectations, and connecting quality and financial data. Those involved in health care are more comfortable with regulatory and database reports. Members of task forces who are involved with defining relevant variables for measurements for clinical improvement initiatives or for inclusion in EHRs now recognize the value of creating databases for monitoring care. Leaders are responding to numbers, especially to publicly reported measurements of care, and are pressuring clinicians to respond as well.

Managing Care for Chronic Illness across the Continuum

Another new challenge for health care professionals is the prevention and management of chronic diseases, which is among the explicit goals articulated in the Affordable Care Act (ACA). Chronic diseases are defined as those conditions that last more than a year and require medical attention or limit activities of daily living. Arthritis, cancer, HIV, and mental and cognitive disorders, such as depression and substance abuse, are considered by the U.S. Department of

Health and Human Services (HHS) as chronic conditions or diseases. People who suffer concurrently from more than one chronic condition—for example, a person who has both hypertension and diabetes—would be considered as having multiple chronic conditions. It is estimated that three out of four Americans over the age of 65 have multiple chronic conditions. Chronic health conditions account for seven out of 10 deaths (Anderson 2010).

The increase in patients with chronic diseases is predicted to cost approximately $4.2 trillion a year by 2023 (Anderko et al. 2012). As part of the ACA, in 2011, the HHS allocated $40 million for surveillance and implementation of prevention and wellness programs targeting such chronic diseases as heart disease, cancer, stroke, diabetes, and arthritis. Many chronic diseases have similar risk factors: issues related to nutrition, physical activity, clinical preventive services, education, and improved management skills for people at high risk for chronic diseases. Education and management processes are being funded by the Centers for Disease Control and Prevention. From a quality management point of view, the challenge is to deliver effective care for chronic diseases in the community rather than solely within a hospital setting.

The Medicare Chronic Conditions Dashboard

In 2013, the CMS developed an interactive web-based tool, the Medicare Chronic Conditions Dashboard, as part of the HHS strategy to coordinate and improve the health of those with multiple chronic conditions. The dashboard displays data on the geographic locations of where multiple chronic conditions occur, what services are required to manage the conditions, and how much Medicare spends on expenses associated with these conditions. The goal of the dashboard is to help health care organizations and communities improve outcomes and lower costs. Although individual privacy is protected, the information on the CMS dashboard is entirely transparent; anyone can access it at: http://www.ccwdata.org/business-intelligence/chronic-conditions/index.htm.

The dashboard represents a step in the CMS commitment to moving from a fee-for-service payer to a value-based purchaser of quality and efficient health care services. Through analytics, the CMS will be able to identify those states, communities, and populations that demonstrate success in caring for and managing Medicare patients with multiple chronic conditions. What exacerbates the cost of treating chronic disease is the high number of hospital readmissions, often because of poor discharge instructions, poor communication and coordination, or no follow-up with health care professionals. Better disease management can reduce readmissions and thus lower costs.

Quality Measures

In 2003, the CMS and TJC developed a set of core measures (care standards or recommended treatment that evidence shows improves outcomes) so that health care organizations could collect and track data and improve care delivery for certain chronic conditions (https://www.jointcommission.org/core_measure_sets.aspx). Among the measures are those related to processes for HF patients, such as whether discharge instructions were given, and for pneumonia patients, such as getting blood culture results within 24 hours of admittance or having tobacco use counseling prior to hospital discharge. According to TJC, those organizations that have implemented core measures have improved care management for these conditions.

The CMS has developed Clinical Quality Measures to monitor and improve the management of chronic disease. For example, to control high blood pressure, the measure collected is the percentage of adult patients who were diagnosed with hypertension and whose blood pressure was adequately controlled during a specific time period. To monitor the use of high-risk medications in the elderly, the measure tracks the percentage of patients 66 years or older who were ordered high-risk medication. And to monitor the efficient use of resources, a measure tracks the percentage of patients with low back pain who did not have an (unnecessary) imaging study done (https://www.cms.gov/regulations-and-guidance/legislation/ehrincentiveprograms/clinicalqualitymeasures.html).

Instituting root cause analyses techniques (see Chapter 6) can help to uncover the causes of readmissions by disease population. Once the cause is identified, the Plan-Do-Study-Act improvement methodology can be used to develop data-driven solutions. If data show that pneumonia patients, for example, are not receiving adequate discharge instructions, another set of measurements can be developed to assess communication and modes of information delivery and to evaluate patient comprehension of the instructions. Only recently have reviews of patient data prior to readmission made the link between discharge instructions (or the lack thereof) and readmission.

Once the association was identified, productive solutions were implemented. Now the measure measures not simply whether discharge instructions were given but whether they were effective. Establishing measurements for effectiveness requires new metrics. Quality management has to incorporate new measures, perhaps census data or demographic data, to help explain the population of patients in the community, to gain insight into their vulnerabilities, and to develop measures to explain their health care behavior.

Monitoring and understanding reasons for readmissions requires an analysis of the entire continuum of care. If data show that readmission from rehabilitation facilities is high, for example, the analysis has to focus on what occurred between hospitalization and rehabilitation to require a patient to be readmitted. The question then becomes: Is there a way to provide appropriate care to the patient in the nonacute facility so as to avoid a readmission? These are new questions, and they require new measurements. Along the same lines, can data be collected and measures developed that would provide information

FIGURE 4.4. RAW HEART FAILURE READMISSION RATE

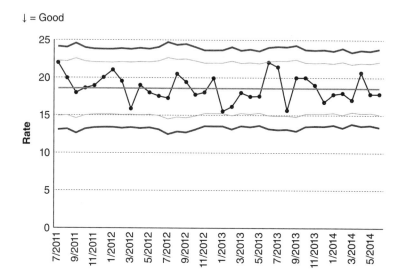

about what kind of care a patient requires to be best managed in a home environment? Measures can determine whether novel approaches (such as telemedicine) are effective.

Case Example: Readmission

The ACA has provisions to reduce payment to hospitals for not meeting reduced readmission targets for acute myocardial infarction (AMI), HF, and pneumonia. In attempting to reduce hospital readmissions, health care leaders are relying on quality management tools to help them discover the root cause of the problem and develop appropriate solutions. A simple run chart or line graph can monitor readmissions by disease over time. Figure 4.4 shows that the actual readmission rate for HF has stayed around 18 percent for three years of observation. If the goal is to reduce that rate to lower, let's say, to 10 percent, leaders might decide to target resources for developing new, more effective management processes.

Managing Aggregated Patient Care Issues

Aggregating data enables patient populations to be better understood and improvements in clinical practice to be targeted and implemented. But certain issues make aggregating data complicated; first and foremost, it is important to carefully define the characteristics of the patient population (i.e., the denominator of the measure) being studied. There are also technical issues. The EHR and the medical record are repositories for storing information. For the record to be meaningful and valuable, professionals have to extract data and create databases from that information. Although it may be more accurate to extract information from computerized data systems than from manual handwritten records, many challenges must be overcome to successfully retrieve data: data silos, organizational barriers, a steep learning curve for professionals, and technological competitiveness.

Health care reform is driving change. Health organizations are expected to collect, report, use, and be evaluated by quality metrics, public health performance variables, and administrative data. Therefore, it is imperative that data be standardized, that analytic techniques for producing meaningful information from aggregated data be established, and that quality measurements be carefully defined and accepted.

Whether in private practice or associated with health organizations, physicians have to rethink the way they provide care. Volume-based reimbursement encourages more care, but with the shift to population management and capitation, where there is a single payment for a defined set of services for enrolled patients, providers have to change from treating sickness to managing wellness. Especially with the push for Accountable Care Organizations, physicians have to manage populations because aggregate results will be rewarded. However, before outcomes can be measured and rewarded, the patient population has to be clearly defined, which is difficult to do because many patients have more than one condition.

Population-Based Measures

Patients, previously viewed as individuals with specific issues, now also have to be considered as members of a group with shared problems and health needs. Quality management professionals think of individuals as members of the numerator of a measure and the population to which they belong as the denominator. Physicians have to both treat individuals and improve collective outcomes. Denominators, or populations, can be defined in highly specific ways—for example, women over 65 with diabetes. Numerators can identify what is being investigated—such as women over 65 with diabetes who receive nutritional counseling. Technological improvements with information systems and more sophisticated quality metrics allow us to measure and compare specific populations and services for successful outcomes and for patterns of utilizations and efficiency.

Population-based measures—that is, measures with carefully defined denominators—can lead to recognition of best practices—high-quality care that is cost effective for a group of patients with similar characteristics. This is especially important in treating chronic diseases, such as asthma, diabetes,

HF, and hypertension. Considering the most effective treatment for large populations requires a different mind-set than thinking about individual treatment plans, and it may require the development of new processes of care. With aggregated data and by using quality management analytics and performance improvement strategies, leaders of health care organizations can devise effective strategies to better manage care, improve outcomes, and control costs.

From a quality point of view, changing processes and improving care for patients with similar characteristics is extremely efficient because the goal is to improve care for as many patients as possible. Physicians have used the rationale that each patient is unique to debunk aggregated data as reflective of another physician's process of care, not their own. However, although each patient is indeed unique, patients may share common characteristics that can be measured and, once measured, improved. And especially when data show that expectations are not being met for an entire population of patients, it is important to be able to analyze and understand what processes are leading to less-than-optimal outcomes.

Denominators, or populations, are defined by shared characteristics. It is important to think carefully about who will be affected by the numerator or which subgroup of the population will be best served by an intervention. The CMS defines the denominator through the exclusion and inclusion criteria for a particular measure and diagnosis. Before there can be quality improvement, health professionals need to understand on which population an intervention will have the greatest impact.

Case Example: Aspirin Administration

For example, the CMS mandates that hospitals administer aspirin to patients who have myocardial infarction, a heart attack. A hospital could easily be in compliance if everyone coming into the emergency department with chest pain was given an aspirin. If everyone gets it, then there is 100 percent compliance, and the numbers reported are perfect. But giving everyone an aspirin is not good medical care and certainly does not match the intent of the measure. The aspirin has to be given to the appropriate patient, which means the denominator has to be clearly defined and the patient has to be accurately diagnosed.

For those who think complying with government measures is a mere annoyance, giving everyone an aspirin or checking off the box each time may seem reasonable. But for those who realize that the measure is based on evidence and that myocardial infarction patients who receive aspirin quickly have better outcomes than those who do not and that, in fact, giving aspirin to everyone may harm some patients, the process of timely diagnosis and appropriate administration of aspirin is good medicine. The measure should be used to improve care. The intent of carefully defining the denominator is to have a positive impact on care.

Microsystems/Macrosystems

Improving care for patient populations may require new paradigms for health care leaders to consider. Thinking about care in terms of macrosystems and microsystems has been encouraged by many organizations, such as the Institute for Healthcare Improvement and the Dartmouth Institute for Health Policy and Clinical Practice.

Macrosystems are composed of microsystems; microsystems are small groups that work together and that, when combined, create macrosystems of organizations and individuals who work together to accomplish a goal. Therefore, the success of any macrosystem is dependent on the success of the individual microsystems of which they are comprised. In a health care organization, a clinical microsystem can be defined as the people who deliver direct care to a specific population of patients, such as a neurosurgery team, with linked processes, information, and outcomes. Microsystems share not only clinical goals but business aims and information.

In the many theoretical discussions about how to transform the complex, expensive, and seriously flawed health care system in the United States, it is not always obvious that the place to begin the change is at the microsystem level. Not only do the microsystems have to be effective and efficient and deliver high-quality care in their own right, but the links among different microsystems need to be seamless, efficient, timely and reliable, and cross the entire continuum of care in order to establish a successful macrosystem.

Microsystems, as part of the larger system, must also be responsive to the goals and vision of the larger organization and work within business and organizational restrictions. The larger organization, in turn, has to be responsive to the needs of the community, the payment and regulatory restrictions in which it functions, and the cultural, legal, political, financial and social milieu in which it is situated.

The Dartmouth Institute for Health Policy and Clinical Practice strongly supports the microsystem approach and has established the Dartmouth Institute Microsystem Academy to help health professionals implement improvement strategies based on microsystems. The Academy focuses on improving the patient experience for a specific condition (clinical microsystem). Clinical microsystems address the issue of whether the care being provided meets the goal of high-quality, high-value, patient-centered care.

The notion is that making changes in microsystems will lead to sustainable change and improvements. Researchers from Dartmouth and the Robert Wood Johnson Foundation analyzed high-performing health systems that used the microsystem approach and identified 10 characteristics that were associated with success (http://tdi.dartmouth.edu/research/intervention/

microsystem-academy) (http://www.dartmouth.edu/~cecs/hcild/downloads/RWJ_MS_Exec_Summary.pdf). Each was crucial to achieving high performance:

1. Strong leadership
2. Great organizational support
3. Focus on staff (professionals)
4. Education and training of staff
5. Interdependence of care team
6. Performance result focused
7. Process improvement focused
8. Patient centered (patient focus)
9. Community and market focus
10. Information and information technology orientation

The microsystem approach resulted in successful improvements in various environments in different kinds of health organizations. For example, at Massachusetts General Primary Care centers, waiting time was reduced to 8 minutes. If the patient had to wait longer than 8 minutes, the copay was waived. At the Shouldice Hernia Hospital in Toronto, Canada, the OR turnaround time was 1.5 minutes as opposed to 90 minutes at other institutions (Huber 2006).

Microsystems and Lean

Lean refers to a set of principles and practices that help to create efficiency and profit. Principles of Lean have been adopted from manufacturing to improve microsystems in health organizations. The goal of Lean is to eliminate waste and focus all efforts on making a product that a customer will want to purchase. Lean identifies 5 Ps to help reach the goal: purpose, process, people, platform, and performance (Institute for Healthcare Improvement, 2005).

As adapted to health organizations, the 5 Ps are targeted to improvements.

1. *Purpose.* In addition to articulating the aim and mission of the project, the purpose also helps identify the appropriate team members for an improvement project. Leadership has to support the purpose for any improvement to be effective. Members of the microsystem should be able to articulate the culture and values of the purpose.
2. *Patients.* Identifying the patients encompasses knowing about the population being targeted for an intervention or improvement. Claims data are good beginnings to describe the population because they provide demographic and general census information. It is important to know the most prevalent diagnoses, secondary diagnoses, average length of stay, comorbidities, mortality rate, age, and so on. Knowing the

patient population can help improve decision making about how best to deliver care.

3. *Professionals.* Microsystems stress teams. The term *professionals* refers to all the staff members who are involved in patient care, and each professional is acknowledged to be an important member of the team. Such respect can stimulate greater engagement in the care process and commitment to improved outcomes.

4. *Processes.* Processes are the activities that make up treatment and the delivery of care. Tasks can be interrelated, serial, redundant, or complementary. Many professionals work in silos and are unaware of what others think, feel, respond to, or understand about the process, their role in it, and the roles of others involved. If a flowchart is developed about patient experiences from admission to discharge, the many people who interact with the process are evident. Sharing knowledge among the team can help to eliminate waste and improve efficiency and effectiveness of care.

5. *Patterns.* Patterns describe the way things are done. For example, patterns can be identified about who talks to whom and how information is communicated. Also, patterns can show what metrics are used and how. Who is accountable for care? What are the clinical data, definitions, and measurements that help to assess and monitor care?

The overall goals of introducing Lean thinking into the organization are to:

- move from the traditional silos of health care institutions to a more collaborative environment;
- improve weak communication structures and establish visible, constant communication among team members;
- move from specialists to teams; and
- change disconnected tasks to a continuous flow of caregiving activities.

Case Example: Total Joint Replacement

In the health care system in which we work, we developed an integrated approach to a care, using a Lean approach for total joint replacement to promote service line efficiency by eliminating waste, encouraging microsystem Lean thinking, especially through defining teams and improving communication. Specifically the joint replacement initiative focused on reducing length of stay, reducing returns to the OR, lowering infection rates, and improving patient satisfaction.

The physician leader of the initiative not only had excellent clinical skills but also brought business and team-building skills to the project. The team

FIGURE 4.5. TACTICS AND TEAM RESPONSIBILITIES

	Initial Office Evaluation	Presurgical Postoperative	Surgery	Postoperative Care	Rehabilitation	Office Follow-up
Surgeon	■		■	■		■
Physician Assistant	■		■	■	■	■
Nurse Educator	■	■	■	■	■	■
Anesthesiologist		■	■	■		
Primary Care Physician		■		■	■	
Physiatrist		■		■	■	■

approach was stressed, with the surgeon, the physicians, physician assistants, nurse educator, nurses, a dedicated orthopedic manager, anesthesiologist, primary care physician, physiatrist, physical therapists, and case manager all understanding their roles and responsibilities in the process, from initial office visit to postdischarge office visit. All activities were overseen directly by the physician director.

Figure 4.5 illustrates the specific responsibilities for each team member. By looking at such a figure, each member can see what is expected of every other team member.

The goal was to minimize variation in the delivery of care to ensure that all patients had optimal care. Therefore, standardized processes were developed for surgical case booking, securing the appropriate implant devices, and articulating specific roles in the OR. After the surgery, each patient received a Patient Friendly Care Map (see Figure 4.6), which outlined what was to be expected, when, and why, such as issues involved in treatment and pain medication. If patients understand the reason for early ambulation or how pain medication is assessed, they are more comfortable, less anxious, and more compliant with the care plan. Understanding the care plan enables patients and families to anticipate, comply, and be actively involved in the surgical plan of care.

Each step in the process was highly defined. For example, before the surgery, each patient went through a series of defined steps to ensure that the team had appropriate information and that the patient had appropriate consultations, such as with a physiatrist, and education about the procedure (see Figure 4.7). The postoperative steps (see Figure 4.8) encouraged physical

FIGURE 4.6. PATIENT FRIENDLY CARE MAP FOR HIP REPLACEMENT SURGERY

This protocol is a general guideline and does not represent a professional care standard governing provider's obligation to patients. Care is revised to meet the individual patient needs.	
BLOOD DRAWING	Blood work may be drawn by the Health Care Team as ordered by your doctor. It may be necessary to draw blood several times during the day in order to check your condition and response to treatment.
TESTS	Additional tests may be ordered by your doctor. The Health Care Team will explain any tests that are ordered.

TREATMENTS

You will have an intravenous line (IV). You will have an abduction pillow (a firm triangle pillow) between your legs while you are in bed to remind you not to cross your legs. A tube will be placed in your bladder to drain urine, it will be removed before you go home. You may have a drain coming from your incision, it will also be removed before you go home. You will have a bandage over your hip, it will be changed as ordered by your doctor. A trapeze will be placed over your bed to make moving in bed easier. Inflatable cuffs will be placed around your legs while in bed to help the circulation.

	be instructed not to cross your legs, to prevent dislocating your new hip. You will be seen by a Physical Therapist and are expected to participate in therapy.
TEAM ACTIVITIES	Members of the Health Care Team will go over the plan of care and answer any questions that you or your family may have. Speak up if you have questions or concerns and if you do not understand ask again.
EDUCATION	You will be taught how to use the pain scale. This will help the staff to understand and manage your pain. You will be taught safety precautions, which will include being

MEDICATIONS and date of birth by the members of the Health Care Team before medications, treatments, procedures or tests. You will be taught how nd cough and use the incentive spirometer to keep your lungs clear. You will be taught about the medication you are taking and the possible side effects.

You may receive antibiotics through your intravenous line (IV) and you may receive medication to prevent blood clots. Your pain medication will be based on your needs, how it is given will be ordered by your doctor. The Health Care Team will explain the medications you are taking and any side effects.

PLANNING	case manager may visit you to talk about your discharge plan. Your nurse will go over your discharge instructions with you and your family before you go home. Your recovery after leaving the hospital will depend on how active you are in your own care and how well you follow directions about the follow-up care and services you need.

activity and appropriate discharge planning. Data were collected, analyzed, and reported to the team about clinical and quality-of-life variables.

By standardizing and monitoring every aspect of the procedure, outcomes improved, infection decreased, and patients indicated improved quality of life. Patients were assessed before the procedure, six weeks after the procedure, and one year after the procedure. In addition, the success of the program resulted in increased volume with concomitant financial gains. Professional and patient satisfaction were increased. Using the microsystem approach with the orthopedic service line as the product and with shared goals for team members, quality and safety were improved, as were efficiency and resource utilization.

FIGURE 4.7. PREOPERATIVE CONTINUUM OF CARE

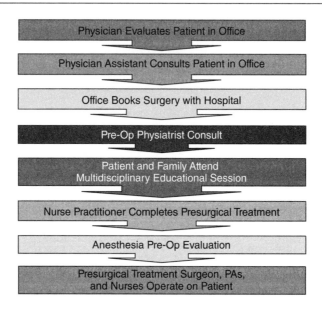

FIGURE 4.8. POSTOPERATIVE CONTINUUM OF CARE

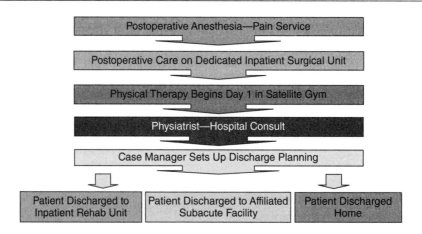

Improving Communication

In today's health care environment, data and HIT are expected to be used in communicating effectively about care. Effective communication strategies have been introduced into health care to improve teamwork, establish improved relationships between physicians and patients, and among professionals for better coordination of care.

Teamwork

Not that long ago, when patients were seen by a single practitioner with perhaps a nurse assisting, communication among caregivers was relatively uncomplicated. Today, when many medical experiences involve not only physicians but also nurse practitioners, physician assistants, nurses, administrators, billers, specialists, pharmacists, technicians, home health aides, and more, new methods of providing effective communication are required to deliver high-quality and safe patient care. Indeed, communication failures are the leading cause of preventable patient harm and must be taken very seriously (Leonard, Graham, and Bonacum 2004, http://www.healthcarebusinesstech .com/communication-patient-harm).

Among the findings of the IOM 1999 report *To Err Is Human* is that success or failure in health care depends on the performance of teams because working in teams promotes communication. The report recommended interdisciplinary team training to increase patient safety and quality health care. TJC, the Institute for Healthcare Improvement, the National Quality Forum, and the Accreditation Council for Graduate Medical Education have all called for implementation of strategies to improve teamwork.

SENTINEL EVENT

According to TJC: "A sentinel event is an unexpected occurrence involving death or serious physical or psychological injury, or the risk thereof." *Serious injury* specifically includes loss of limb or function. The phrase "or the risk thereof" includes any process variation for which a recurrence would carry a significant chance of a serious adverse outcome. Such events are called "sentinel" because they signal the need for immediate investigation and response.

Source: http://www.jointcommission.org/assets/1/6/camh_2012_update2_24_se.pdf

---

Each caregiver among the multiple caregivers who deliver services to a single patient may be most comfortable working independently of others, with the unfortunate consequence of causing the care to be quite fragmented and the communication disconnected. With individuals working alone, sharing information about a coherent and comprehensive plan of care is difficult and requires specific efforts in collaboration (Leasure et al. 2013). The importance of communication among multiple caregivers has given rise to the notion of teams, where professionals work together, communicate effectively, and provide patients with coordinated care. Some teams work together for years, such as highly specialized orthopedic teams or cardiac surgery teams, and some teams are formed for a specific purpose, such as a quality improvement initiative on a specific project. But many teams are ad hoc: caregivers who address the problems of a particular patient during a particular episode of illness or hospitalization.

Regardless of whether the teams are of long or short term, communication is crucial for effective care to be accomplished. Teamwork is difficult because many medical professionals are trained independently, are from different disciplines with specific cultures, and have had various educational training and experience; they may also have distinct personal and cultural communication styles. Yet they are all expected to cooperate and coordinate activities while performing their specific required tasks.

As important as teamwork is in the complex health care setting, simply installing or labeling members of different disciplines a "team" does not mean that the outcome will be coordinated care. There has to be a shared mind-set, a willingness to cooperate and communicate effectively with the common goal of improving quality and safety for the patient. Health care is not team friendly, which is why special and specific training is required to promote effective teamwork. Health care organizations have a hierarchical culture, which often hinders effective communication among caregivers, especially nurses and physicians. For this reason, standardized communication tools, such as TeamSTEPPS, SBAR, and checklists, have been developed.

TeamSTEPPS

TeamSTEPPS is an acronym for Team Strategies and Tools to Enhance Performance and Patient Safety. Developed in 2006 for the aviation industry by the Department of Defense and the Agency for Healthcare Research and Quality (AHRQ) to improve the quality, safety, and efficiency of health care, it is an approach to effective teamwork and communication. Its evidence-based toolkit is designed to train providers in enhanced communication and teamwork skills (King et al. 2008). TeamSTEPPS has been implemented successfully in the military health care system, and the AHRQ is attempting to support the implementation of TeamSTEPPS nationally for health care organizations. In addition, TeamSTEPPS is a training and educational program focused on developing skills and competencies in leadership, situation monitoring, mutual support, and effective communication.

The goal of TeamSTEPPS is to deliver high-quality, safe patient care through the use of teams that will have the capacity to use information and resources in a collaborative way to achieve optimal outcomes for patients. Members of the teams are expected to be aware of their individual roles and responsibilities as well as the collective goal for the patient. Information sharing is key, as is conflict resolution. The curriculum focuses on three phases: assessment, training, and implementation. Specifics of the training can be found at http://teamstepps.ahrq.gov/about-2cl_3.htm. TeamSTEPPS, which is usually offered by aviation trainers or other consultants, hopes to create an atmosphere where all team members feel comfortable speaking up when they suspect a problem. Human fallibility, including fatigue and forgetfulness, is often rejected as a normal issue to be addressed in avoiding adverse events.

For several reasons, TeamSTEPPS has not been universally implemented in health care settings. One reason is that training for TeamSTEPPS requires resources of time and a financial commitment to release staff for the training, and not all leaders are convinced that the resource drain will pay off. Although TeamSTEPPS has been shown to be useful in military and aviation settings, no substantial body of research proves its successful adaptability to health care. Also, variations in organizational structure and culture are not accounted for in the general curriculum, and so the training may not be appropriate for all settings.

Case Example: Improving Cardiac Mortality

When one of the flagship hospitals in the health care network in which we work determined to improve its cardiac morality rate, leaders supported an improvement initiative that involved many changes, among them introducing TeamSTEPPS, adopting **Collaborative Care Councils** and other TeamSTEPPS strategies. Collaborative Care Councils foster shared mental models, communication, mutual trust, and a team approach to patient care. The goal of fostering patient-centered care through high-functioning, frontline interdisciplinary teams could be met through the interdisciplinary team structure of the councils, which would be a more collaborative and effective approach than the existing provider-centric, siloed, and hierarchical model.

The goal of the initiative, supported by the system's Institute of Nursing, was to create a culture of safety and a sustainable teamwork strategy to reduce errors. In addition to the vision of zero tolerance for errors, the system hoped to empower staff at every level to speak up to improve safety. The training stresses effective communication tools, such as SBAR (discussed next), multidisciplinary team engagement, mutual trust, a shared model of safety, and a framework for conflict resolution.

Leaders endorsed the model for improved safety, and although physicians expressed some initial skepticism, once the initiative was launched and the outcomes were successful, professional enthusiasm and pride overcame the initial reluctance. The team learned a problem-solving technique that reinforces care plans or adjusts them appropriately, and the method was very effective in breaking down silos. Huddles and handoffs—the transfer of information during transitions in care, which includes the opportunity to ask questions—are now routinely used in the ORs, intensive care units, and postoperative care areas of all the hospitals in our multihospital health care system and facilitate direct communication among the frontline care providers. The initiative resulted in reducing mortality rates, lowering infection rates, and promoting greater provider and patient satisfaction.

SBAR

SBAR, an acronym for Situation, Background, Assessment, and Recommendation, refers to a communication tool or framework that was adapted from the military to health care for the purpose of structuring appropriate and timely communication among members of a patient's health care team. Its highly structured format and formalized outline are especially useful to communicate patient status and clinician expectations during shift changes and handoffs, and it has been incorporated into TeamSTEPPS.

The SBAR technique attempts to overcome individual communication and personal styles so that communication follows an expected path and contains specific elements. Often clinicians have different perceptions of care expectations, and the SBAR format helps to ensure that everyone is on the same page. Because it is so formalized, it also helps overcome hierarchical issues that result from not all caregivers feeling equally safe to speak, especially about patient safety and perceived potential harm.

Different modes of communication are common in medical training. Nurses are taught to offer general narratives of clinical situations while physicians are trained to be very concise and specific. Nurses are taught that it is not their job to make diagnoses, but they are usually the first line of defense in a patient safety situation. SBAR can help eliminate stylistic differences and mitigate established hierarchy patterns of communication. A common mental model and recognized critical thinking language can help caregiving teams to function well.

When using SBAR, the clinician describes specific elements to other team members:

• *Situation*, which refers to a brief explanation of what is happening at the present time. Because clinicians understand that a brief assessment is expected, they hone their critical thinking skills. Elements to be described include the identification of the person you are speaking to; identifying yourself; identification of the patient by name, date of birth, age, sex, and reason for admission; and the issue with the patient.

- *Background,* which describes what led up to this situation and includes the patient's presenting complaint and a brief summary of the patient's medical history.
- *Assessment,* which includes the speaker's view of what is going on in the situation and includes the patient's vital signs (heart rate, blood pressure, temperature, oxygen saturation), pain scale and level of consciousness. If any of the vital signs are outside of the normal parameters, the professional states his or her clinical impression of the patient's condition.
- *Recommendation,* which is where the professional explains what is required and how urgently, offers suggestions of actions to be taken, and clarifies what action is expected to be taken (http://www.jointcommission.org/at_home_with_the_joint_commission/sbar_%E2%80%93_a_powerful_tool_to_help_improve_communication/).

With the complexity of care and the myriad caregivers involved in a patient's treatment across the entire continuum of care, precise, concise, and structured information helps to avoid gaps and inefficiencies in information transfer (Clancy and Tornberg 2007). Nurses trained in SBAR learn to synthesize information and think critically about their recommendations for action. The technique also provides novice nurses with direction. SBAR is especially useful for informing physicians who are covering, subspecialists, or others who are not entirely familiar with a case what is the status, the problem, and a suggested plan of action. In addition, this kind of cogent, concise, and coherent information helps to get the provider to the bedside when necessary. If the nurse recommends that the patient be seen, the physician understands that the situation may be urgent.

Checklists

Checklists are ubiquitous. We all use them in various settings, for shopping lists, to-do lists, organizing trips and dinner parties, and so on. And there is no shortage of checklists in health care. There are surgical checklists to ensure proper procedures, CEO checklists to promote values and goals, checklists for caregivers to deal with specific conditions, checklists for emergency preparedness, preoperative checklists, anesthesia checklists, checklists for patients to prepare for procedures, among many others. As with most tools, they are useful under certain conditions and are not as effective in others.

Checklists, simple interventions that have been used very successfully, are designed to assist memory. They are used in the aviation industry to great success, standardizing the steps in a process, and formalizing expectations about what is to occur and in what sequence. In the health care setting, checklists help to encode the necessary steps in a process and prevent crucial steps from being forgotten or overlooked. Checklists are particularly effective when routines have become automatic. In those cases, when one is on autopilot, distracted, tired, or simply bored, it is easy to forget a step in a process. Checklists provide standardization of processes and insurance that all steps are accomplished; they can help to reduce variability that might result in poor performance.

Checklists are easy to use, ensuring that communication is not idiosyncratic or capricious. There are steps to follow; everyone has the same expectations of behavior. Not only do checklists encourage shared expectations, but they eliminate communication style differences that can lead to patient harm. Checklists, then, serve as a kind of translation tool so that different specialists with different training have access to identical information (Winters et al. 2009).

Checklists were enthusiastically endorsed by government agencies involved in improving patient safety. The "Keystone ICU" project, which was funded by the AHRQ, involved more than 100 Michigan intensive care units. The initiative involved adopting an evidenced-based infection control checklist to reduce the incidence of bloodstream infections associated with central lines (Pronovost et al. 2006). The intervention used five strategies recommended by the Centers for Disease Control and Prevention:

1. Wash hands with soap.
2. Clean patient's skin with chlorhexidine antiseptic.
3. Put sterile drapes on the entire patient.
4. Wear sterile gown and mask.
5. Put sterile dressing over the insertion site.

Not rocket science or high tech, by any means. The intervention was remarkably successful in eliminating these infections almost entirely in all the intensive care units, and the improvement was sustained over an 18-month period. After this success, these checklists were launched nationally, with successes reported.

The World Health Organization also began recommending checklists in 2007 to improve surgical safety, avoid infections, and encourage better communication (http://www.who.int/patientsafety/implementation/checklists/en/). It enlisted an international multidisciplinary panel of experts to create a surgical safety checklist. The checklist was piloted and validated in various setting across the world. The success of the surgical safety checklist was reported in *The New England Journal of Medicine* (Haynes et al. 2009) and showed that deaths and complications from surgery were reduced by 36 percent.

Many studies of checklists report successes. Therefore, the interesting question is: With so many reported successes, and with so much government support, and such commonsense positive attributes, why aren't checklists universally used in health care? The answer, as it almost always is, is culture.

Developing appropriate and evidence-based checklists is difficult and requires time and research. But the real problem is implementation. Simply handing caregivers a checklist does not address the problem. They need to be motivated to use it, to change the way they do things, to incorporate it, to use it consistently, and to understand its value with regard to safer outcomes. Checklists are merely tools, and ones that require constant updating as new information comes to light. Patient safety involves establishing a culture of safety, perhaps using such tools. But cultural commitment is essential for any tool to be successful. The hierarchical structure of medical care, and perhaps especially in the OR during an emergency, needs to be modified in order to empower nurses, for example, to question physicians who are not following a checklist.

Many physicians resist using checklists because they feel that checking off a list will not improve care delivery or avoid mistakes. Also, physicians are trained to think independently, to rely on their training and experience and not to reach for cognitive aids during an emergency. Critical thinking in an emergency cannot and should not be overridden by a checklist. Professionals know their job and do not want to be confined to someone else's notion of how their job should be accomplished. Checklists that are poorly designed or have not achieved physician buy-in may actually complicate tasks and be inefficient.

Summary

Health care professionals face many new challenges in the reform environment. Administrators and clinicians need to become familiar with:

- the evolution and use of multiple measurements in improving care;
- various techniques for monitoring and improving patient satisfaction;
- the value of relying on data and dashboards to prioritize resources and improvement efforts;
- techniques that have developed to improve care in the community and better manage disease populations; and
- various techniques to improve communication between caregiver and patient and among caregivers.

Key Terms

best practices, Collaborative Care Councils, deciles, patient populations, patient satisfaction, performance measures

Quality Concepts in Action

The hospital that you are associated with has a 24 percent rate of readmission for HF patients. CMS data indicate that the rate should be lower and is lower for comparable hospitals. The medical staff explains that these patients cannot cope with treatment at home for different reasons, are noncompliant with their medication management, do not come for follow-up visits, and therefore go into crisis that requires hospitalization. As a senior administrator, what approach would you take? Would you:

- reevaluate the competency of caregivers and the adequacy and effectiveness of their treatment and discharge instructions?
- examine the problem from the process point of view and analyze throughput, intake, discharge, and follow-up procedures?
- do a Plan-Do-Study-Act assessment for performance improvement to develop new and better processes?
- hire external consultant experts to examine the process and offer advice for improvements?

Argue the merits and disadvantages of each of these approaches.

References

Ajami, S., and T. Bagheri-Tadi. 2013. "Barriers for Adopting Electronic Health Records (EHRs) by Physicians." *Acta Informatica Medica* 21(2), 129–134.

Anderko, L., J. S. Roffenbender, R. Z. Goetzel, F. Millard, K. Wildenhaus, et al. 2012. "Promoting Prevention through the Affordable Care Act: Workplace Wellness." *Preventing Chronic Disease* 9: 120092.

Anderson, G. 2010. *Chronic Care: Making the Case for Ongoing Care*. Princeton, NJ: Robert Woods Johnson Foundation.

Clancy, C. M., and D. N. Tornberg. 2007. "TeamSTEPPS: Assuring Optimal Teamwork in Clinical Settings." *American Journal of Medical Quality* 22: 214–217.

Committee on Quality of Health Care in America, Institute of Medicine. 2001. *Crossing the Quality Chasm: A New Health System for the 21st Century*. Washington, DC: National Academies Press.

Dlugacz, Y. 2006. *Measuring Health Care: Using Quality Data for Operational, Financial, and Clinical Improvement*. San Francisco: Jossey-Bass.

Ezzati, M., A. B. Friedman, S. C. Kulkarni, and C. J. Murray. 2008. "The Reversal of Fortunes: Trends in County Mortality and Cross-County Mortality Disparities in the United States." *PLoS Medicine* 5 (4): e66.

Gregg, E. W., Q. Gu, Y. J. Cheng, K. M. Narayan, and C. C. Cowie. 2007. "Mortality Trends in Men and Women with Diabetes, 1971 to 2000." *Annals of Internal Medicine* 147 (3), 149–155.

Haynes, A. B., T. G. Weiser, W. R. Berry, S. R. Lipsitz, A.-H. S. Breizat, E. P. Dellinger, T. Herbosa, et al. 2009. "A Surgical Safety Checklist to Reduce Morbidity and Mortality in a Global Population." *New England Journal of Medicine* 360: 491–499.

Huber, T. 2006, September 18 and 25. "Micro-Systems in Health Care: Essential Building Blocks for the Successful Delivery of Health Care in the 21st Century." Presentation to the CCHA CCS NICU Improvement Project.

Institute for Healthcare Improvement. 2005. "Going Lean in Health Care." IHI Innovation Series White Paper. Cambridge, MA: Institute for Healthcare Improvement.

Jha, A. K., T. G. Ferris, K. Donelan, C. DesRoches, A. Shields, S. Rosenbaum, and D. Blumenthal. 2006. "How Common Are Electronic Health Records in the United States? A Summary of the Evidence." *Health Affairs* 25 (6): w496–w507.

King, H. B., J. Battles, D. P. Baker, A. Alonso, E. Salas, J. Webster, L. Toomey, et al. 2008. "TeamSTEPPS™: Team Strategies and Tools to Enhance Performance and Patient Safety." In: Henriksen, K., Battles, J.B., Keyes, M.A., Grady, M. (eds.) *Advances in Patient Safety: New Directions and Alternative Approaches (Vol. 3: Performance and Tools).* Rockville, MD: Agency for Healthcare Research and Quality.

Kohn, K. T., J. M. Corrigan, and M. S. Donaldson. 1999. *To Err Is Human: Building a Safer Health System.* Washington, DC: National Academies Press.

Leasure, E. L., R. R. Jones, L. B. Meade, M. I. Sanger, K. G. Thomas, V. P. Tilden, J. L. Bowen, et al. 2013. "There Is No 'I' in Teamwork in the Patient-Centered Medical Home: Defining Teamwork Competencies for Academic Practice." *Academic Medicine* 88 (5): 585–592.

Leonard, M., S. Graham, and D. Bonacum, D. 2004. "The Human Factor: The Critical Importance of Effective Teamwork and Communication in Providing Safe Care." *Quality & Safety in Health Care* 13(Suppl. 1): i85–i90.

Lindenauer, P. K., P. S. Pekow, K. Wang, D. K. Mamidi, B. Gutierrez, and E. M. Benjamin. 2005. "Perioperative Beta-Blocker Therapy and Mortality after Major Noncardiac Surgery." *New England Journal of Medicine* 353 (4): 349–361.

Pronovost, P., D. Needham, S. Berenholtz, D. Sinopoli, H. Chu, S. Cosgrove, B. Sexton, et al. 2006. "An Intervention to Decrease Catheter-Related Bloodstream Infections in the ICU." *New England Journal of Medicine* 355: 2725–2732.

Rossouw, J. E., G. L. Anderson, R. L. Prentice, A. Z. LaCroix, C. Kooperberg, M. L. Stefanick, R. D., et al. 2002. "Risks and Benefits of Estrogen Plus Progestin in Healthy Postmenopausal Women: Principal Results from the Women's Health Initiative Randomized Controlled Trial." *JAMA: The Journal of the American Medical Association* 288 (3): 321–333.

Winters, B. D., A. P. Gurses, H. Lehmann, J. B. Sexton, C. J. Rampersad, and P. J. Pronovost. 2009. "Clinical Review: Checklists—Translating Evidence into Practice." *Critical Care* 13: 210.

Suggestions for Further Reading

AHRQ Conference on Health Care Data Collection and Reporting. 2007, March. *Collecting and Reporting Data for Performance Measurement: Moving Toward Alignment.* Report of Proceedings. Chicago: AHRQ Publication No. 07-0033-EF.

Batalden, P., and M. Splaine. 2002. "What Will It Take to Lead the Continual Improvement and Innovation of Health Care in the Twenty-First Century?" *Quality Management in Health Care* 11 (1): 45–54.

Gawande, A. 2007, December 10. "The Checklist: If Something So Simple Can Transform Intensive Care, What Else Can It Do?" *The New Yorker*, pp. 1–8.

Institute of Medicine Roundtable on Value & Science-Driven Health Care. 2010. "Clinical Data as the Basic Staple of Health Learning: Creating and Protecting a Public Good." Workshop Summary. Washington, DC: National Academies Press.

Joint Commission on Accreditation of Healthcare Organizations. 2004, June 29. "Sentinel Event Statistics." www.jcaho.org/accredited+organizations/ambulatory+care/sentinel+events/sentinel+event+statistics.htm

Lingard, L., G. Regehr, B. Orser, R. Reznick, G. R. Baker, D. Doran, S. Espin, et al. 2008. "Evaluation of a Preoperative Checklist and Team Briefing among Surgeons, Nurses, and Anesthesiologists to Reduce Failures in Communication." *Archives of Surgery* 143: 12–18.

Merlino, J. I., and A. Raman. 2013, May. "Health Care's Service Fanatics." *Harvard Business Review*: 108–116.

Mohr, J., P. Batalden, and P. Barach. 2004. "Integrating Patient Safety into the Clinical Microsystem." *Quality* & S*afety* in *Health Care* 13 (Suppl. 2): ii34–ii38.

Nelson, E. C., P. B. Batalden, T. P. Huber, J. J. Mohr, M. M. Godfrey, L. A. Headrick, and J. H. Wasson. 2002. "Microsystems in Health Care: Part 1. Learning from High-Performing Front-line Clinical Units." *Joint Commission Journal on Quality Improvement* 28 (9): 472–493.

Nelson, E. C., P. B. Batalden, M. M. Godfrey, L. A. Headrick, T. P. Huber, J. J. Mohr, and J. H. Wasson. 2001, November 30. "Executive Summary for Health Care Leaders: Microsystems in Health Care: The Essential Building Blocks of High Performing Systems." Robert Wood Johnson Foundation, RWJ Grant Number 036103. http://www.dartmouth.edu/~cecs/hcild/downloads/RWJ_MS_Exec_Summary.pdf

Thomas, E. J. 2011. "Improving Teamwork in Healthcare: Current Approaches and the Path Forward." *BMJ Quality & Safety* 20: 647–650.

Thomas, L., and C. Galla. 2013. "Building a Culture of Safety through Team Training and Engagement." *BMJ Quality & Safety* 22: 425–434.

Writing Group for the Women's Health Initiative Investigators. 2002. "Risks and Benefits of Estrogen Plus Progestin in Healthy Postmenopausal Women: Principal Results from the Women's Health Initiative Randomized Controlled Trial." *JAMA* 288 (3): 321–333. doi: 10.1001/jama.288.3.321

Useful Websites

http://www.ahrq.gov

http://www.ashpfoundation.org/lean/CMS9.html

http://www.ccwdata.org/business-intelligence/chronic-conditions/index.htm

https://clinicalmicrosystem.org/

http://www.cms.gov/Medicare/Quality-Initiatives-Patient-Assessment-Instruments/HospitalQualityInits/HospitalHCAHPS.html

https://www.cms.gov/regulations-and-guidance/legislation/ehrincentiveprograms/clinicalqualitymeasures.html

http://www.cms.gov/Research-Statistics-Data-and-Systems/Statistics-Trends-and-Reports/Chronic-Conditions/

https://www.framinghamheartstudy.org/about-fhs/history.php

http://www.hcahpsonline.org/files/HCAHPS%20V9.0%20Appendix%20A%20-%20Mail%20Survey%20Materials%20(English)%20March%202014.pdf

https://www.health.ny.gov/statistics/chac/indicators/

http://www.healthcarebusinesstech.com/communication-patient-harm/

http://www.hhs.gov/ash/initiatives/mcc/#_edn3

http://www.jointcommission.org/assets/1/6/camh_2012_update2_24_s.pdf

https://www.jointcommission.org/core_measure_sets.aspx

http://www.jointcommission.org/patient_blood_management_performance_measures_project/

http://www.jointcommission.org/the_view_from_the_joint_commission/core_measure_success_sharing_lessons_learned/

http://www.jointcommission.org/at_home_with_the_joint_commission/sbar_%E2%80%93_a_powerful_tool_to_help_improve_communication/

http://www.jointcommission.org/sentinel_event.aspx

http://www.medicare.gov/hospitalcompare/About/Timely-Effective-Care.html

http://www.medicare.gov/hospitalcompare/Data/Overview.html

http://www.mhqp.org

http://www.ncbi.nlm.nih.gov/books/NBK54296/

http://iom.edu/~/media/Files/Perspectives-Files/2012/Discussion-Papers/BPH_Ten_HLit_Attributes.pdf

http://library.ahima.org/xpedio/groups/public/documents/ahima/bok1_033940.pdf

http://pediatrics.aappublications.org/content/124/Supplement_3/S315.long

http://teamstepps.ahrq.gov/about-2cl_3.htm

CHAPTER FIVE

IMPROVING PATIENT SAFETY

Chapter Outline

Understanding Medical Errors and Adverse Events
High-Reliability Organizations
The Role of Quality Management in Promoting a Safety Culture
Prioritizing Improvements
Expanding Data Sources: Partnerships to Develop Best Practice
Leading Organizational Improvements
The Role of Nursing Leaders in Promoting Safety
The Role of the Medical Staff in Promoting Safety
Promoting Safety through Effective Communication
Summary
Key Terms
Quality Concepts in Action
References
Suggestions for Further Reading
Useful Websites

Key Concepts

- Understand issues involved in establishing a patient safety culture.
- Recognize contemporary thinking about adverse events.
- Analyze the role of clinical, administrative, and nursing leadership in promoting culture change.

- Discuss monitoring patient safety with quality data.
- Describe how effective communication improves care across the continuum.

Most discussions about improving health care include the importance of establishing a "culture of safety" in health care institutions. Although "Do No Harm," the fundamental principle for physicians, is often quoted, patient safety has not always been central to organizational strategy. In the early days of quality assurance (QA), leaders focused on identifying problems that tended to be associated with crises or incidents that resulted in patient harm. These incidents were reported to regulatory agencies and the hospital's medical board, and the hospital's legal department addressed the problem in order to reduce or eliminate the risk of malpractice claims. Problems were not defined as clinical safety issues but as financial risk issues. However, as government and regulatory agencies have become more involved in defining adverse outcomes, sentinel events, incidents, and never events, patient safety issues have been emphasized (https://psnet.ahrq.gov/primers/primer/5/safety-culture, http://www.ihi.org/resources/Pages/Changes/DevelopaCultureofSafety.aspx).

Understanding Medical Errors and Adverse Events

Often, gaps in patient safety come to the attention of leaders because reportable **medical errors** have occurred with serious consequences. Unless errors of all these types are documented, however, the extent or prevalence of the problem remains unknown. Because the reporting of errors is so central to identifying flaws in health care delivery, the Institute of Medicine (IOM) has recommended that errors be reported in a systematic and standardized manner. The federal government has recommended that the National Quality Forum define serious reportable events, referred to as never events. The idea is that mandatory reporting of serious health care errors will improve patient safety and promote accountability.

TERMS FOR MEDICAL ERRORS

Several terms are used in discussing medical errors and patient harm.

- **Medical errors** are preventable mistakes or failures in the process of care which are almost inevitable in our complex health care delivery system. They can be harmful but often do not result in a patient injury. For example, not giving medication on time, even an aspirin, is considered an error. Usually such an error does not lead to injury and simply gets corrected with little or no documentation. Medical errors that do not result in harm are often labeled **near misses,** close calls, or simply mistakes.

- Occasionally, however, medical errors lead to **adverse events** (AEs). According to the Committee on Quality of Health Care in America and Institute of Medicine (IOM) (2001), an adverse event is associated with unintended harm to the patient due to an error (either of commission or omission) rather than from the underlying disease or condition of the patient.
- The Joint Commission (TJC) has labeled certain AEs **sentinel events,** so called because they should sound an alarm that a process is deeply flawed. Sentinel events cause serious physical or psychological injury to patients and are not related to the natural course of a patient's illness. Examples of sentinel events include infant abduction, surgery performed on the wrong body part, and retention of a foreign body after surgery.

Clearly there are overlaps among these terms.

Reporting Patient Safety Issues

The public expects oversight of such serious patient safety issues and looks to the government to supply it. The Agency for Healthcare Research and Quality (AHRQ) describes reporting patient safety issues as comparable to reporting train derailments or plane crashes (Kizer and Stegum 2014). The provider is expected to report on AEs and the oversight agency is expected to investigate and impose standards of safe care. In addition to the reporting requirements of the federal government and accrediting agencies, many states have mandatory reporting requirements.

Mandated reporting and assigning accountability for errors are relatively new. Traditionally, if an error were reported, a file would be opened and, more often than not, a nurse would be rebuked, reeducated, or, in extreme cases, fired. Incident reporting was on a case-by-case basis, and because of the punitive result of the reporting, few professionals were eager to report incidents, especially if no serious patient harm occurred. If a medication was given and the patient had a mild reaction, such as a rash, no one rushed to report it as an incident. Rather, allergy medication was administered, and the incident was not documented. If an incident had to be reported because there was patient harm, the process was tedious, full of paperwork, human resource meetings, and disciplinary actions. Error reports were not used to spur performance improvements.

Systems Errors

Dr. Lucian Leape, one of the foremost early proponents of the patient safety movement, was able to transform the discourse on medical errors and patient safety to encourage a nonpunitive and systems-based approach. His landmark article, "Error in Medicine," published in *JAMA* in 1994, focused attention for the first time on the extent of and danger from preventable medical errors. In his article, he offered data on the extraordinarily high error rate in medicine, saying that 180,000 people die every year in the United States from preventable medical mistakes. The extent of the problem was not realized by either the medical community or the public because of a lack of documentation. Leape's work influenced the landmark 1999 IOM report, *To Err Is Human*, to which he contributed. Physicians may think their individual experience of errors is unusual or uncommon, and since most do no harm, they consider errors as a normal consequence of highly complex treatment.

Dr. Leape was among the first patient safety advocates to target medical culture as the culprit in poor safety. Traditionally physicians are trained that mistakes are unacceptable. Physicians are expected, and expect themselves, to be infallible. and therefore errors are not admitted or discussed, even among themselves. "Physicians typically feel, not without reason, that admission of error will lead to censure or increased surveillance or, worse, that their colleagues will regard them as incompetent or careless. Far better to conceal a mistake or, if that is impossible, to try to shift the blame to another, even the patient" (Leape 1994, 1852). The culture, including threats of malpractice claims, isolates physicians who cannot admit or discuss their mistakes with colleagues and certainly not use them as opportunities to understand a problem and improve it.

Although most clinicians recognize that this notion of infallibility is unrealistic and that errors do occur, error prevention traditionally was achieved through education and punishment; for nurses, this included a "rigid adherence to protocol" (Leape 1994, 1852) and for physicians, improved knowledge. A culture of individual blame for errors or mistakes has always been pervasive in health care settings. Errors are considered to be the result of someone's fault. Leape argued that the only way to reduce errors in health care was to change the way professionals think about errors, and move from an individual blame approach to a systems approach, where care delivery systems and processes are examined for potential errors.

Institutionalizing Error Prevention

Most important, error prevention has to become institutionalized, part of a new culture and a new way of thinking, based on the notion that errors are inevitable and the result of system flaws rather than individual character flaws. According to the AHRQ, until blame and shame are eliminated and until employees know they will not be punished for reporting errors or near errors, reporting rates will not be accurate (http://www.ahrq.gov/professionals/quality-patient-safety/patient-safety-resources/resources/advances-in-patient-safety/vol4/Kizer2.pdf). Ideally, data have to be collected about errors as part of the normal daily routine so that the type and scope of the problem can be identified and root causes—the underlying system failures—can be explored.

Many of the principles of quality management incorporate techniques to document and analyze errors:

- Statistical quality control
- Data collection documenting variation from the standard
- Recognizing errors as opportunities for improvement
- Root cause analysis
- Developing system modifications to improve processes that are vulnerable to errors

Leape pointed out that unless leaders support patient safety as a major goal, fundamental changes could not take place and succeed. Interestingly, although Leape's insight——that medical errors are the result of systems and that medical culture needs to change before safety can be addressed and improved——has been accepted as accurate, individuals are still being blamed decades after his article and the IOM report.

Even with the recognition that most errors result from complex systems that have weak points, and even with the understanding that culture plays a critical role in changing attitudes and practice, change has not come easily. Medical care continues to be paternalistic and hierarchical, with different groups working in independent silos. Fear of censure continues to undermine accurate error reporting, although most caregivers realize that unless the gaps in safety can be identified, problems cannot be adequately addressed. Communication among caregivers remains poor, and not solely because systems are complex and information is easily lost. Culture change is difficult. The importance of medical culture in reducing threats to patient safety cannot be stressed enough. Recognizing that errors are underreported and that therefore safety risks exist, regulatory agencies, the government, and medical organizations began to formulate processes to encourage improved safety practices.

AHRQ PATIENT SAFETY SURVEY

In 2010, when the AHRQ surveyed caregivers about patient safety, it asked whether they felt free to discuss errors. Very few respondents said they did.

Questions asked in the survey include those listed next.

Feedback and Communication about Error

- We are given feedback about changes put into place based on event reports.
- We are informed about errors that happen in this unit.
- In this unit, we discuss ways to prevent errors from happening again.

Communication Openness

- Staff will freely speak up if they see something that may negatively affect patient care.
- Staff feel free to question the decisions or actions of those with more authority.
- Staff are afraid to ask questions when something does not seem right.

Frequency of Events Reported

- When a mistake is made, but is caught and corrected before affecting the patient, how often is this reported?
- When a mistake is made, but has no potential to harm the patient, how often is this reported?
- When a mistake is made that could harm the patient, but does not, how often is this reported?

Nonpunitive Response to Errors

- Staff feel like their mistakes are held against them.
- When an event is reported, it feels like the person is being written up, not the problem.
- Staff worry that mistakes they make are kept in their personnel file.

The AHRQ identified nonpunitive responses and error reporting as clear opportunities for improvement across the county.

Source: http://www.ahrq.gov/professionals/quality-patient-safety/patientsafetyculture/hospital/index.html

The Necessity of Culture Change

Although professionals know what to do to avoid errors, patient safety is still an issue. For example, reducing falls has long been established as a measure of safe quality care, so much so that falls are considered never events, and financial penalties are associated with them. Many hospitals have implemented fall prevention programs, developed over time and with effort, yet patients continue to fall at almost the same rate as before these efforts went into effect. According to the AHRQ: "Falls are the second most common adverse event within health care institutions following medication errors, with inpatient fall rates ranging from 5.09 to 6.64 per 1,000 patient days across the nation" (https://innovations.ahrq.gov/profiles/fall-prevention-toolkit-facilitates-customized-risk-assessment-and-prevention-strategies?id=3094#1).

The government's definition of never events is punitive; funding is reduced or eliminated for errors that should never occur, including falls, hospital acquired pressure injuries, wrong-site surgery, and so on. The government hopes that financial punishment will encourage culture change, but, thus far, there is little indication that change is occurring.

The question, then, is what will encourage or force organizations to change? It is not enough for the government to shake its financial fist at hospitals or for TJC to require increased compliance or suffer lower accreditation scores. Even leadership support is insufficient if the frontline staff is not educated and involved in improvement efforts.

Culture change has to occur at every level of the organization and at every step of the process, following Deming's principles and modeled on the Cleveland Clinic's Patient Satisfaction Initiative (see Chapter 4). Leaders, administrators, unit managers, frontline workers, ancillary professionals—everyone has to be involved in safety efforts. In the system in which we work, patient safety rounds were initiated to try to encourage involvement. The goal is for a multidisciplinary team to become more patient focused, identify problems in real time, and implement improvements.

Errors, even seemingly trivial ones, need to be reported before flaws can be identified and addressed. Traditionally, professionals react to the occurrence of an adverse event. But this retrospective approach is too late. Flaws should be identified and corrected *before* patient safety is compromised. Encouraging the reporting of near misses requires a culture change so that those who report have no fear of censure (either formal or informal), open communication among everyone involved in the patient experience is the norm, and analysis of errors or potential errors, with a root cause analysis, is systematic and standardized. In this way, processes can be evaluated and systems of care assessed to target whether revisions or improvements are required.

Simply put, we need to change the way we do business. As much as we talk about open communication, as the AHRQ survey shows, caregivers do not feel as if open communication is welcome. We know that information is lost during shift changes, and many attempts have been made to improve communication, such as TeamSTEPPS (see Chapter 4), which explicitly routinize the transfer of information, yet information is constantly lost. We need to creatively adopt new ideas for how to work.

High-Reliability Organizations

Addressing safety issues is, of course, not unique to health care. Other industries, especially those with potentially catastrophic consequences from gaps in safety, such as nuclear power plants, airlines, wildfire stations, and the military, have recognized that anticipating mistakes can help avoid them. High-reliability organizations (HROs), as these organizations or industries are called, stress safety by promoting a mindfulness mind-set that has staff constantly alert to potential safety gaps.

Concepts of high reliability provide a way to *think* about safe processes and a safe environment and to establish a culture focused on reducing mistakes, failures, and errors. It is not a mechanistic tool but rather a cognitive approach that can help organizations reach the ultimate goal of providing an environment in which processes can be predicted, harm can be prevented, and a safe environment can be created.

Guiding Principles

HROs are based on five principles:

1. Sensitivity to operations
2. Preoccupation with failure
3. Deference to expertise
4. Resilience (ability to recover from and maintain stability in the face of setbacks)
5. Reluctance to simplify

The first three principles are useful in detecting potential errors; the final two help with the response to an error (Weick and Sutcliffe 2007).

Being sensitive to operations means keeping vigilant attention to possibilities of risk, danger, and the unreliability of operational systems and processes. HROs encourage a blame-free culture where individuals can speak up without fear of censure or retaliation.

Being preoccupied with failure means being constantly focused on—that is, mindful of—its possibility and aware that even small failures can add up to big ones with disastrous consequences. Therefore, HROs encourage reporting of near misses (potential errors) and take steps to imagine where mistakes might occur before they happen. Any deviation from reliability can lead to failure; therefore, HROs have a concentrated focus on "what if?"

HROs realize that rigid hierarchies in decision making may lead to mistakes and that expertise is not necessarily coupled with organizational titles or positions. Especially in high-risk environments, authority for decisions should be flexible and easily shifted to those people most expert in particular fields, regardless of rank, reporting structure, or the table of organization. In an HRO, staff are trained to think creatively and draw on varied expertise when necessary.

A commitment to resilience means that the organization has developed mechanisms to respond dynamically to situations, including errors, and in the midst of stress so that the inevitable problems that occur do not disrupt and disable the organization. Since mistakes often occur when unanticipated, flexibility of reaction is essential to reduce unwanted consequences.

HROs stress complexity and develop processes to incorporate subtleties. They are skeptical of simplicity, and welcome diverse opinions and insights.

They are reluctant to accept the common tendency to provide simple answers to complex problems. Simplification runs the risk of covering up important information.

ADOPTING HRO PRINCIPLES

Organizations that adopt HRO principles explicitly and deliberately embrace concepts that emphasize:

- continuous vigilance about risk, where reports of flawed processes can be made without fear of censure or retribution;
- efficient and respectful teamwork, where all functions are equally valued, especially when facing a crisis;
- effective communication that is democratic and respectful;
- situational awareness, understanding the potential dangers involved in various processes and functions; and
- ongoing education and training.

Becoming a High-Reliability Organization

For health care organizations to become HROs, leaders must understand and work to overcome the unique challenges involved in changing entrenched organizational habits. For example, health care organizations traditionally tolerate provider autonomy. But autonomy can lead to variability, and variability can lead to unreliability and can endanger patient safety (Dlugacz and Spath 2011).

Many experts believe that national and regional benchmarks for quality and safety are not set high enough and that leadership commitment to change ongoing practices is often weak; also, resources for change may be scarce. In a 2013 survey of the American College of Healthcare Executives, for example, 85 percent of chief executive officers (CEOs) said their top concern was with financial challenges and 28 percent said their concerns were medication errors and public reporting of outcomes data (https://www.ache.org/pubs/Releases/2014/top-issues-confronting-hospitals-2013.cfm).

A culture change is necessary in order for health care organizations to become HROs. The mindfulness that is central to HRO principles requires transformed values, redefined roles, changed expectations, and a deliberate focus on danger. The challenge to health care organizations to standardize safe practices involves increasing reliability in highly variable, unpredictable, and heterogeneous environments. Some organizations attempting to incorporate HRO practices reward staff financially for promoting good outcomes and for reporting near misses, but the best road to success is to adopt the mind-set of an HRO and remain focused on reliability.

To change the health care culture, it is also important to link quality and finance and to engage chief financial officers, using data, to make the business case for improving reliability and safety (Dlugacz 2010). It is essential for health care leaders to understand how resources are allotted to programs in order to make sustainable changes. Transforming a health care organization into an HRO has the added benefit of providing a competitive advantage; it is good for business to be a safe and reliable organization with good outcomes and few adverse events.

The Role of Quality Management in Promoting a Safety Culture

Developing a culture of safety involves more than a new policy handbook; it involves integrating new ideas, such as high reliability and near-miss reporting, into everyday practice for everyone involved in patient care. This change of mind-set is not easily achieved; it is time consuming and expensive, and it requires reorientation and reeducation of physicians and other professionals. Without a changed mind-set, however, there is no change in culture.

In past decades, accountability for the delivery of care was localized. In a QA model, each incident was considered unique. No one believed that errors signaled a larger problem and needed to be investigated. If a patient's medical record did not contain a history and physical, for example, this was a problem because the gap was not in compliance with regulations. Today it would be considered a problem because it has an impact on patient safety and might reveal a general problem about the process of care. Moving from a QA model of problem identification toward an integrated quality management culture of safety involves every layer of the organization.

As new questions are being asked by clinical and organizational leaders —such as how incidents can be prevented and how patient care can be improved, or who is accountable for problems that lead to incidents—the role of quality management in designing methods to monitor, assess, and improve processes is also being redefined. Questions such as these have moved quality management toward performance improvement, focusing on process redesign and prevention, to better define "good," "safe," "quality" care. Promoting a safe environment for patients—that is, a culture of safety—has become a central concern for hospital leaders.

Using Quality Data to Promote Safety

Increasingly, quality management is using evidence, in the form of data and databases, to convince physicians that the underlying processes and structures in the delivery of care might be flawed and require improvement. Traditionally when outcomes were poor or when adverse advents occurred, physicians often argued that individual (in)competence or particular circumstances were involved and that corrective actions should involve (re)education or disciplinary action. With quality management data and a better understanding of systems, these traditional values, behaviors, and beliefs are beginning to change.

The common physician and nursing complaint that quality was "just paper" (i.e., documentation) is slowly being replaced by an awareness that the relationship between good processes and good outcomes needs to be monitored with quality data. In the health care system in which we work, a board committee was established and charged with overseeing issues related to patient safety. Quality management leaders used data to educate the CEO and the board of trustees about the relationship among processes of care, outcomes of that care, identification of problems, and improvement efforts. The goal was to target systemic process flaws, which, once identified, could be addressed through performance improvement initiatives.

Today, since leaders are concerned about publicly reported measures of care, regulatory deficiencies, and denied claims from insurers, they support a strong quality structure to understand, monitor, and improve the delivery of care. Data are basic to monitoring care, targeting accountability, and improving communication. Use of comparative databases, measuring performance along **service lines**, and providing quality education to clinical staff are opportunities to improvement and to reduce variability. (A service line is a model of care management that establishes coordinated care in a horizontal patient-centered way for all services involved in a specific disease or condition.) When performance data are reported to leaders, accountability for gaps in care can be identified.

Data should be the basis of making decisions, of targeting improvements, and of changing behaviors. Collecting and reporting data for regulatory reasons, as was the case for many years, is different from monitoring the efficiency and efficacy of care (even though the two might lead to similar results). Quality data should be used to assess care, define the scope of care, meet the expectations of the patient population, respond to the needs of the community, understand adverse events, and evaluate improvements. Leaders must direct which data should be collected and define priorities of analysis.

Case Example: Monitoring Falls

For example, data about falls with injuries from across the health system in which we work are collected, aggregated, analyzed, and reported to system leaders. (Each individual hospital has its own reports as well.) Figure 5.1 displays falls injuries over an almost three year period that is the aggregate for all hospitals in the system. The graphic shows that there is normal variation over this period of time and that falls are in statistical control (see Chapter 7). But statistical control is different from clinical control; and although there does not

FIGURE 5.1. FALLS WITH INJURY

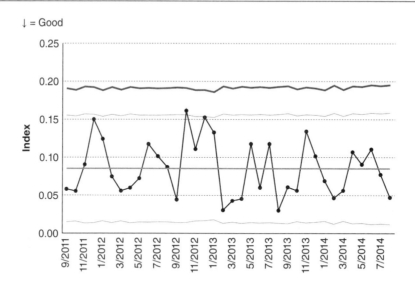

seem to be any red flag to investigate further, if leaders' goal is to reduce falls with injury to zero, data show that there has been no real reduction. From this data report, the caregivers and managers can focus their efforts on developing processes to lower the number of falls and attain sustainable improvements.

Monitoring with Measures

Databases are being created to help senior leaders make critical decisions about their organizational priorities. These databases aggregate information about quality measures of efficiency (such as length of stay [LOS], turnaround time), clinical quality indicators (such as mortality, readmission), and patient satisfaction, and try to define "value" for the organization and for the patient population.

Health care organizations monitor over 70 hospital measures and a similar number for outpatient services, nursing homes, and home care. This ever-expanding production of measures can become overwhelming. In addition, the population being measured, or the denominator for the measure, may be different depending on who is doing the measuring. The Centers for Medicare and Medicaid Services (CMS) measures are different from those used by insurance companies. For an organization to manage these measures and use them to improve safety and prioritize change requires sophisticated analytics, knowledge of statistics, and reports to leaders.

Data-based reports are the end result of careful data and variable construction, development of numerators and denominators for quality indicators

FIGURE 5.2. ANALYTICS AND INTERPRETATION

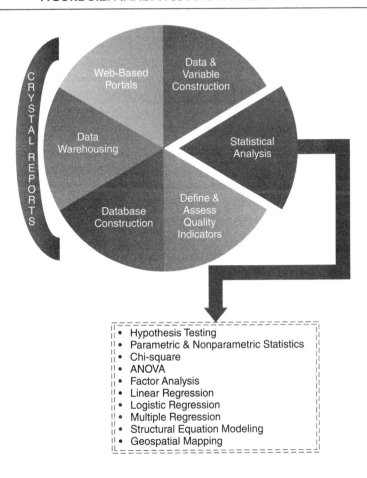

(which would define the population), constructing databases for tracking and trending, comparisons among organizations or units, and storing the data for aggregation. Once the data have been organized, various statistical analytical processes are used to provide sophisticated information for data interpretation (see Figure 5.2). Obviously leaders do not have to know how to perform linear regressions or geospatial mapping themselves, but they do need to have statisticians on staff who can. However, because these analytic positions do not directly provide patient care, they are often undersourced. It is critical that leaders commit resources to these positions in order to build a data-driven environment for decision making.

In our system, analysts have developed quality and safety measures consistent with the leadership goal of being in the top decile in quality and safety in the country. The innovative dashboard reports that are generated graphically present monthly performance metrics and offer leaders of individual organizations the ability to access reports on demand and monitor trends based on the most currently available data. By monitoring consistent measures across the health system, performance can be easily evaluated, best practices can be shared among organizations, and gaps in care can be identified quickly. The common platform allows for benchmarking, and statistical tools are used to ascertain whether improvement efforts and interventions are effective.

Managers at every level of the organization need to understand the importance of data and its value in providing the tools to analyze the dynamics of care. Analytics also objectively explain which systems are actually working successfully, with few errors and greater patient satisfaction, and which ones are not. Analysis of data helps establish whether an intervention or initiative has resulted in the desired improvements.

Ever since New York State introduced risk-adjusted mortality for cardiac surgery patients and as the CMS and others have made data more available and transparent, hospital administrators and clinicians have feared being ranked poorly or looking as if their care is flawed. This is understandable. Therefore, many people are becoming more familiar with examining data, and the process is being integrated into leadership discussions. Some organizations have increased accountability by charging medical directors to focus on data to improve daily operations.

Case Example: APACHE

When care decisions are in fact rooted in data, safety and efficiency improve. For example, **APACHE** (an acronym for Acute Physiology, Age, and Chronic Health Evaluation) is a data management system developed to provide objective and consistent information about intensive care unit (ICU) care, the most expensive resource in the hospital.

Data from APACHE provide descriptive and clinical information about patient demographics, severity of illness, appropriate levels of care, and patient outcomes.

When APACHE was introduced into the system in which we work many years ago, the rich data it provided led to specific improvements. Data on patient acuity revealed that physicians were assigning patients to the ICU because they wanted to be assured that their patients would be carefully monitored or while they were awaiting tests, not because they required the highly sophisticated technology of the ICU. Admission criteria were developed, and the data convinced physicians to use the ICU more appropriately. ICU admissions were reduced by half, which enabled a more efficient allocation of staff resources.

Based on the information provided and communicated, other new policies and protocols were established, such as weaning protocols for removing patients from ventilators. Step-down units, where patients could be cared for appropriately, were established. These improvements in care and efficiency were based solely on data rather than on impressions or individual physician practice, and they resulted in improvements in both quality, safety, and efficiency (Lustbader et al. 2001).

Now more than ever before it is critical that health care professionals learn to use and trust data and statistical analysis of data. The electronic health record (EHR) can be used by analysts to develop meaningful databases. The new generation of health professionals is expected to be familiar with basic statistics and data analytic techniques so that monitoring clinical care and organizational efficiencies are maximized.

Prioritizing Improvements

The mission and vision of a health care organization is more than words; the statements should define the relationship between the organization and the patient. If sufficiently explicit, the mission and vision can inform what data should be collected to reach specific goals. Of course, priorities may and should change as conditions change and goals mature. Information about a specific issue or process can be more important at some times than at others. Once priorities are established, quality management, along with clinical leaders, can develop performance improvements, including appropriate databases, that will monitor specific variables. Those databases, reviewed by leaders, can establish areas for further improvement efforts. The point is not to fly blind but to have information with which to make decisions and then to collect information to assess whether those decisions resulted in improvements.

It seems obvious that all the data available to leaders must be organized into some kind of order. One way to organize data is for administrative, clinical, and quality leaders to define criteria to determine the relative importance, or priority, of specific issues. As resources are limited, choices have to be made about which issues to improve and which data to collect. Prioritization is a challenge because it involves understanding the interrelationships of services and meeting multiple and sometimes conflicting expectations. Leaders have to juggle and, it is hoped, balance strategic, clinical, and organizational goals with personnel, budget, risk, satisfaction, safety, clinical outcomes, and adverse events.

In years past, TJC recommended that priorities be linked to high-risk, high-volume, and problem-prone issues—that is, serious issues that have an impact on many patients. Today's leaders have to make decisions based on many other organizational and regulatory requirements as well, especially meeting CMS measures and Accountable Care Organization demands. The CMS provides benchmarks and financial incentives for low rates of readmission, mortality, infection, and will not reimburse organizations for never events. Clearly, since leaders cannot make all aspects of care top priorities, focus on everything simultaneously, or allocate resources to all problems equally, there needs to be some **prioritization criteria**, and that prioritization must rely on accurate data and data analysis (Tromp and Baltussen 2012).

Using Data to Define Priorities

In the system in which we work, by examining the various dashboards that quality management has developed as a response to leadership goals, leaders can look at information and determine the appropriate direction for the system's improvement efforts and for individual hospitals. The specific indicators that comprise the dashboard reflect the interests and priorities of the C suite. The dashboards provide leaders with the information they need to monitor the quality of care being delivered and its efficiency. Information from dashboards can target specific goals, and depending on those goals, variables can be defined to monitor progress.

THE C SUITE

The *C suite* is a shorthand expression to collectively refer to an organization's most important senior executives. Generally, senior leadership titles begin with the letter *C* for chief, as in chief executive officer (CEO), chief operating officer (COO), chief medical officer (CMO), chief nursing officer (CNO), chief financial officer (CFO), chief information officer (CIO), and others.

For example, if among the goals of leaders is satisfying customer expectations, with the patient always the primary customer, information needs to be gathered, through surveys, focus groups, and interviews, about customer expectations, and then the variables that help to define those expectations need to be developed. If patient surveys reveal that the emergency department (ED) is overcrowded, and patients are leaving without being seen and evaluated, or complaining about long waits, data should be collected to determine what processes contribute to the overcrowding or the bottlenecks.

Figure 5.3 shows monthly data for the ED in a community hospital. The data tracks the number of patients admitted and discharged and the number of patients transferred into and out of the ED (A–E). The tracking of volume can help leaders understand how to best allocate resources. The figure also tracks patients who left before being seen (F), perhaps because of long waits, and those who left against medical advice (G), as well as mortality and unplanned readmissions (H–K). Monthly reports such as these offer real insight into what is often a chaotic and overcrowded busy department.

FIGURE 5.3. MONTHLY EMERGENCY DEPARTMENT DATA

Volume Statistics New Record	
A. Number of patients **registered** (volume) in ED (includes B, C, E, F, G, H)	
B. Number of patients who were **admitted** into the hospital	
C. Number of patients who were treated and released (**discharge**)	
D. Number of patients who were **transferred into** ED	
E. Number of patients who were **transferred out** of ED	
F. Number of patients who left ED without being evaluated (**LWOBE**)	
G. Number of patients who left ED against the medical advice of the physician (**AMA**)	
H. Number of **ED mortalities** (patients who were registered but **not admitted**, including DOA status, patients who arrive by ambulance in arrest, receiving ACLS or BLS, etc)	
I. Number of **ED deaths within 24 hours** of admission	
J. Number of **unplanned returns within 72 hours**	
K. Number of **unplanned returns within 72 hours** who were **admitted or transferred** to another hospitals or facilities	
L. Total hours that the ED is on **Ambulance diversion** for this month	

Pediatric Volume

Total reg volume [   ]   # of admissions [   ]   # of treat & release [   ]   # transferred [   ]

Psych Volume

Total reg volume [   ]   # of admissions [   ]   # of treat & release [   ]   # transferred [   ]

Leaders might want to define who is in charge of gatekeeping and thus accountable and to assess whether there are clear criteria for admission to the ED. Are radiological and other consultations occurring in a timely way, and if not, why not? Is the staff well trained, sufficient, and competent? Is there an efficient process to move admitted patients to appropriate beds in the hospital? All these processes can and should be measured so that leaders can understand and evaluate the process for flaws. With information, decision makers can determine where the problem exists and develop possible solutions; once developed, leaders can track whether improvement efforts have the desired impact.

If leaders are committed to zero infection (a cultural shift from finding some defects acceptable), data and information can be collected about types of infections, places in the hospital where there is more or less infection, sterility procedures in the operating rooms, and policies developed to monitor catheterization and wound sites.

Figure 5.4 graphs the mortality rate for sepsis and septic shock over a six-year period. The data reveal a steady decrease in mortality. The decrease reflects changes in care and interventions, such as issuance of guidelines, a

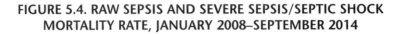

FIGURE 5.4. RAW SEPSIS AND SEVERE SEPSIS/SEPTIC SHOCK MORTALITY RATE, JANUARY 2008–SEPTEMBER 2014

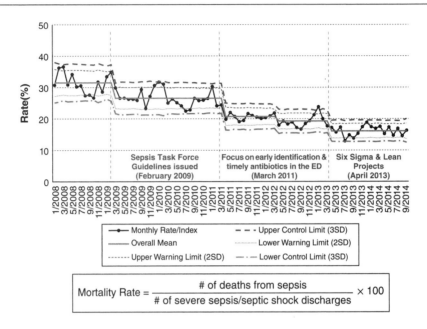

focus on early identification, timely antibiotic administration, and targeted Six Sigma/Lean projects to reduce mortality from sepsis. Without these data and reports of this kind, it would be difficult to assess the success of these improvement efforts.

Case Example: Understanding Suicide

In collaboration with leaders, quality management professionals can help to analyze care and to create databases to expose relationships. For example, patient suicide is one of the five primary sentinel events reported to TJC (http://www.jointcommission.org/assets/1/23/jconline_April_29_15.pdf). Although recognized as a serious problem, it is not obvious what variables should be tracked to better understand and monitor suicide in the inpatient hospital population. Perhaps patients on certain medications or who have certain diagnoses might be more susceptible to risk than others.

The health system at which we work undertook a series of performance improvement efforts to identify suicide risk factors and maximize patient safety in medical/surgical units and in the ED. Quality management convened a task force to try to analyze the causes of 17 attempted and completed suicides. Data revealed that inadequate patient assessment, poor communication, and staff knowledge deficits were factors.

Most striking, data uncovered information revealing that patients at risk for alcohol withdrawal were at greater risk for suicide attempts than others. This information allowed us to develop improved assessment (especially for alcohol use), using a central intake model and a transfer summary form from acute care to behavioral health. Also, a continuous suicide risk assessment tool was incorporated into the inpatient behavioral health care rounds. Data resulted in improved care management (Dlugacz et al. 2003).

Defining Priorities Locally

Obviously, each organization has to determine its own priorities, and leaders of different departments or units can and should define their own priorities and goals. An ED manager might want to improve the triage process or waiting time while, on a neurological unit, the manager might want to understand what forces have an impact on LOS. On a surgical unit, infection and nutrition might be issues. On a psychiatric unit, the treatment plan might be most important to patient management.

For example, when health system leaders where we work realized that follow-up care for heart failure patients after hospital discharge was less than optimal, they determined to address the situation. A standardized tool for follow-up phone calls was developed (see Figure 5.5). Nurses were trained to ask questions, such as: "Did you weigh yourself today?"; "Has your coughing increased?"; "Did you take your medication?"; and so on. Then, depending on the patient's response, the nurses could provide information and implement appropriate care. The standardized tool has not only improved patient safety but also has helped to reduce hospital readmissions since care coordination and health risks are immediately addressed. When patients require physician appointments or other outpatient services, the follow-up care nurses organize appointments and transportation.

Case Example: Implementing Prioritization

The daily management of a unit, department, organization, or practice is under siege from data. Hospitals collect data and report on such measures as: outcomes (such as mortality), patient experience (on the Hospital Consumer Assessment of Healthcare Providers and Systems [HCAHPS]), never events, budget, operations, staffing and efficiency, TJC and CMS. They also collect data and report on many measures internal to the organization, such as blood utilization, infection control, and incidents. In order for managers to manage so much data, regular meetings should be convened to examine the data, identify trends, and establish improvement goals. A deliberate approach to evaluating data and prioritizing for improvement based on data is crucial.

Depending on the organizational structure of your organization, there may be many levels of priorities. In the health care system in which we work,

FIGURE 5.5. DISCHARGE FOLLOW-UP INFORMATION HEART FAILURE

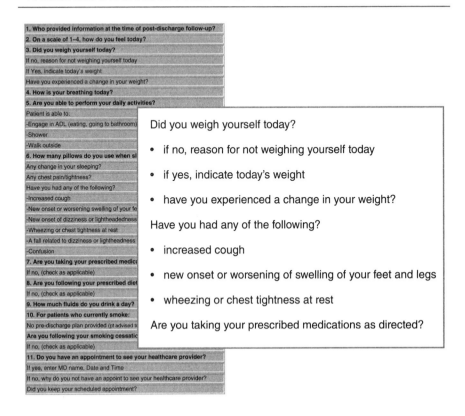

there are system priorities, individual hospital priorities, and individual unit priorities. Middle management, unit directors, and department heads may have their own priorities and require improvements based on their specific local data. They need data to make intelligent decisions about staff ratios and education and also respond to senior leadership prioritization goals.

A useful tool for managers is to create a **prioritization matrix** to assist in evaluating which data are most useful for improvement efforts. The matrix should include rankings for questions, such as: Does this measure:

- have an impact on patient safety;
- increase resource efficiency;
- conform to the strategic plans of the organization and further the goals of leaders;
- improve the delivery of care; and
- meet established benchmarks?

FIGURE 5.6. PRIORITIZATION MATRIX

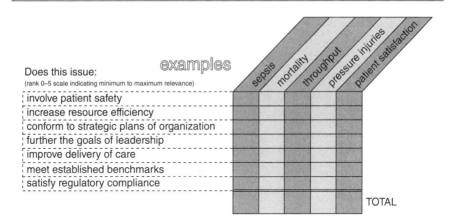

Managers should meet with their teams to determine the relative rankings of these concerns. In this way, managers can assess their performance and their improvement needs in light of their objectives and goals.

Rather than waiting for senior management to dictate how the data should be used and what improvements should be made, using a matrix to evaluate data encourages a proactive approach to prioritization (see Figure 5.6). Working with data in this way encourages a new style of quality management, where the status of care is constantly challenged and objective information is used to override clinical opinion. Ongoing data evaluation may illustrate gaps in care and help to correlate process or interventions with outcomes, such as reasons for high mortality.

To develop a matrix, begin by establishing evaluative criteria, such as the questions posed earlier: patient safety, efficiency, meeting organizational goals, compliance, and others. If there are many elements, rank them as primary, secondary, tertiary, and so on. Then list potential (and competing) areas for improvement across the top of the matrix, such as sepsis mortality, pressure injuries, patient satisfaction, and throughput. These improvement concerns change over time. Using a 0–5 scale to indicate minimum to maximum relevance, the team or manager can rank each issue according to the criteria. Does the issue affect patient safety? Does the issue require extensive resources or staffing or time? Is the issue required for the CMS or TJC reporting?

After ranking each issue, the numbers can be totaled to indicate which issues are top priority and which are less so. Making choices as to what to improve, based on quantifying one concern over another, helps to objectify and clarify decisions. The objectification removes emotional or subjective judgments. When priorities change, or when the data reveal new issues, a new or modified matrix can be developed.

Expanding Data Sources: Partnerships to Develop Best Practice

It is not unusual for an organization to partner with other organizations to combine data resources to better understand and improve their delivery of services.

Case Example: Collaborations to Promote Patient Safety

The hospital system in which we work is involved in several collaborations that promote sharing data and best practices.

For example, leaders in our large multihospital system have reached out to partner with the Institute of Healthcare Improvement (IHI) to take advantage of its resources and learn from it. The IHI has identified measurements for certain conditions, such as measures that explain population health (risk status, chronic conditions), the patient experience (likely to recommend), end-of-life care, and treatment for specific conditions, such as sepsis. For example, the IHI recommends that within three hours of a patient presenting with severe sepsis, an organization should measure serum lactate levels, obtain blood cultures prior to antibiotic administration, and administer broad-spectrum antibiotics among other processes.

Measuring these variables enables an organization to understand how well it is performing in regard to sepsis care. The strategic partnership between the IHI and our system has helped us to reduce our sepsis mortality rate.

Figure 5.7 graphs improvement in the care of sepsis patients at one of the system hospitals over time. This measure has improved dramatically. Serum lactate levels are an indicator of how much oxygen is available in blood. When the level is low, lactic acid levels rise; high levels can be an indicator of septic shock. By testing the blood within a short time frame of entering the ED, treatment for sepsis and septic shock can be administered effectively. Bringing measures such as these to the attention of leaders has helped to prioritize improvement efforts and provided patients with better care.

Another collaboration exists with the Dartmouth Institute for Health Policy & Clinical Practice collaborative, which focuses on the high cost of care; the goal is to develop payment models that increase safety and reduce costs. Other health systems involved in this collaborative (Mayo Clinic, Denver Health, Intermountain Healthcare, Dartmouth-Hitchcock, Cleveland Clinic, etc.) will share data on patient care, costs, and outcomes on nine conditions: (1) total knee replacement, (2) diabetes, (3) asthma, (4) hip surgery, (5) heart failure, (6) perinatal care, (7) depression, (8) spine surgery, and (9) weight-loss surgery. Having more data and information enables better decisions and better programs.

FIGURE 5.7. SERUM LACTATE ORDER TO RESULT WITHIN 90 MINUTES FOR SEVERE SEPSIS/SEPTIC SHOCK IN THE EMERGENCY DEPARTMENT

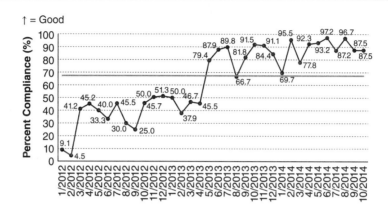

Our health system is also associated with TJC's Center for Transforming Health Care to address safety concerns. Projects in this collaboration include reducing sepsis mortality, increasing hand hygiene, decreasing surgical site infections, preventing heart failure rehospitalizations, and improving communication during hand-offs.

Leading Organizational Improvements

Leaders have to take an active role in understanding issues related to quality and safety. To do so, leaders must: be more involved in hospital medical/clinical operations; understand measurement systems that include not only clinical variables but also operational measures for supply chain, efficiency, turnover, throughput, and so on; and be responsive to community expectations. The new challenges for CEOs include maintaining improvements, reducing incidents and adverse outcomes, staying abreast of CMS measures and those of insurance companies, and promoting efficiency and reducing waste.

Leaders are also responsible for prioritizing areas for improvement in an efficient and effective manner, reducing costs and balancing financial issues. Simply put, leaders need to promote an organization that provides value to the patient at a reasonable cost and communicates its commitment to safety and quality so that every member of the organization is involved.

Today's CEOs realize that they are responsible for the provision of care, not just the financial viability of the organization, as in the past. More important, CEOs understand that maintaining high standards of quality and using quality methods to evaluate and improve care benefit the organization financially and increases patient satisfaction. Quality management has moved out of its metaphorical basement office to become an important component of the strategic planning process.

Supporting Quality Data

Recognizing the need for change, leaders at most health care organizations have increased their support for quality management methodology and expect all staff to work within a quality management framework, to use and interpret data, and to make improvements based on data. Quality committees, performance improvement coordinating groups, and physician safety champions define policy, set goals, and communicate concerns and prioritization needs. Various disciplines and multidisciplinary teams should meet regularly as task forces to interpret quality data available from internal or external sources.

Supervisors and managers are expected to know the specifics of the patients on their unit, be able to identify problems to understand their nature and frequency, define their scope of care, determine if errors reveal process problems, and develop safety nets—all based on data. Unit leaders are responsible for identifying common factors that influence care on their units or departments, establishing appropriate indicators and developing methodologies to collect and communicate data; they need to determine and implement solutions to problems as well. In other words, everyone is expected to work within a quality framework. Without data, decisions are subjective and even capricious; with data, decisions are based on objective facts.

It makes no sense in today's reform environment to separate financial and operational data from quality and clinical data. And with the EHR and the government's support of health information technology (HIT), the challenge for organizations and their leaders is to convert data into information that can be used for decision making and analyzing processes of care. Today's problem is not to acquire data but to understand what it means, interpret it for useful change and improvement, prioritize improvement initiatives and resource expenditure from the analyzed data, and present it in meaningful formats to the board of trustees, to the frontline workers, and everyone in between.

Business Intelligence

With data central to understanding care, it is not surprising that leaders are responding to the challenges of health care reform by developing **business intelligence** data platforms to meet quality benchmarks that reflect best practices for patient safety, and that have an impact on reimbursement and satisfaction. Data platforms are also useful for determining the value of business and financial initiatives, including marketing, cost efficiencies, and regulatory compliance. Especially under the pay-for-performance and bundled payment model of care and reimbursement, senior leaders need to understand how to deliver cost-effective quality care. Clinical outcomes and business outcomes are connected. Therefore, data need to be at the forefront of all business decisions.

Health care business intelligence can provide organizations with the ability to use their data to improve quality of care, increase financial efficiency and operational effectiveness, conduct innovative research and satisfy regulatory requirements. Business intelligence (BI) refers to a collection of computer-based techniques used in extracting, identifying, and analyzing data, providing current and predictive views of business operations through the use of data reporting, using online analytical processing, data mining, and more. Its aim is to support better business decision making and, as a result, a BI system can also be known as a decision support system (DSS).

Many of the upcoming expectations of health care reform require sophisticated analytics and merged databases. For example, to avoid being penalized with reductions in Medicare reimbursement for avoidable readmissions, large merged databases can help leaders understand the delivery of care by tracking and trending variables associated with readmissions and creating real time reports on patient issues. Patient satisfaction issues will also be related to reimbursement fees, and satisfaction data, such as HCAHPS, need to be analyzed for improvement initiatives and marketing campaigns. Meaningful use of health information technology and the EHR will result in large databases for analysis as well. Computerized provider order entry has been mandated and safety and errors need to be monitored via data.

The goal is to turn data into useful information. Meaningful reports are based on aggregating data from diverse data sources, such as billing, clinical data, the EHR, and other sources, such as the AHRQ safety measures, and then interpreting the data and presenting reports that leaders can make use of. Data are also collected from Premier, a health care performance improvement alliance of approximately 3,600 U.S. hospitals, which has created a comprehensive database of best practices and cost reduction strategies, and from Press Ganey, an organization that collects data on the patient experience and compares individual hospitals to a national database. Quality management gathers data from these various sources and stores them in a data warehouse. Then the data are combined and analyzed for reports to leaders (see Figure 5.8).

Business intelligence combines these databases and develops analytics to define care along service lines. If a hospital's neurosurgery unit is not among the top ranked, why not? From a marketing point of view, something needs to change, and developing a single platform with merged data helps leaders understand and improve processes. Business intelligence models force

FIGURE 5.8. INTEGRATING DATA/GENERATING REPORTS

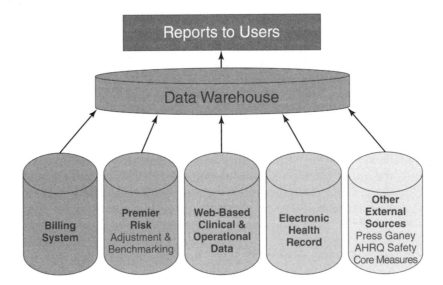

collaboration among departments, much as a general practitioner organizes specialists and consultations for a single patient. Analysts and leaders need to know how each piece of the organization affects other pieces, which individual variables are associated with each other, and which are not compatible.

The Role of Nursing Leaders in Promoting Safety

Nurse executives have a crucial role in promoting patient safety. They are involved in changing the culture and ensuring that the organization's priorities are met by developing strategies for improving the delivery of care. For example, if the system has prioritized reducing heart failure readmissions, nursing leaders have to oversee changes that would lead to good discharge planning, timely social work consults if appropriate, and follow-up care, and they must be sensitive to health literacy and social and/or cultural factors that may impair care after discharge. If the CEO prioritizes patient safety and quality, then the nurse executive and nursing leaders have to figure out how to operationalize that goal at the bedside. The nurse executive has to understand how to allocate resources for optimal delivery of services and to define competency that would enable the staff to carry out the strategy.

Today's challenges require that nurses and in particular nurse leaders acquire and use new skills. In the past, the head nurse would know the patients on her or his unit and measure whatever was required by TJC. Traditionally nurses were expected to address what are called **nursing-sensitive measures**, such as pressure ulcers or falls, conditions that good nursing care should be able to avoid. Nurse managers would have the responsibility of ensuring that whatever protocols were in place were followed. They were also accountable for tracking the length of stay of patients on their unit, managing transfers from the ED, and collecting census information about the patients on the unit.

Today, in addition to those responsibilities, nurse managers have to be trained in data entry, the EHR, checklists and be able to work effectively in teams. They need to be adept at SBAR and TeamSTEPPS (see Chapter 4), and they are encouraged to get advanced professional training and degrees. Nurse leaders have to do more than ensure appropriate staffing or supervise the education and competency of the workforce. Today, because health care quality is so data-driven and nurse leaders have so much more data available to them, they are expected to address more complex issues, such as efficiency, the continuum of care within the hospital and into the community, patient education, and discharge planning. Nursing leaders are expected to use analytics to make decisions. For example, if data show that urinary tract infections are a problem, nursing has to analyze the problem (perhaps too much time on a catheter) and then develop solutions to improve.

The government expectations for nursing leaders and nursing functions has also increased. For example, the **B-Care Tool**—Bundled Payments for Care Improvement Continuity Assessment and Record Evaluation—requires an in-depth nursing evaluation and documents not only the patient's presenting problem but also other variables, such as mental status and social support. The tool is a streamlined version of the Continuity Assessment and Record Evaluation (CARE) Item Set, developed by the CMS, which is a "standardized patient assessment tool which measures medical, functional, cognitive, and social support status across acute and postacute settings, such as long-term care hospitals, rehabilitation facilities, skilled nursing facilities, and home health agencies" (http://www.cms.gov/Medicare/Quality-Initiatives-Patient-Assessment-Instruments/Post-Acute-Care-Quality-Initiatives/CARE-Item-Set-and-B-CARE.html). Specific information is gathered from patients, such as about skin integrity.

Communication Strategies

It is the nurse leader who monitors participation and success of the microsystems and assesses how the team is functioning. In the past, leadership silos eliminated any crossover between administrative leadership goals and nursing executive goals. Today's patient-focused care requires that everyone be on the same page, that effective communication strategies be implemented between physicians and nurses, and that all clinicians share responsibility for the accuracy and completeness of the EHR and for monitoring data.

The changes encourage collaboration and team building. With information centralized in the EHR, it is much easier for different professionals to review and analyze the same information. With the management of chronic disease a focus for the nation, nurses and physicians need to share decision making and communicate effectively about how to provide services to improve the delivery of care. The entire workforce of a service line has to march in step and be committed to working together to ensure optimal outcomes. Without coordination, it would be difficult if not impossible to design efficient and effective care by service line.

In this environment, quality measures are the lynchpin for communicating information about the delivery of care. Leaders react to the measurements and make policy decisions based on them. If the safety of the environment of care, for example, is below a benchmark, leaders—administrative, clinical, environmental service personnel—have to share responsibility about what is needed to improve. The chief nursing officer (CNO) might want to reassess the process of care if, for example, falls are a problem. That would mean devising measures to monitor the continuum of care, not just on one unit. As medical and surgical units dwindle and more procedures are being performed on outpatients in ambulatory centers, new metrics for quality and safety will be developed to ensure good care. Perhaps for the first time, the CNO stands on an equal footing with other members of the leadership team. The CNO has to figure out data requirements and how to provide effective and efficient interdisciplinary care.

Nurse managers need new skill sets and competencies, including improved business and communication skills. They should be familiar with **Magnet** standards, the gold standard for excellent nursing care, and figure out how to integrate evidence-based medicine into daily bedside care as well as be familiar with credentialing standards. Today nurse managers are integrally involved in operations, are more analytically oriented, and understand metrics.

Integrating New Responsibilities

Today's nurse manager is the CEO of the unit and on duty 24/7. These managers are responsible for safety, the budget, and patient and employee satisfaction, and are no longer solely caregivers but administrative leaders as well. They have to understand the policies of the human resource office as well as understand the basics of quality management and performance improvement, and be familiar with system priorities and government and regulatory issues and expectations. Good nurse managers know everything on the floor and rely on data to be informed. They understand elementary statistics and have to know how to use the information from data to create change. They cannot demand certain kinds of behavior under threat and expect success. But using reason and showing data might be effectively persuasive. Head nurses rely on good data to plan programs, deal with budgetary concerns, and maintain excellent care.

With so many responsibilities and so much required of nurses, leaders have to be effective. It is easy to be overwhelmed with tasks to do and not to think strategically and plan for change and improvement. Today's nurse leaders need to be sophisticated in managing information, daily and for the future. Decisions have to be data driven, objective, and clear to influence behavior. Ideally, nurses should have an internship in quality management and take classes in statistics. Everyone needs to be able to function in a data environment, be sophisticated in small-group dynamics, value interdisciplinary teams, and know the responsibilities of caregivers across the continuum of care.

Transformational Leadership

It is undisputed that effective nurse leadership is a necessary factor in achieving optimal outcomes for patients and increased satisfaction for staff. For over two decades nurses have embraced a theoretical framework called transformational leadership, where visionary, intelligent, and charismatic leaders influence and motivate others to work for the greater good and inculcate high ideals and moral values. Transformational leaders create a motivating vision for followers and communicate that vision effectively and with enthusiasm. These leaders create a strong sense of loyalty to the organization. Expectations for performance are high.

Rather than relying on negative feedback or focusing on tasks or even providing rewards for extra effort, transactional leaders inspire a shared vision that motivates others to think about more than self-interest and the desire to excel. They do this by setting an example and building rapport with teams. Responsibilities are shared by all. The idea is that staff are more satisfied and that turnover is reduced in the work environment created by a transformational leader. These leadership qualities are very similar to qualities described in Magnet hospitals. Leaders who operate as transformational leaders not only are associated with improved job satisfaction but also with a stronger organizational commitment and increased productivity (Hutchinson and Jackson 2013).

Case Example: Monitoring Patient Safety

At one of the flagship hospitals in the system in which we work, Kerri Scanlon, the CNO of the hospital and the deputy chief nurse executive for the system, has developed data tools to improve patient safety, nursing care, and accountability as part of a "New Nurse Quality Program."

Figure 5.9 shows some of the data elements that comprise the patient outcome monitoring tool. The tool, which measures patient assessment, pain, falls risk, effective communication, and other relevant variables, is completed by

FIGURE 5.9. PATIENT OUTCOME MONITORING TOOL

❏ Patient Care Assessments and Reassessments
❏ Pain Assessments and Reassessments
❏ Fall Risk Assessments
❏ Restraint Management
❏ Effective Communication—Limited English Proficiency and Hearing-Impaired Patients
❏ Patient/Family Education
❏ Planning Care, Treatment, and Services
❏ Providing Care, Treatment, and Services
❏ Coordinating Care, Treatment, and Services

the nurse manager and quality management patient safety leader on a weekly basis. The form is accompanied by a **tracer**, a methodology that reveals exactly how the staff cared for the patient. This monitoring tool increases accountability and provides nurse leaders with crucial information about patient care, staff competence, and educational opportunities.

The Role of the Medical Staff in Promoting Safety

Medical leaders also have new responsibilities in relation to working with quality metrics. In the past, the responsibilities of the CMO were defined by regulatory agencies, such as TJC, which dictated that the credentialing and appointment process be overseen by the medical leader. The CMO was also often involved in peer reviews in terms of QA issues. The role was more administrative and regulatory than one of clinical leadership—that is, it provided direction for priorities and made changes for improvements. Clinical leadership was in the hands of the medical directors and chairs of departments, who usually reported directly to the CEO (bypassing the CMO). In a managed care environment, the medical director was concerned with data and standards and communicated information to the medical professionals who were part of the insurance company.

Today, medical leaders have to be well versed in statistics because they are working in a data-heavy world. They have to be able to interpret data and illustrate that their delivery of care is successful and that changes in care from improvement efforts are sustained. Today, as quality management has evolved and as data are more plentiful and available and as measurements of operations, processes, and outcomes are evaluated by insurance agencies and the CMS, the expectations of medical directors have changed. They now have the authority or legitimacy to actually oversee the delivery of physician care processes.

Typically a physician interacted with quality management only if an adverse event, a sentinel event, or an incident was reported. Then the medical director would supervise the involved physician and, if necessary, recommend education, or corrective actions, or even disciplinary measures. The focus was on reviewing the process of care.

Providing Education to New Physicians

However, today, the medical director is responsible for educating the medical staff on quality because the Accreditation Council for Graduate Medical Education (ACGME) requires it. By requiring residents to "systematically analyze practice using quality improvement methods, and implement changes with the goal of practice improvement" (https://www.acgme.org/acgmeweb/ Portals/0/PFAssets/ProgramRequirements/CPRs2013.pdf), the ACGME has established that residents need to learn the fundamentals of quality management and performance improvement.

Further, the ACGME has developed the CLER program to educate new physicians, residents, and fellows about providing patients with safe, high quality care. CLER stands for Clinical Learning Environment Review, a program designed to provide U.S. teaching hospitals, medical centers, health systems, and other clinical settings with periodic feedback that addresses: patient safety; health care quality; care transitions; supervision; duty hours and fatigue management and mitigation; and professionalism (http://www.acgme.org/ acgmeweb/portals/0/pdfs/cler/cler_executivesum.pdf).

Case Example: Resident Education Program

As a response to the new requirement, the Krasnoff Quality Management Institute offers educational programs to residents, physicians, and health professionals both within the health system in which we work and elsewhere. The goal of the education is to familiarize health professionals with quality management skills so they can flourish in a data-driven health care environment and learn fundamental principles of population management. The program teaches them to focus on process and outcomes, to identify gaps in the efficient and effective delivery of care, and to develop improvement strategies.

Participants receive training in the fundamentals of quality management and in advanced research methods. In the fundamentals curriculum, residents are exposed to an overview of quality management principles, philosophy, and history as well as such tools and techniques as the Plan-Do-Study-Act (PDSA) cycle for performance improvement, how to conduct a root cause analysis, and the importance of public reporting of measures. They learn how to use data for assessing, evaluating, and monitoring health care processes and services. Residents learn about the use of measures of effectiveness to resolve a clinical problem or issue.

The education about public reporting highlights how these reports have a direct impact on health care delivery systems. Public reporting venues, methods, and information dissemination are discussed. Data transparency, measurements for improvement and accountability, and value-based purchasing are reviewed in relation to the use of quality measures, public reporting, and their financial implications in today's health care environment.

In the more advanced module, education focuses on using data to conduct quality research, with information about basic statistics, data collection, sampling, and analytic techniques. The advanced module focuses on how to conduct research activities that improve quality of care, increase efficiency, and reduce costs. Participants in this educational program learn about the relationship between process and outcome and the complexity of research methodology.

The course finishes with an introduction to data collection techniques and an overview of statistical analyses. Topics include probability and non-probability sampling techniques used in research, creating a data collection goal and plan, understanding various data sources where information can be obtained, and tips and techniques for determining what type of statistical analysis to use. (For more specific information about quality management educational modules, go to http://www.thekqmi.org/wp-content/uploads/2013/10/iLearn-Description.pdf.)

Residents who have successfully completed quality management education have introduced important performance improvement activities into their daily work, taking theory and applying it effectively to the delivery of care. Rather than examining a process on a case-by-case or individual patient basis, they learn how to identify common factors in a process or problem and how to collect data to illuminate the problem for others.

For example, a pediatric resident realized that the electronic systems in labor/delivery were incompatible with those in the neonatal intensive care unit. She developed a simple checklist so that crucial information, such as membrane rupture or diabetic status of mother, was not lost in transfer. Another pediatric resident realized that inefficiencies in the discharge planning process exposed his young vulnerable patients to increased days in the hospital. He established special rounds where social work and case managers would be informed of the estimated day of discharge at admission and develop processes to further timely discharge.

Geriatric residents have investigated projects related to dietary supplements in the elderly population, health literacy and advanced directives, and tele-health. Training new physicians to use data to investigate problems in the delivery of care and to develop improvements that they track with data has resulted in improved quality and safety for patients and more efficient care.

Promoting Safety through Effective Communication

Data, data analysis, database development, control charts—all aspects of quality management—need to be effectively communicated to caregivers and administrators for patient safety to be monitored and optimized. The new health care environment relies on administrative and clinical leaders to be proactive about preventing errors. A unit manager has to collect data to understand types of problems that occur, the extent of problems, the patient population affected by the problems, the daily processes and activities that may contribute to the problems, and the resources involved in managing the problems. The more data collected and analyzed, the better problems are understood. The better understood problems are, the less likely it is that an error will occur.

For example, pressure ulcers can be a marker of poor-quality care and be expensive to treat; putting processes in place to reduce pressure ulcers makes good sense, both in terms of quality and finance. The first step to reducing pressure ulcers is to have information about the scope of the problem, which should be garnered by collecting data on volume and severity; then the process of care should be analyzed to locate weak points; then improvements should be developed, implemented, and monitored for sustainability.

Another example: A unit manager should be able to analyze which of the patients on the unit develop hospital-acquired pneumonia. Do those patients have any common characteristics, either demographic or clinical variables? Data are required to answer that question. How long is the length of stay of those patients who acquire pneumonia as opposed to others with similar characteristics who do not? What is the cost to the organization in terms of length of stay, staffing, and treatment? When senior leaders inquire as to why the rate of pneumonia is high, they expect objective information about a problem and potential solutions. Once relevant variables are defined, a database should be developed to understand relationships in the process of care.

Breaking Down Silos

Problems can be interpreted differently depending on one's position. The medical point of view may be different from an administrative one and still different from a quality management one. A physician may ask why a particular patient developed pneumonia: Was there anything in the clinical condition that predisposed the patient? Physicians may look to the medical literature to offer explanations. Typically, physicians do not involve themselves with process improvement or outcomes analysis. To succeed in today's health care environment, however, they will need to learn to do so.

Quality managers may look at the same problem from another point of view. They may target a system problem, perhaps delays in antibiotic delivery or the timeliness of radiological reports, and institute performance improvement activities. Unfortunately, these points of view do not always overlap, which reinforces the silo mentality and shows the cultural variation embedded in the health care delivery system. Ideally these different approaches to care processes should be merged.

Quality care means that everyone involved in care, from the board of directors to the bedside worker, should feel responsible to the patient and the organization. Since so often the activities of one person are interconnected with those of others, effective communication is essential. To deliver quality care, an organization requires a culture of open communication. Poor communication can result in hours of rework, errors, or complaints. Poor communication harms patients and is expensive.

Communication is not solely about transferring information but about a culture that shares the goal of excellence in patient care. With excellent communication, leaders and managers of units or departments can ensure that patients' expectations are met, that physicians and nurses understand each other, that consultants effectively relay information to others, and that the staff understands the department's and the organization's goals and priorities.

Most organizations have a communication structure that helps to move information across the institution and from the bedside caregiver to the board of trustees. In the health care system in which we work, unit managers report quality care indicators to their managers, who report to the hospital quality director, who meets with directors from other hospitals in the system to define goals and priorities. Committees comprised of administrative and medical leaders, quality management professionals, and senior executives meet to review the quality reports of each hospital.

Depending on its type, information needs to be transmitted to medical boards, administration, or external agencies. It must also be focused so that it explains clinical phenomena in a way that promotes accountability for excellent delivery of services. All the information helps to guide decision making, from the unit to across the entire system and into the community, to identify problems and formulate improvements. In this way, information is translated into action.

Case Example: Reducing Length of Stay for Stroke Patients

The new bundled payment system, the wave of the future, requires that leaders analyze efficiency. They need to know whether the resources that are being expended on each patient are too much, too little, or just right. Understanding the process of care across the continuum allows for targeted analysis of any point in the process.

When leaders in the hospital system in which we work prioritized reducing the LOS for stroke patients, they did so because they realized that a shorter LOS would be good for both patients and the organization. Before reduction strategies could be implemented, however, the process of care, across the entire continuum, had to be analyzed and understood.

The care of a stroke patient could be influenced not only by the way the acute hospital phase was managed but also by many other factors, such as the availability of rehabilitation services, how the patient responded to treatment and medication, transfer issues moving the patient to another level of care, family support, discharge planning, and home care issues. If clinical processes, social work, utilization management, discharge planning, and home care (all involved in LOS) are independent and working in silos, poor communication is inevitable and LOS increases. The process of moving the patient along the continuum has to be managed. If the LOS is longer than expected, communication issues need to be analyzed and processes must be improved.

In our system, in an attempt to understand the process, quality management looked at the common denominator of the majority of patients rather than the outliers. The idea was that if the process could make an impact on many patients, we could reduce LOS and meet payer expectations. The communication process was examined from admission through discharge and defined the many people and services involved in an episode of hospitalization (see Figure 5.10). Potentially, information could be lost at any point in this complex process that involves many people.

Once the specifics of how a patient moves across the continuum were understood, from preadmission, the admitting process, the treatment cycle, to discharge, individuals were identified to be accountable for each point in the process.

Comparing our data to those of other hospitals and establishing benchmarks, using our own analysis and those of the CMS, we were able to define appropriate LOS. Quality management leaders made use of external guidelines to define and standardize care. Risk-adjusted models were developed to control for variation in clinical symptoms and comorbid conditions. We searched for commonalities in the delivery of care.

For example, a stroke patient's discharge planning should begin when the physician orders a change in medication, from intravenous heparin to oral warfarin. We asked what were the criteria physicians used to determine when a patient was ready to switch medications. Aggregated data show that most stroke patients had normal blood levels and were ready to switch medications after four or five days. The clinical literature supported this time frame as well.

FIGURE 5.10. COMMUNICATION ACROSS THE CARE CONTINUUM

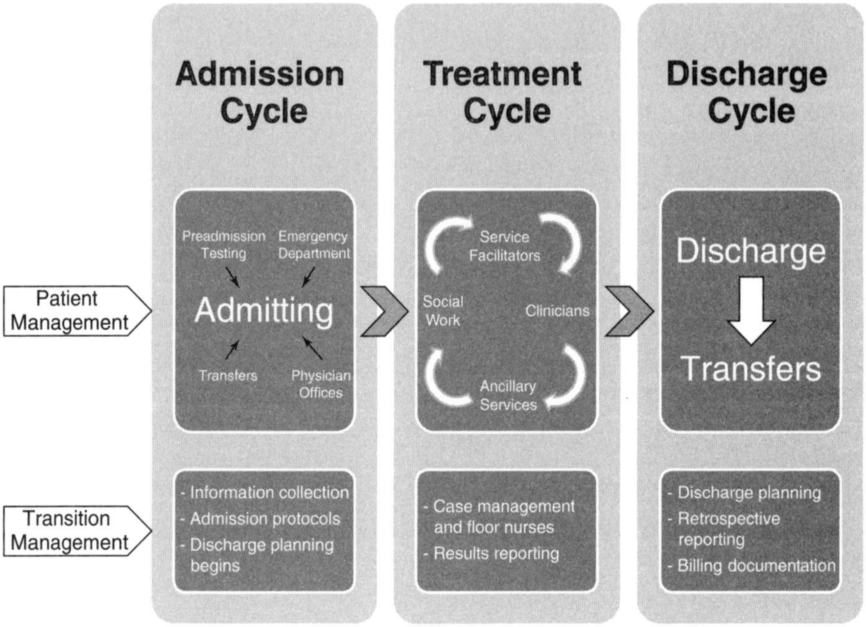

However, physicians treating individual patients, one at a time, had no access to this aggregated information. Once quality management showed them the data, however—data that had been collected over a period of time, risk-adjusted and benchmarked against similar hospitals—they were better able to anticipate resource utilization.

We also discovered that there were not only clinical determinants to the decision to switch medication. Information from the laboratory that showed a patient's readiness for the switch did not always reach the nurse or physician in a timely way. Therefore, the patient's LOS was affected by inefficiencies in communication, not medical need. If social work could not ensure that a patient's home environment was safe for aftercare, the patient might remain in the hospital until a suitable placement could be found. But if that were the case, it was possible and more efficient to move the patient to a lower level of care. The point is until the analysis was made, there could be no improvements to the process. Each department was working in isolation, not in a coordinated patient-centered way. Once the communication flow was improved and multidisciplinary teams were established, LOS and patient safety improved.

Summary

Changing traditional medical culture to establish a culture of safety in order to improve patient care involves adopting new ideas and incorporating quality management tools and philosophy into every level of the health care organization. Specifically, a culture of safety involves:

- understanding the role of data in performance improvement activities;
- developing programs to address system flaws that result in errors, events, and patient harm;
- establishing priorities using data and dashboards;
- using quality data to improve communication among caregivers across the continuum of care;
- educating medical staff in using quality management principles to monitor and improve care; and
- eliminating traditional silos and creating a patient-centered team approach to care.

Key Terms

adverse events, APACHE, B-Care Tool, business intelligence, Magnet, medical errors, near misses, nursing-sensitive measures, prioritization criteria, prioritization matrix, sentinel events, service lines, tracer

Quality Concepts in Action

The C suite and senior leaders of a health care organization often find it difficult to juggle the competing priorities of quality and safety with financial responsibilities. Often the CEO prioritizes financial needs before addressing quality and safety concerns. However, today, with pay for performance (i.e., payment for safe, quality care and penalties for poor outcomes), these concerns need to be merged successfully. As a quality administrator faced with a traditional CEO who prioritizes finance, would you:

- attempt to pressure the clinical staff (physician and nursing) to support and prioritize quality, hoping to influence the administration?
- use data analytics to illustrate to the C suite that meeting benchmarks results in financial rewards and that poor care puts finances at risk?

- keep a low profile and offer small steps toward improving quality so as not to invoke backlash from finance?
- combine staff education with administrative analytic reports to try to influence everyone at once to prioritize quality/safety?

Argue the relative effectiveness of each of these approaches to influence the attitudes and behaviors of senior leaders.

References

Committee on Quality of Health Care in America, Institute of Medicine. 2001. *Crossing the Quality Chasm: A New Health System for the 21st Century.* Washington, DC: National Academies Press.

Dlugacz, Y. D. 2010. *Value Based Health Care: Linking Finance and Quality.* San Francisco: Jossey-Bass.

Dlugacz, Y. D., A. Restifo, K. A. Scanlon, K. Nelson, A. M. Fried, B. Hirsch, M. Delman, et al. 2003. "Safety Strategies to Prevent Suicide in Multiple Health Care Environments." *Joint Commission Journal on Quality and Safety* 29 (6): 267–278.

Dlugacz, Y. D., and P. L. Spath. 2011. "High Reliability and Patient Safety." In P. L. Spath, ed., *Error Reduction in Health Care: A System's Approach to Improving Patient Safety,* 2nd ed. pp. 35–56. San Francisco: Jossey-Bass.

Hutchinson, M., and D. Jackson. 2013. "Transformational Leadership in Nursing: Towards a More Critical Interpretation." *Nursing Inquiry* 20 (1): 11–22.

Kizer, K. W., and M. B. Stegun. 2014. "Serious Reportable Adverse Events in Health Care." *Advances in Patient Safety* 4: 339–352.

Kohn, K. T., J. M. Corrigan, and M. S. Donaldson. 1999. *To Err Is Human: Building a Safer Health System.* Washington, DC: National Academies Press.

Leape, L. L. 1994. "Error in Medicine." *JAMA* 272 (23): 1851–1857.

Lustbader, D., E. Hussain, M. C. Jacobs, E. Cohn, Y. Dlugacz, L. Stier, and A. Greenwood. 2001, December. "Methodology for Improved ICU Resource Utilization and Quality of Care Across a Large Health Care System." *Critical Care Medicine* 29(12): A79–A79.

Tromp, N., and R. Baltussen. 2012. "Mapping of Multiple Criteria for Priority Setting of Health Interventions: An Aid for Decision Makers." *BMC Health Services Research* 12: 454.

Weick, K. E., and K. M. Sutcliffe, K. M. 2007. *Managing the Unexpected: Resilient Performance in an Age of Uncertainty,* 2nd ed. San Francisco: Jossey-Bass.

Suggestions for Further Reading

Dlugacz, Y. D. 2004. *The Quality Handbook for Health Care Organizations: A Manager's Guide to Tools and Programs.* San Francisco: Jossey-Bass.

Dlugacz, Y. D., L. Stier, D. Lustbader, M.C. Jacobs, E. Hussein, and A. Greenwood. 2002, August. "A Quality Approach to Critical Care." *Joint Commission Journal on Quality Improvement.* 28:8, 419–434.

Fenter, T. C., and S. J. Lewis. 2008. "Academy of Managed Care Pharmacy Pay-for-Performance Initiatives." *Journal of Managed Care Pharmacy* 14 (6, Suppl. S-c): S12–S15.

Langley, G. L., R. D. Moen, K. M. Nolan, T. W. Nolan, C. L. Norman, and L. P. Provost. 2009. *The Improvement Guide: A Practical Approach to Enhancing Organizational Performance*, 2nd ed.. San Francisco: Jossey-Bass.

Naessens, J. M., J. M. Campbell, Huddleston, B. P. Berg, J. J. Lefante, A. R. Williams, and R. A. Culbertson. 2009. "A Comparison of Hospital Adverse Events Identified by Three Widely Used Detection Methods." *International Journal for Quality in Health Care* 21 (4): 301–307.

Resar, R., F. A. Griffin, C. Haraden, and T. W. Nolan. 2012. *Using Care Bundles to Improve Health Care Quality*. IHI Innovation Series white paper. Cambridge, MA: Institute for Healthcare Improvement.

Thomas, L., and C. Galla. 2013. "Building a Culture of Safety through Team Training and Engagement." *BMJ Quality & Safety* 22 (5): 425–434.

Useful Websites

http://www.acgme.org/acgmeweb/portals/0/pdfs/cler/cler_executivesum.pdf

https://www.acgme.org/acgmeweb/Portals/0/PFAssets/ProgramRequirements/CPRs2013.pdf

http://www.ahrq.gov/professionals/quality-patient-safety/patientsafetyculture/hospital/index.html

http://www.ahrq.gov/professionals/quality-patient-safety/patient-safety-resources/resources/advances-in-patient-safety/vol4/Kizer2.pdf

http://www.ahrq.gov/research/findings/final-reports/pscongrpt/psini2.html

http://www.cdc.gov/HAI/pdfs/bsi/checklist-for-CLABSI.pdf

http://www.cdc.gov/homeandrecreationalsafety/falls/adultfalls.html/riskassessment-and-prevention-strategies?id=3094#1

http://www.cms.gov/Medicare/Quality-Initiatives-Patient-Assessment-Instruments/Post-Acute-Care-Quality-Initiatives/CARE-Item-Set-and-B-CARE.html

http://www.ihi.org/resources/Pages/Tools/SevereSepsisBundles.aspx

http://www.ihi.org/knowledge/Pages/WIHIPartnershiptoReduceDeathsSepsis.aspx

http://www.ihi.org/resources/Pages/Changes/DevelopaCultureofSafety.aspx

http://www.jointcommission.org/assets/1/18/UP_Poster.pdf

http://www.jointcommission.org/assets/1/23/jconline_April_29_15.pdf

https://www.jointcommission.org/standards_information/up.aspx

http://www.nursecredentialing.org/default.aspx

http://www.usnews.com/pubfiles/BH_2014_Methodology_Report_Final_Jul14.pdf

http://www.ahrq.gov/professionals/systems/hospital/fallpxtoolkit/index.html

https://psnet.ahrq.gov/primers/primer/5/safety-culture

PART TWO

APPLYING QUALITY TOOLS
AND TECHNIQUES

CHAPTER SIX

WORKING WITH QUALITY TOOLS AND METHODS

Chapter Outline

Identifying a Problem
Describing Information
Variability
Making Use of Data
Using Quality Tools and Techniques to Improve Safety
Clinical Pathways or Care Maps
Improving Performance: Plan-Do-Study-Act
Summary
Key Terms
Quality Concepts in Action
Suggestions for Further Reading
Useful Websites

Key Concepts

- Define the appropriate steps involved in investigating a problem.
- Understand the value of quality tools, such as cause-and-effect diagrams and flowcharts.
- Identify appropriate graphics to display quality information.
- Learn basic statistical methods of describing data.
- Improve the delivery of care through root cause analysis of problems and failure mode and effects analysis of potential problems.

- Describe the advantages of clinical guidelines to the organization and to the patient.
- Understand the PDSA methodology for implementing improvements.

Statistical tools offer reliable and effective ways to assess and process information and to make data meaningful and useful. Administrative and clinical leaders are becoming more familiar and comfortable with seeing displays of quality data and making use of that information for performance improvement. Quality tools help to: communicate information about the delivery of care; analyze issues, incidents, or problems with the delivery of care; and develop care methodologies and algorithms to reduce variation in care.

Various tools and methods have been developed to work with quality data and measures. We have mentioned many of these tools in previous chapters—in particular, control charts, run charts, checklists, and the Plan-Do-Study-Act (PDSA) methodology—that help to track and trend quality information. This chapter focuses on the properties of these tools and how best to use them to improve care and efficiency.

Identifying a Problem

Let's begin with tools and techniques that help to define a problem. As an example of a problem, consider falls. If a leader wants to understand why the rate of patient falls is high or has not decreased to acceptable levels (zero?), then the first step is to gather a **multidisciplinary team** of stakeholders who can offer ideas from their particular fields of expertise. The team might have representatives from housekeeping, who are responsible for maintaining the rooms, and from materials management, who are responsible for call bells. People from the environment of care who are responsible for lighting, as well as physicians, nurses, aides, and other direct caretakers, should also be part of the team. These are the frontline workers who will have to implement changes.

Once the team is formed, it considers various questions, such as:

- Is housekeeping staff aware of safety risks, such as preventing patients from slipping on wet floors or having obstructions in the rooms?
- Are the rooms and bathrooms hazard free?
- Are nurses responding quickly to call bells, or is there some bottleneck?
- Are they responding to call bells as a priority, or are they experiencing **alarm fatigue**, when an overload of noise causes alarms to be ignored?
- Is medication causing patients to fall?

Pharmacists should also be involved, since some medications can make patients unstable, drowsy, or have to urinate frequently. Involving the different experts on the team has the further advantage of increasing buy-in to the improvement process.

The team should then develop a set of variables to quantify falls: frequency, location, time of fall, outcome of fall by severity. Data can be collected from many sources: medical record reviews, incident reports, patient complaints, observation, and so on. The goal of the data collection is to create consistency in accurately describing rates of falls and to standardize the definition of falls so that all clinicians who may be affected by the data understand why improvements may be necessary. Although fall prevention programs are numerous and well established, their impact is limited due to poor data collection, lack of uniform definition, poor variable construction, and therefore a poor analysis of how interventions make an impact on fall prevention.

Cause-and-Effect Diagram

With many theories being floated as to possible causes for falls, data analysis is important. However, at times an incident analysis is required; if the team can identify issues for one specific incident of a fall, it may point to a weakness in the process or system, which can be improved.

A cause-and-effect diagram, also called a **fishbone diagram**, or an Ishikawa diagram, named after its inventor, Kaoru Ishikawa, is used to illustrate the various factors that have an impact on an outcome. A cause-and-effect diagram helps analysts target the causes of a problem, especially useful for complex problems. The underlying assumption is that many factors have an impact on an outcome and that some factors perhaps are more salient than others. A multidisciplinary team of stakeholders identifies possible causes of the poor outcome. Once those potential causes are defined, they can be bucketed into categories, which then become the labels for the large "bones" of the diagram. The diagram also clarifies the different processes and roles involved in an incident and exposes the interaction between the two.

Figure 6.1 shows a cause-and-effect diagram of a patient fall. These categories—characteristics of the patient, the environment, policies, equipment, and personnel involved in patient falls—are specific to this analysis. Another problem or even another fall might have different categories, and then the fishbone would have different categories.

The specific elements under the major categories should be examined for which factors could be improved. If the environment is not appropriate, improvements can be instituted. Perhaps the handrails are loose or the lighting is insufficient or the food tray has been left out of reach of the patient's bed. The multidisciplinary team examines each of the subheadings on the main categories and evaluates whether they were implicated in the fall. Once specific

FIGURE 6.1. FALLS CAUSE-AND-EFFECT DIAGRAM

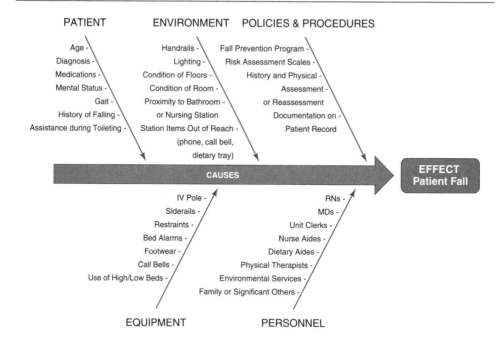

issues are identified as causes of the fall, and there is usually more than one cause, steps can be taken to make improvements.

Flowchart

Another valuable tool for understanding the elements of a process is a flowchart. A flowchart is a graphical representation that diagrams the sequence of events, and the decision points in a process, with the goal of identifying inefficiencies, bottlenecks, or gaps in care. Most flowcharts follow the convention of using a rectangle to chart activities and a diamond shape to show decision points in the process.

Figure 6.2 is a flowchart of the steps involved in analyzing and reporting an adverse event, such as a fall. If the fall resulted in harm to the patient, the arrows point to a case review to determine whether the standard of care was met. If a multidisciplinary team determines the standard of care was not met, then official reports are made to appropriate agencies, such as the Department of Health or The Joint Commission (TJC). If no harm came to the patient, then the process is reviewed by the hospital's quality committee and medical boards and reported to committees of the board of trustees. If it is found that any

FIGURE 6.2. FLOWCHART

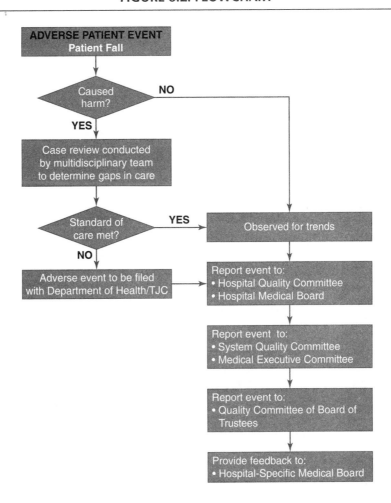

point in the process should be improved, a team is convened to begin a PDSA process.

Checklist

A checklist is a set of ordered steps developed to ensure that every step in a process has been effectively accomplished. Checklists are used to ensure maximum patient safety. Originally modeled on the checklists used in other high-risk situations, such as airplane takeoffs and landings, checklists in health care have been adopted to reduce or eliminate risk to patients.

FIGURE 6.3. TIME-OUT CHECKLIST

RESPONSIBLE PARTIES			
Nurse	Step 1	Begin time-out	❏
	Step 2	Surgeon and anesthesiologist confirm time-out	❏
	Step 3	Members of surgery team are present	❏
	Step 4	Surgery team is introduced	❏
Surgeon	Step 5	Patient name identified	❏
	Step 6	Patient date of birth confirmed	❏
	Step 7	Site of surgery confirmed	❏
	Step 8	Side of surgery confirmed	❏
	Step 9	Patient position checked and confirmed	❏
	Step 10	DVT prophylaxis contraindications checked	❏
	Step 11	DVT prophylaxis given if not contraindicated	❏
	Step 12	All special equipment and required tools are present	❏
Anesthesiologist	Step 13	Radiological studies are present and confirm previous steps	❏
	Step 14	Informed consent is confirmed	❏
	Step 15	Allergies are checked	❏
	Step 16	Name of antibiotic and time given stated	❏
	Step 17	Need and availability of blood products confirmed	❏
Circulator	Step 18	Everyone verbally agrees that all precautions are taken and if unsafe situation, then everyone is responsible	❏
	Signature:		
	Verification Signature:		

Figure 6.3 is a checklist for **time-out** in surgery. TJC and the Centers for Medicare and Medicaid Services has mandated time-out procedures to ensure that the correct surgery is being performed on the correct patient. Unfortunately, wrong-site surgery and misidentified patients occur. Therefore, taking a moment to ensure that everyone in the operating room (OR) agrees that the correct procedure is being performed on the correct patient seems a very reasonable precaution. The clinical staff is supposed to check off and sign that all the steps on the checklist have been followed. The checklist also enhances accountability by identifying the clinician responsible for certain parts of the procedure.

In this example, the nurse circulator, who is responsible for ensuring the patient's safety during surgery, (steps 1–4) is responsible for introducing the time-out, and ensuring that all members of the team are present and know each other's role. The surgeon ensures that the patient is correctly identified (steps 5, 6), that the site of the surgery is articulated and confirmed (steps 7, 8), and that the patient and the room are properly prepared for the surgery (steps 9–12). The anesthesiologist confirms that radiological studies are present, that the informed consent is signed, that allergies are noted, and that medication is given in a timely way (steps 13–16). If the patient requires blood products, that too is checked (step 17). Finally all members confirm that they are responsible for patient safety (step 18).

The details of this and other checklists serve not only as memory aids but also as reminders to the entire team to work together for safety. These particular checks were developed because of incidents where the wrong patient has been operated on or surgery was done on the wrong site, radiological studies were absent, there was no informed consent, and others. Using checklists to ensure that the procedure is done properly seems like simple common sense, but in fact many clinicians resent being told they need to follow a "recipe" and often avoid doing the checklist properly. It should be noted that the checklist does not cover all eventualities or potential problems. Clinicians need to integrate a commitment to patient safety for errors to be reduced.

Run Chart

Various graphical tools help to display data. Many of these tools are quite familiar, such as charts, tables, and graphs. Visual or graphic representations of data enable leaders to oversee care and make informed decisions about resources. Different tools are more or less appropriate for communicating different types of information.

A useful tool to help understand the delivery of care is the run chart. A run chart is simply a line graph that tracks or trends a specific variable over a period of time.

Figure 6.4 is a line graph (or run chart or trend chart) that shows the number of newborn deliveries over a one-year period. The X- or horizontal axis labels the time period, in this case, the months of the year, and the Y- or vertical axis shows the number of deliveries. The graph shows that some months (March, June, October) have a greater number of deliveries than others. The variation might suggest that further monitoring be done, perhaps looking back a number of years so that leaders can respond to patterns and more effectively allocate resources.

Histogram

Figure 6.5 shows a bar chart, also called a histogram, of waiting time for emergency department (ED) triage (the order of treatment based on urgency). This form of display is particularly useful for continuous variable data, such

FIGURE 6.4. NEWBORN DELIVERIES RUN CHART

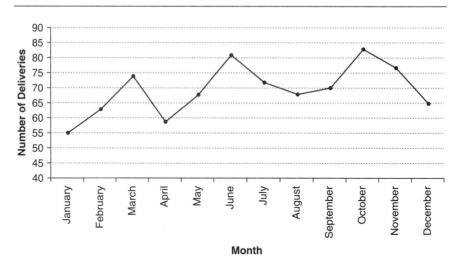

FIGURE 6.5. WAITING TIME FOR EMERGENCY DEPARTMENT TRIAGE

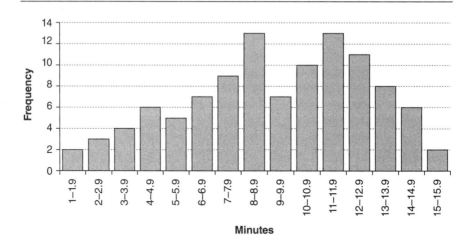

as time. The lengths of the vertical bars represent a defined group, here minutes. A quick glance at this chart shows what kind of variation exists in the process and the most frequently occurring value in the data. The bars of the histogram show the data at intervals, and the height of the bars shows how many data points fell into that interval.

The chart shows waiting time in the ED separated into one-minute intervals (on the X-axis) with the number of patients charted on the vertical

(Y-) axis. If there was a normal distribution (see discussion under "Bell Curve" later in the chapter) of waiting time, we would see the largest bar at 8 minutes (the mean), but these data show that many patients wait 11 minutes, which may indicate a bottleneck that may be disrupting the process. Leaders may want to investigate further. Without the aggregated data displayed in this chart, it would be more difficult to communicate this information.

Describing Information

In order to be useful, data must be analyzed and described. It is important to understand what the data mean and how the information provided by the data can be used productively. Most of us are familiar with numerical data and can interpret it. For example, weight is numerical, and we have norms for what is "normal" weight and what is considered overweight and underweight. Cholesterol levels are also numerical, as are glucose levels. Physicians interpret these numbers as high or normal or low and then treat accordingly. But there are also other kinds of data, such as categorical, questions that can be answered as yes/no or on a scale of like/dislike. Regardless of the type of data, understanding the average of data helps users identify the norm, the outliers, and the range of the distribution.

We are all familiar with **averages**: The average outdoor temperature for a certain month is often given, the average well temperature of a person is known, the average height and weight of a population can be calculated, the average income of families living in certain locations, and so on. The average value helps represent the entire set of data, serving as a kind of quick summary of what is typical. Knowing these averages can provide a quick glimpse into whatever the topic is.

There are three typical ways of characterizing averages: mean, median, and mode. Each of these contributes a specific piece of information and is useful in specific circumstances.

Mean

The mean is the typical value in a range of values. It is calculated simply by adding up all the values in a dataset and then dividing the result by the number of values in the dataset. When students want to know their grades on tests, for example, they add up all their test grades and divide by the number of tests to get their average or mean grade (assuming each test carried the same weight). Mathematically, the mean is the sum, often symbolized as the Greek letter sigma, $\sum$, divided by n, the number of values:

$$M \text{ (mean)} = \sum / n$$

If you have a dataset of, for example, test grades that consist of 95, 92, 87, and 63, your sum total or $\sum$ is 337. The mean is calculated as 337 divided by 4 (the number of grades), giving you an average grade of 84, or a B. You know that the lowest grade of 63 is pulling down your grade (skewing the results). The mean is sensitive to every piece of data, including the outliers, such as the 63.

Physicians do a similar calculation with many variables. If your systolic blood pressure reading, which records the amount of pressure in a person's arteries when the heart muscle contracts, is 120, 122, 118 at various readings, the mean of 120 is normal, and no steps to adjust blood pressure need to be taken. However, if over several months your pressure varies and the readings range from 120, 135, 142, then the mean rate is 397/3, or 132, which is above normal. Therefore, a physician may prescribe medication to lower blood pressure.

Median

Another way to calculate an average is to locate the median. The median is the midpoint of a dataset, meaning that 50 percent of the data are above that point and 50 percent are below. The median is not influenced by outliers that skew the mean. The value of the median average is that you get a sense of what is "normal" because the data are not skewed.

For example, inpatient hospital length of stay (LOS) is very important to managers and administrators; they need to know how many beds are filled for how many days and for what departments and floors/units in order to effectively manage and allocate resources. LOS varies greatly. People admitted for rehabilitation can stay for weeks, and others may be discharged after only 24 hours. Therefore, the data can be skewed in either direction, on both ends. In this case, knowing the median offers information about the norm, or what is most prevalent, rather than the average, or mean.

To calculate the midpoint, organize your data points from low to high or high to low, and then count and find the middle point. If you have 11 patients and you want to calculate the median LOS, you order the numbers. Let's say their LOS was: 6, 3, 7, 16, 2, 4, 3, 6, 8, 1, and 19 days. You order the numbers: 1, 2, 3, 3, 4, 6, 6, 7, 8, 16, 19. To locate the midpoint, count and you see that 6 is the median because there are 5 numbers below and 5 higher.

It does not matter what the numbers are once they are ordered. If your dataset has an even number of data points, then find the two in the middle and calculate the mean. The calculations of median and mean are different and often result in different numbers; the calculation you use depends on what you are looking for, the norm (median) or the mean, which takes all data into account, including outliers.

Mode

It is sometimes useful to know the value that occurs most frequently in a dataset (i.e., the mode). The mode is especially useful in describing a high-volume population. Unlike either the median or the mean, the mode can describe categorical data. If you wanted to find the most frequent condition in your population or the most frequent type of surgery, you would calculate the mode. If 20 patients have pneumonia, 10 have heart failure, and 40 have diabetes, the modal condition would be diabetes because it occurs most frequently in the data. Identifying the mode might have ramifications for knowing how to staff a unit or buy supplies or create efficient processes.

To summarize, what measure of central tendency you use depends on your goal—that is, what it is you are interested in describing. The mean is generally thought of as the average, but when extremes of data, or outlying data points, skew the data, you might be better served by calculating the median. If you want to know the most prevalent item in the data, then look for the mode.

Variability

It is often informative to understand the variability of your data, which is to say, how different each data point is from another. Take a group of numbers, 7, 6, 3, 3, 1. This group has some variability; the mean of the data is 4. Another set of data, 3, 4, 5, 5, 4, also has a mean of 4 but has less variability (i.e., less difference in the distribution). Yet a third set, 4, 4, 4, 4, 4, also has a mean of 4 and no variability at all. You can see that knowing the mean of a dataset might not always offer a description of the data that is sufficient for your purposes.

Range

It may be useful to know the range of your data, which means how widely dispersed the data points are. The calculation is simple: Subtract the lowest number from the highest. So, for example, if your stock has gone from $50 a share to $75, the range (in this case, profit) would be $25. Or if the temperature in December "ranged" from 23 degrees to 53, the range of the temperature variation would be 30 degrees.

Standard Deviation

Although the range may give you a sense of the big picture—that is, the dimensions of a problem or issue—it is extremely general. If you want to fine-tune the range, which is to say, to learn more specifically how much a set of data varies from the mean, you can calculate the standard deviation (SD). The SD is the average distance from the mean. The larger the SD, the farther away the data point is from the mean. By knowing the SD of a dataset, you know what is normal, or standard, and what is high and low, or large and small.

STANDARD DEVIATION

There is a formula for calculating the SD, but today computer programs and calculators make it quite easy for the novice statistician to do.

The formula in Figure 6.6 is like a recipe (instructions to do certain steps in a certain order). Since the point of knowing the SD is understanding variation from the mean, the first step is to calculate the mean. Next subtract each item in the dataset from the mean ($X - \overline{X}$) and square the result. Add together all the squared deviations—that is, take the sum—and divide that by the number of data points minus 1 ($n - 1$). Take the square root of that number (having squared the sums, you now unsquare them, or take the square root). The resulting number is the SD. Again, calculators and computers make this task manageable, but it is worth knowing at least superficially what is involved in the calculation of the SD.

In a set of data, knowing the SD tells you about variation. If the SD is small, let's say .4, that means that the data points are only .4 units away from the mean, and therefore they are more uniform than varied. However, if the SD is 3, then each data point is, on average, 3 units away from the mean, which indicates a great deal of variation of the values. For example, if the SD for LOS is large,

FIGURE 6.6. STANDARD DEVIATION FORMULA

$$S = \sqrt{\dfrac{\Sigma \, (X - \overline{X})^2}{n - 1}}$$

where: S is the standard deviation

Σ (sigma) tells you to find the sum of what follows the symbol

X represents each data point

$\overline{X}$ (called X-bar) is the mean of the dataset

n is the number of data points being analyzed

that indicates that the patients' stay is very long or short (away from the mean in either direction) and may need to be studied further. Leaders can assess patterns and trends with information about SD.

Bell Curve

Many phenomena are normally distributed: height of population, body temperature, blood pressure, blood sugar levels, and others. When these data are graphed, with the data on the X- (horizontal) axis and the amount of data on the Y- (vertical) axis, a symmetrical bell-shaped curve results (see Figure 6.7). The central peak at the midpoint of the curve shows the mean or median, which are the same in a normal distribution. Fifty percent of the data lie on either side of the mean. Extremes fall at either end of the curve. The average, where most results are, is in the middle. Most normal distributions fall 3 SDs from the mean. Therefore, if you know the mean and the SD, you can compute 3 SDs in each direction on a graph, and normal data will fall within this range.

Bell curves are useful in representing large sets of data. If you want to study populations, such as hundreds or thousands of pneumonia patients, you can use a bell curve to reliably identify the norm.

Figure 6.7 shows the distribution of diastolic (the pressure in the arteries between heartbeats) blood pressure in a group of patients. Normal diastolic (the lower number) blood pressure is around 80, according to the American

FIGURE 6.7. BLOOD PRESSURE BELL CURVE

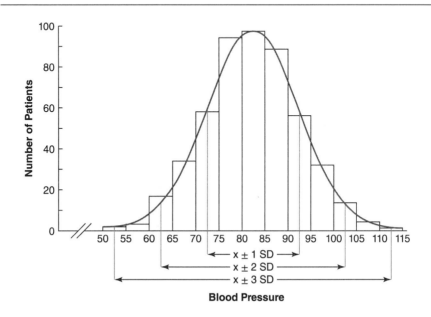

Blood Pressure

Heart Association. As shown on the figure, most of the patients in this group (about 95 percent) fall near or a little higher than normal.

Making Use of Data

Data can and should be used for performance improvement and research. Many excellent texts explain in detail research fundamentals and statistics. This section highlights only a few major points. Research should begin with a **hypothesis**, which means an assumption that can be tested. Usually a hypothesis involves the investigation of a relationship, say, the relationship between increased age and falls or sedentary lifestyle and obesity. The assumption is that one factor has an impact on the other. Any characteristic, attribute, or phenomena that can have different values is a variable. A research hypothesis may investigate how one variable influences another.

Let's hypothesize that patient falls are related to LOS. The hypothesis is that the more falls on a unit, the greater the LOS will be for patients on the unit. The underlying assumption is that falls (the independent variable) prolong LOS (the dependent variable), due to complications. You start with a **null hypothesis**, which assumes that there is *no* relationship between these variables (i.e., there is no relationship between patient falls and LOS). Research and objective evidence is used to confirm or disprove this assumption. Therefore, your research hypothesis will posit a relationship: Patient falls are related to LOS or, more specifically, if patients fall and sustain serious injuries, they will require services/treatment that will prolong LOS. A research hypothesis is really an educated guess; you don't pluck ideas from thin air.

Once you develop your quality or performance improvement research question based on your hypothesis (do patients who fall have longer LOS?), you need to test it, which involves collecting data. Depending on the number of patients you want to study, especially if it is a large group, you may want to do research on a **sample** population, finding instances of individuals who have characteristics that represents the larger group. The idea is that if the sample represents the group, the research results from the sample can be generalized to the entire group. Calculating the sample size is important because if it is too large, you can waste time and resources, and if it is too small, the results may be inaccurate.

If, for example, someone is doing research on the exercise habits of adolescents, it would be impractical to attempt to gather data from every adolescent in the country, city, or even region. But it is not unreasonable to research a small number of people who have characteristics typical of the entire group. If you want to study urban teens who attend public high school in a particular city, then you gather a subset of that group to study. You might want to take a **random sample** of this group—that is, simply choose teens whose names are listed on every 10th line of a high school roster of students. Sample size is determined by formula once you know your population size, the margin of error you are willing to tolerate, how confident you need to be in your analysis, and how much variability (SD) you expect.

Significance

If you discover a relationship between your variables, the next step is to evaluate whether the relationship is meaningful—that is, whether the results are **statistically significant**. That term means that the connection between the variables is not due to chance or random occurrence but is, in fact, meaningful. Significance level can be calculated and reported as a **p value**. If the data show a p value of <.05, that means there is a 1 in 20, or 5 percent, chance that the relationship is merely the result of chance.

Let's take as an example the hypothesis that intensive care units that have intensivists, that is, physicians who specialize in critically ill patients in the ICU, have fewer self-extubations (patients who remove their own ventilators rather than having the tube removed by a health professional) than those units without intensivists. You collect data from intensive care units that do and do not have intensivists and collect data over time about the rates of self-extubations. You discover a difference between these two populations, but is it significant? That is, is the presence of the intensivist what makes the difference, or is some other variable responsible, perhaps nursing staff or sunlight or noise? The level of significance informs you about whether you have made the wrong assumption. Good research should have no more than a p<.05 or 5 percent chance of making a spurious connection.

Using Quality Tools and Techniques to Improve Safety

In addition to revealing information about the delivery of care, quality tools such as these can be used to analyze serious problems or to understand the cause of adverse events that result in patient harm. They can also be used to proactively anticipate whether a gap in care could lead to patient harm. Analysis of adverse events can help to identify vulnerabilities in safety. Regulatory bodies, such as TJC, require that adverse events be analyzed for root causes and that corrective actions be developed to prevent the same or similar errors from occurring in the future. Many states require root cause analysis (RCA) as well.

Root Cause Analysis

RCA is a highly structured approach to analyzing incidents, events, or variation from the standard of care. Originally developed as a tool for industrial incidents, it has been adapted and adopted for error analysis in health care and is incorporated into medical training as part of the Common Core Requirements of the Accreditation Council for Graduate Medical Education (https://medicine.umich.edu/sites/default/files/content/downloads/CPRs2013.pdf). The goal is to identify underlying problems in systems or processes rather than blame any individual for the incident. In fact, RCA assumes a system failure rather than one of an individual's performance.

The model focuses on prevention rather than punishment and identifies the problems in the system that led to the event (such as poor communication), human factors (such as fatigue), environment (such as ineffective sterile procedures) and policies (education of new staff). The specific algorithm of analysis follows the pattern of collecting information to understand the sequence of events leading to the error. TJC and other organizations, such as the Agency for Healthcare Research and Quality, provide templates for conducting RCAs; see, for example, https://www.jointcommission.org/framework_for_conducting_a_root_cause_analysis_and_action_plan/.

The RCA is a retrospective tool—that is, it is used after an incident has occurred, looking back at what happened to attempt to find the cause. It takes a very commonsense approach, defining what happened, why it happened, and what can prevent it from happening again. The U.S. Department of Veterans Affairs suggests that the following questions be asked about an incident (http://www.patientsafety.va.gov/professionals/onthejob/rca.asp):

- What happened?
- Who was involved?
- When did it happen?
- Where did it happen?
- How severe was the harm (actual or potential)?
- What is the likelihood of the event recurring?
- What were the consequences?

Another common mode of analysis is to ask "why" five times, which should provide five different possibilities, with each response more specific than the last, drilling down, so to speak, from each answer. It is important to conduct a RCA as quickly as possible after the event and to interview everyone involved so that memories do not fade and details become lost. Administrative leaders have to support the time and effort involved in taking staff away from their daily routines to be involved in an RCA.

Once questions and answers are asked and reviewed, a cause-and-effect diagram (fishbone) can be created to categorize the responses into larger categories. A flowchart should be used to outline what happened first, second, and so on, with the hope of identifying where there were safety gaps in the process.

When errors occur, RCA usually reveals that poor communication is among the primary causes of patient harm. A surgical team is a classic example of how various specialists have to function effectively as a unit to best care for a patient. An aloof and uncommunicative or arrogant surgeon can break the necessary line of communication and put the patient at increased risk. If a nurse recognizes an error but is afraid to speak out because of the traditional hierarchy in place, especially in an OR where the surgeon is the ruling monarch, the patient is again at risk. Like arrogance, fear or intimidation also can cause communication failures. It is the role of leaders to create an environment that encourages effective and open communication and teamwork and reduces intimidation. Only in this way can a patient-centered safety culture be maintained.

Case Example: Sepsis Mortality

To offer an example of a root cause analysis, let's use a hypothetical case of sepsis mortality. A 38-year-old man in good health required cardiac surgery to replace a heart valve. The surgery was uneventful. However, on the third day after surgery, it was discovered that his sternal (breastbone) wound was oozing and infected. Steps were taken to immediately remedy the situation: infection control consultations, appropriate antibiotic delivery. However, the patient had to undergo multiple trips to the OR to reopen the wound to attempt to clean it and eliminate the infection. Despite all the efforts made to control the infection, the patient developed sepsis and died. An RCA was conducted to investigate what happened to compromise this patient's safety.

A multidisciplinary team examined various aspects of the process of moving a patient successfully through surgery. The RCA uncovered multiple gaps in care. The main issues were grouped into the general OR environment, failed adherence to sterility protocols and procedures, the current OR practices, and, finally, the sterility of the instruments. Drilling down, it was found that these larger categories had multiple issues that could be identified. For example, the OR was overcrowded with instruments—in fact, so overcrowded that some of the equipment was stored in the (unsterile) hallway. Sterile equipment was left close to the doorway, against protocols, because as many people came in and out of the room, the sterility of the room was compromised.

Perhaps because the surgery was somewhat routine, there was found to be a breakdown of vigilance. Procedures that should have been perfect were found to be acceptable as "good enough." Shortcuts were taken that compromised the patient. For example, the anesthesia carts were found to be not cleaned appropriately. The cleaning was supposed to be the responsibility of the anesthesia technician, but he was unaware of this responsibility. The antibiotic used to prepare the skin, betadine, requires sufficient time to dry to be effective. It was discovered that the drying time in this case was insufficient. There were fewer instruments than required, and therefore the sterilization was done on a "flash" (i.e., brief) cycle because there was pressure to turn over the OR quickly. Generally speaking, sterility was not maintained because there was no oversight, and no one felt responsible; when a responsibility is everyone's, in practice, it often becomes no one's. These are just a few instances of what was outlined on the cause-and-effect diagram.

There were so many breaches of proper sterility protocols and procedures that it was difficult to determine which of the many infractions led to this patient's surgical wound infection. A reasonable conclusion is that the culprit in this case was the culture of safety or, rather, the lack of it. There was poor vigilance, poor adherence to procedures, poor responsibility, and finally what looked like a total breakdown of proper protocols. Physicians and staff had become complacent and therefore not careful. The analysis of the tragic consequence of this breakdown resulted in new protocols, education of staff, redesign of the ORs, improved vigilance, assignments of responsibility, and increased monitoring of all safety and sterility protocols.

Failure Mode and Effects Analysis

RCA is, as we said, a retrospective tool. A team analyzes what has already occurred. But it is also wise to assess systems, especially those being developed, or new ones, *before* something harmful occurs; that is, to take a proactive approach to see whether there are potential vulnerabilities that might lead to serious incidents if they are not identified and improved. An RCA analyzes *why* something occurred; the failure mode and effects analysis (FMEA) asks, *what if* this happened? (See Figure 6.8.)

Just as with the RCA and other tools, the FMEA was developed for industry and adapted to health care. The goal is to proactively identify the risk of failure and/or harm in systems or processes in order to make improvements before an incident occurs. Since most errors are caused by good people who are well trained and well intentioned, flawed processes and systems are the focus of both tools. The emphasis for the FMEA is on prevention; this analysis is especially useful when considering a new process, which can then be designed to prevent those failures.

In an FMEA, you also track the specific steps in a process and ask whether something could go wrong; that is, you ask whether any step in the process might be vulnerable to failure. Once you identify what might potentially fail, you ask why it would fail. What would be the causes? Then you ask what the consequences (effects) of the failure would be. If a serious threat to patient harm is identified, even if it is only theoretical, the process should be improved. The American Society for Quality, the Institute for Healthcare Improvement, the Institute for Safe Medication Process, and other organizations provide health care professionals with tools and examples of how to conduct an FMEA (http://asq.org/learn-about-quality/process-analysis-tools/overview/fmea.html).

The general steps or procedures for conducting an FMEA are prescribed. The failure mode begins with establishing a multidisciplinary team with diverse

FIGURE 6.8. COMPARING RCA AND FMEA

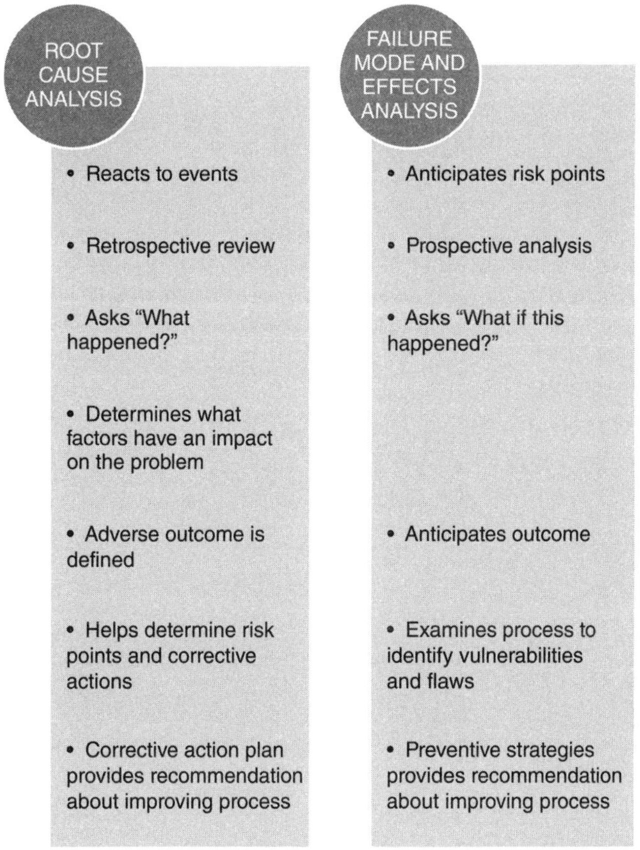

ROOT CAUSE ANALYSIS	FAILURE MODE AND EFFECTS ANALYSIS
• Reacts to events	• Anticipates risk points
• Retrospective review	• Prospective analysis
• Asks "What happened?"	• Asks "What if this happened?"
• Determines what factors have an impact on the problem	
• Adverse outcome is defined	• Anticipates outcome
• Helps determine risk points and corrective actions	• Examines process to identify vulnerabilities and flaws
• Corrective action plan provides recommendation about improving process	• Preventive strategies provides recommendation about improving process

expertise about the process or system being investigated. Flowcharts are used to identify each of the steps in the system and to communicate the diverse steps to all team members (who might be familiar only with their part of the process). The team analyzes the function or purpose of each step in the system or process and projects potential failures of each.

For each potential failure, the consequences to the system and the patient are outlined so that the team can explicitly identify what happens if this failure occurs and the likelihood of the failure occurring. If the failure could be serious, harmful, or catastrophic, and if it is likely to occur, it becomes a high priority for improvements. Once the failure modes—the most risky steps in the process—have been identified, then a root cause analysis is conducted, based on the team's experience, and possible causes for the potential failure

FIGURE 6.9. TRANSFUSION FLOWCHART

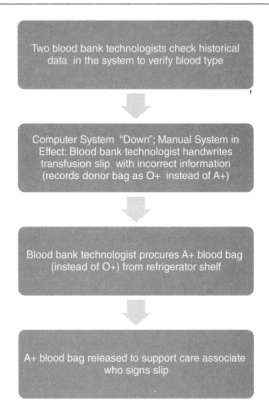

are listed. Once the causes are identified, new processes and systems can be developed to prevent harm and failure.

Case Example: Blood Transfusion

An FMEA of the complex blood delivery process can unearth potentially serious problems and develop solutions proactively.

Figure 6.9 illustrates the process flow of releasing a transfusion bag from the blood bank. The flowchart shows a vulnerability in the system if the computer is down and a technician needs to handwrite information about the blood. If the technician makes an error and the patient receives the wrong blood type, that error could cause very serious, even fatal, harm to the patient.

Because an FMEA located this potential vulnerability in the system, processes were put in place that before the blood is released, whether from computer-generated or handwritten information, two independent technicians have to verify and confirm that the transfusion bag matches the blood type of the patient.

Thinking about potential vulnerabilities reveals various other possibilities for error. In the blood transfusion example, imagine a scenario where a very experienced and capable nurse put a vial of blood into her pocket while she waited for the computer-generated label to be produced. For some reason the label was delayed, and she forgot about the vial until later in the day. An FMEA might target timing of blood draw and computer printout as potential areas of risk and address the issues.

As with the RCA and the PDSA methodology, the FMEA can be a time-consuming, lengthy, and resource-intensive process; therefore, it requires the support and commitment of leaders. With both the RCA and the FMEA, the end result is an action plan for improvements in the process. Mistakes happen—good people make errors, smart people forget vital parts of a process. By confronting issues head on rather than ducking them or assuming the error was a one-time slip-up that will not happen again, intelligent leaders can avoid serious consequences to patient safety. Unless you use a deliberate methodology, such as RCA or FMEA, to analyze processes, it is not obvious how to make the necessary improvements. Errors provide opportunities to understand the vulnerabilities and flaws of a process in order to safeguard the future.

Clinical Pathways or Care Maps

Identification and improvements of gaps in care have a positive impact on patient safety. Standardizing care so that variation is limited also promotes safe practices. Standardization is especially challenging because patients, providers, treatments, and outcomes have tremendous variability. Even with attempts at standardizing processes and procedures and recommending that caregivers follow evidence-based guidelines, variability remains.

Hospitals manage a broad variety of services and a diversity of diagnoses, treatments, patients, units, and treatment options, with individual patients requiring individual plans of care that depend on many factors, including disease, comorbid conditions, and psychosocial issues. To deal effectively with the enormous complexity of requirements, a tool, such as a pathway, care map, or guideline that reduces variation and reinforces uniformity, is extremely useful to the manager, clinician, and administrator.

A care map is an interdisciplinary standardized plan of care for specific diagnoses or procedures with explicitly detailed interventions and outcomes to be accomplished on a time line. Figure 6.10 shows a section of a care map for hip replacement surgery. It outlines the treatment for day 4: for example, what tests are expected, what needs to be assessed, what treatments are involved, medications to be administered, and so on.

FIGURE 6.10. HIP REPLACEMENT CARE MAP

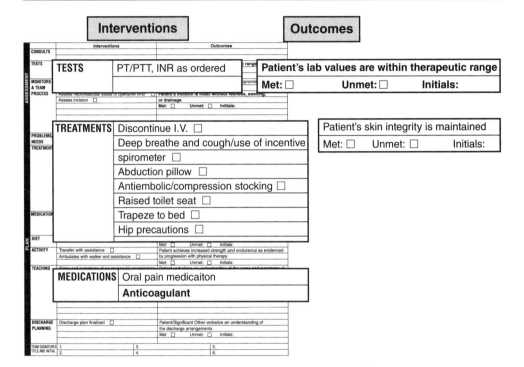

Care Map Characteristics

The use of a clinical pathway or care map helps to decrease variability and to coordinate care among professionals and across the continuum of care, from preadmission to after discharge, for specific patient populations. The care map includes medical demographics, such as allergies, advance directives, medical history, medications, and contact information, as well as what consultations, tests, and procedures were ordered and completed with dates. The interventions include both assessment and treatment plan, including information about diet, activity, treatments, and discharge plan. The outcomes noted address not only clinical and physiological outcomes but also psychosocial, education, and comfort/pain.

Outcomes are expected to be measureable, realistic, and highly specific to each intervention. The interdisciplinary team evaluates the outcomes daily, determining whether the desired outcome was met or not met. If it was not met, the team assesses what is needed and determines treatment to address the problem. The care map functions as a baseline: what should be done during what time frame, generally speaking. It is a way to distill what interventions are necessary and what outcomes are desirable.

Pathways help to create efficiencies in resource consumption and decrease length of stay. Every action is planned in advance, and all caregivers understand what is supposed to occur on each day of the patient's hospitalization. Care maps reinforce interdisciplinary communication and specify accountable professionals as well as create a systemwide common culture. Patient individuality is preserved because the care map is only an outline of care, with key clinical markers noted.

Care maps are developed by physicians and approved by medical boards. The time lines are based on evidence and on benchmarks provided by the Centers for Medicare and Medicaid Services. The treatment outlines are flexible and based on diagnosis; if the original diagnosis changes within the first 24 hours, the care map is changed accordingly. For example, if a patient is admitted with pneumonia and placed on the pneumonia care map and the next day a chest X-ray reveals that the patient has congestive heart failure rather than pneumonia, the nurse changes the care map from the pneumonia one to the heart failure one. Or if a patient is admitted with a myocardial infarction and is placed on a myocardial infarction care map, after surgery for a coronary artery bypass graft, the patient is put on a new care map for the bypass graft.

Variance

Data about variance from the expected plan are collected and used to analyze individual issues (perhaps an infection prevented an intervention) and also to communicate specific information to the rest of the team. If the expected intervention or outcome does not occur, that fact is documented on the variance form. If variation is noted, then the nurse or physician documents what did occur or why some intervention did not occur and why, and what should be done about it, by whom and when.

Figures 6.11 and 6.12 are examples of how variance is tracked and reported from the community-acquired pneumonia care map. Figure 6.11 shows how specific outcomes are checked off on specific days for an individual; the expected outcomes are either met or unmet. This example shows that on day 3 of treatment, the patient was able to take oral medication and had a normal respiratory rate but not normal pulse oximetry (pulse oximetry is the measure of oxygen in the blood and should be above 90). The caregivers are able to see at a glance from the care map what may be of concern about the patient's situation and respond appropriately.

Figure 6.12 shows aggregated data from all the outcomes data for a year. The graph shows that the outcome that is unmet most often involves discharge instructions. If patients do not understand the discharge instructions or if they were not educated effectively on the discharge instructions, they may have to be readmitted or may have other problems. By reviewing the aggregated variance data from the care map, leaders know what gaps in care need improvement efforts.

FIGURE 6.11. VARIANCE ANALYSIS: CAP CHART

MET	UNMET		COMMUNITY-ACQUIRED PNEUMONIA OUTCOMES
✓		Day 1	Oxygenation assessment (*ABG or pulse oximetry*) within 24 hours of arrival
✓		Day 2	Exhibits decreased respiratory effort
✓		Day 3	Patient is afrebrile
✓			Patient can take oral medication
✓			Respiratory rate < 24
	✓		Pulse oximetry > 90 or pO2 > 60 mm
✓			Patient pulse < 100
✓			Baseline mental status
	✓		Patient safely increases activity level
	✓	Day 5	Patient verbalizes discharge instructions (*signs and symptoms of complication to report to MD, understanding of vaccines*)

FIGURE 6.12. VARIANCE ANALYSIS: CAP OUTCOME BAR CHART

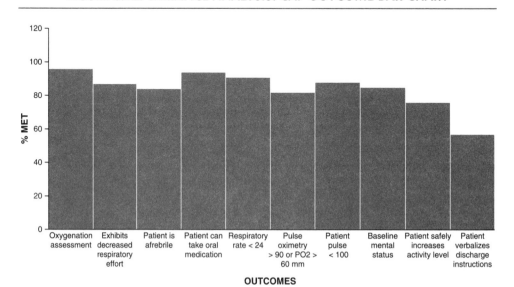

Improving Efficiency

Managers of units find guidelines especially helpful because guidelines can help them organize the many different plans of care they are responsible for. Guidelines help unit administrators manage their unit more efficiently and effectively. Also, guidelines can improve efficiency and cost savings.

For example, a pneumonia patient is expected to have a five-day LOS, changing antibiotic delivery from intravenous (IV) to oral (PO) at day 3; the appropriateness of this changeover should be assessed on day 2 (see Figure 6.13). Under the Plan section of the pneumonia guideline for day 2, clinicians are reminded to assess readiness. A check box is provided so that on day 3, the clinician knows the assessment was indeed made. Once the medication change is made, discharge planning should be finalized.

If a pneumonia patient is sent home too early or remains in the hospital beyond what is necessary (i.e., has excess days), that is not profitable to the organization, nor is it good for the patient. Being discharged too early might result in complications and require readmission. Optimal quality care lowers costs and serves the patient and the organization well.

To improve safety and efficiency, then, caregivers have to be alert to the antibiotic delivery change at day 3 and begin the discharge planning process (see Figure 6.14). Underuse or overuse of hospital resources is financially and clinically inefficient. If the switchover to oral medication is made on day 3 and discharge planning is begun at that time, the patient is appropriately discharged on day 5. Although these issues may seem easy to implement, in practice, the complexity of care often results in inefficiencies. Guidelines can help to alert staff to the sequence of events and serve as reminders of what should occur on which day.

Case Example: Creating Guidelines

Clinical professional organizations publish guidelines for disease management, based on evidence, describing how best to deliver care for specific conditions or for specific procedures. Individual hospitals also develop their own guidelines, tailored to meet the needs of their specific patient population. The methodology that the health system in which we work used to develop guidelines suggests how the process works (see Figure 6.15).

As with any important process that is introduced, leadership support is essential for success. Once leaders prioritize the creation of the care map, a multidisciplinary team is formed to research the most up-to-date clinical literature on the topic, disease, or procedure and to develop consensus on what should be the standard of care.

In the system in which we work, pathways are reviewed by the department chair or director, the hospital medical board, the quality performance improvement coordinating group (PICG), and the nurse executive. Once the guideline is approved, education about how to implement it takes place

FIGURE 6.13. QUALITY IMPROVEMENT THROUGH CARE PATHWAYS

Pneumonia

DAY 2 DATE: ____/____/____

ASSESSMENT		Interventions		Outcomes	
	CONSULTS				
	TESTS				
	MONITORS & TEAM PROCESS	Daily assessment/reassessment ☐		2. Patient exhibits depressed respiratory effort, i.e. no dyspnea or use of accessory muscles on exertion and controlled respiratory rate	
		Vital signs every: _____			
		Aspiration precautions ☐			
		Intake and output ☐		Met: ☐ Unmet: ☐ Initials:	
		Assess skin ☐			
	PROBLEMS/ NEEDS	1.	3.	5.	
		2.	4.	6.	
	TREATMENTS	Deep breathe and cough/use of incentive spirometer ☐		Patient demonstrates ability mobilize secretions by coughing	
				Met: ☐ Unmet: ☐ Initials:	
		Oxygen as ordered: _____			
		IV access: _____			
		Encourage fluids (if not contraindicated) ☐		**Trigger: Assess IV to PO Antibiotic switch**	
		DVT prophylaxis ☐			
		Pulse oximetry: _____ ☐			
PLAN	MEDICATIONS	IV antibiotics		Patient's pain is effectively managed	
		Inhalation therapy		Met: ☐ Unmet: ☐ Initials:	
		Pain management			
		Assess clinical readiness for switch from IV to Oral antibiotics. ☐			
	DIET	As ordered: _____			
	ACTIVITY	As ordered: _____			
	TEACHING	Reinforce plan of care, disease process, and safety precautions ☐		Patient/significant Other verbalize an understanding of the disease process	
				Met: ☐ Unmet: ☐ Initials:	
	DISCHARGE PLANNING	Assess support system ☐			
		Establish discharge plan ☐			
	TEAM SIGNATURES AND TITLE	1.	3.	5.	
		2.	4.	6.	

FIGURE 6.14. IMPROVED EFFICIENCY AND THROUGHPUT

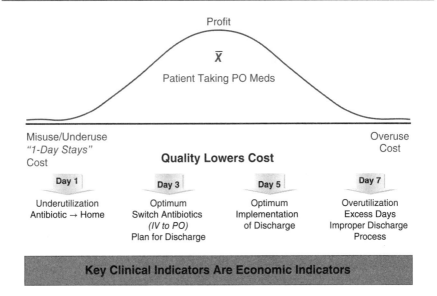

through direct education, in-service training, webinars, and so on. Clinicians implement the guidelines as part of patient care rounds, and, if reassessment is necessary, changes are made. Patient outcomes are monitored as part of the implementation process. The guidelines are also used by patients so that they understand their care plan. Clinicians use them to reduce variation and resource consumption, improve patient satisfaction, and, most important, deliver best practice.

Improving Performance: Plan-Do-Study-Act

Shewhart's and Deming's practical PDSA cycle of performance improvement has been used extensively since the 1980s. The approach was endorsed by TJC because the methodology is based on quality measurements and uses a multidisciplinary team approach to improvements. It is hoped that the PDSA method would help to eliminate the traditional silos in which health care functions and by doing so improve the process of care. The PDSA has also been adapted by the Institute for Healthcare Improvement as a preferred **performance improvement methodology**.

Generally, someone in a leadership position, such as a manager, is charged with overseeing improvement initiatives, which may involve Planning

FIGURE 6.15. CLINICAL GUIDELINES CREATION METHODOLOGY

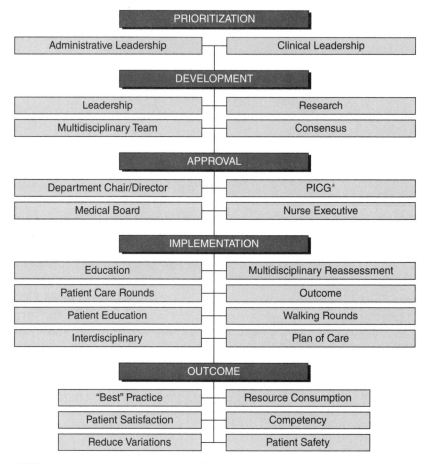

*PICG—performance improvement coordinating group

improvements, actually implementing or Doing the improvement, checking or Studying and evaluating the improvement, and then Acting to implement the change in the organization. This robust performance improvement methodology is used to continuously evaluate performance and standardize processes; eliminate errors, waste, and rework; and reduce variation.

The PDSA cycle (see Figure 6.16) is especially useful for testing changes in practice in a real world/work setting. Several elements have to be in place before an organization embarks on a performance improvement initiative. First and foremost, leaders have to support the quest for improvement,

FIGURE 6.16. PDSA CYCLE

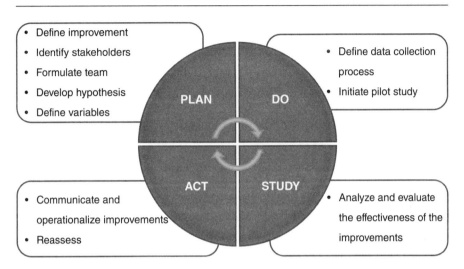

- Define improvement
- Identify stakeholders
- Formulate team
- Develop hypothesis
- Define variables

PLAN

DO

- Define data collection process
- Initiate pilot study

ACT

STUDY

- Communicate and operationalize improvements
- Reassess

- Analyze and evaluate the effectiveness of the improvements

allocating resources and prioritizing the effort. Most important, the organizational culture has to be one that is ready for change. Traditionally quality management personnel conduct the PDSA assessment once the board of trustees or the chief executive prioritizes an improvement initiative. Leaders set goals for the hospital in keeping with its vision and mission and may suggest a threshold for what they ideally want to result from the improvement.

Plan

The Plan stage is the most critical and also the most time-consuming part of the process. During Plan, the vision of the improvement is defined, which is to say, a sense of what an improved process might be and how it would ideally work is explicitly articulated. The stakeholders in the process need to be identified as they are the ones affected by the proposed change and input from them is crucial. The multidisciplinary team comprised of quality and clinical experts formulates an assumption about the process (i.e., develops a hypothesis). For example, a working hypothesis could be that patients who receive antibiotics prior to surgery have fewer infections than patients who are not given medication. In addition to developing a hypothesis, the scope of the effort in terms of people, resources, time, and money has to be defined and then allocated to the process improvement effort as well.

Along with the stakeholders and the frontline workers who make up the improvement team, when identifying what the improvement should be, the voice of the patient (customer) should be taken into account. Information about how patients experience their hospitalization and how they feel about their health care interactions is available from Press Ganey surveys and the Hospital Consumer Assessment of Healthcare Providers and Systems (HCAHPS) surveys. It is important to understand improvement efforts in terms of the patient experience because one of the goals is to satisfy the patient.

Focus groups can also be used to talk to the patients and professionals who have a stake in the process under investigation. The more multidisciplinary the stakeholders are, the more you'll learn about the process improvement effort, including what barriers may have to be overcome. Another way to plan how to improve is to bring the goal of the improvement effort to the medical board and elicit members' input about the strengths and weaknesses of the existing process and their ideal goals for an improved one. In order to really understand the improvement process, you should ask, and be able to answer: who, what, when, where, why, and how much?

Once you understand what has to be changed and improved, you must define relevant variables and develop a database that can assess whether your improvements have made an impact.

Do

In the Do phase, a pilot study for the proposed change should be developed in order to ensure that the changes are practical and to identify problems. The mechanics of the data collection process need to be clearly defined: who will be responsible for collection, how, with what method; who will receive data reports, in what form; who will analyze the data, and over what time period and with what statistical tools? If appropriate, relevant literature can and should be reviewed for established data collection methodologies and analytic techniques. Existing professional literature can also provide benchmarks for established standards of care.

Study

The Study phase is the evaluation and assessment part of the process. Statistical analysis is used to study the results of the improvement effort and observe lessons learned from the pilot. If modifications need to be made, a new pilot is launched. New measures may need to be developed as well.

Act

Once the improvement process has been analyzed and understood, the change has to be communicated and operationalized on a larger scale. A database or table of measures can be developed to ensure the sustainability of the improvement effort. It is important for the improvement team and leaders to review the results of the changed and improved process. It is very easy to return to old ways of doing things once the initial enthusiasm for the change wanes.

Case Example: Workplace Violence

Workplace violence is a serious problem for health care workers. Research shows that the ED has the highest rate of violence in the hospital and that nearly half of all workplace violence occurs in the health care setting (https://www.osha.gov/SLTC/healthcarefacilities/violence.html). That the ED should be vulnerable makes some sense. EDs are often crowded, even chaotic, and can be understaffed because volume is not always predictable. Unless people are frisked at the door, they can carry in weapons. People with substance abuse and mental health problems use EDs, as do criminals, when they need medical attention. Abuse and violence have an impact on staff and patient safety, not only on their physical well-being but also on morale and workplace satisfaction. Workdays can be lost due to injury, and compensation may have to be paid.

To investigate the seriousness of the problem with violence in the EDs, a multidisciplinary team was formed to assess the situation. The team was comprised of ED nurses, administrators, physicians, security personnel, the environment of care staff, and quality management. They collected baseline data on the number of reported injuries due to assault over the past 12 months, how many times the security code/alert was called, what time of day/shift had the most injuries and calls, what the staffing ratios were during the time of injuries, what was the chief diagnosis or complaint, and how many patients had to be restrained. Staff members were surveyed about their workplace satisfaction, with questions about their feelings of safety. When the data were collected and reviewed, leaders determined that the rate of workplace violence was too high and that an improvement initiative was needed. The team determined that a PDSA analysis would be the most useful improvement methodology.

In the Plan stage, members of the team researched the relevant literature for benchmarks and best practices. Once they were educated about best practices, they began to plan their improvements. The plan included education for security personnel, nurses, and other caregivers. There are many robust certified training programs in managing workplace violence, and violence in the health care setting; and people who receive the education become trainers and return to their organization to train others.

It was also determined that an improved assessment was needed to evaluate patients for potential violence and to identify patients with substance abuse issues and mental health problems. Communication markers, such as red flags on curtains and/or in the EHR, would be used to alert staff of the potential for violence or disruptive behavior. Orientation for new personnel would include education about violence. The team recommended, and the literature review supported, that more guards be hired during the hours that the data revealed were most dangerous.

In the Do stage, multiple interventions were made. Education was provided to the caregiving staff to better alert them to potentially violent patients and how to best react in a dangerous situation. Security personnel were trained for improved communication tactics. Patients who were identified as potentially violent were housed in private rooms/spaces. Caregivers were trained to approach potentially violent patients with a partner. Security guards were instructed to make extra rounds. Staff worked with emergency medical services so that if patients were admitted as a result of gang violence, patients from different gangs were separated and taken to different hospitals.

In the Study stage, data were collected on the number of assaults reported since the interventions and compared to the same time period the previous year. Data on the number of restraints necessary, lost workdays, and police reports were also collected. Data showed that the interventions made a difference: Violence was dramatically reduced and the staff members who were surveyed expressed more satisfaction and less fear of workplace violence. In the Act phase, these successful interventions were formally adopted by the medical board and introduced into all the EDs in the system, and other trauma units.

Summary

Understanding how to make use of quality tools, techniques, and methods can improve the process of care and promote efficiency. Health care professionals should have a working knowledge of analyzing and interpreting problems and improving care through:

- cause-and-effect diagrams, flowcharts, and checklists;
- graphical displays of information, such as run charts and bar graphs;
- basic statistical understanding of data, such as averages, distribution, and significance;
- root cause analysis techniques;
- failure mode and effect analysis techniques;
- clinical pathways; and
- PDSA methodology.

Key Terms

alarm fatigue, averages, fishbone diagram, hypothesis, multidisciplinary team, null hypothesis, p value, performance improvement methodology, random sample, sample, statistically significant, time-out

Quality Concepts in Action

The PDSA methodology for performance improvement results in changed processes. It can also be used to enhance or modify a piece of a larger process. Sometimes referred to as Rapid PDSA, the results are more immediate and the impact is successful in the short term. Once improvements are made, a more deliberate PDSA can be developed over time.

Say you are the leader of a busy ED who wants to improve the identification of sepsis patients so that treatment can be more timely and thus effective. Patients who present in the ED with symptoms of sepsis need to have laboratory tests to confirm the diagnosis. and you believe that the information between the laboratory and the ED is not being transferred either efficiently or quickly. You want to implement a Rapid PDSA to improve this situation. In developing your PDSA, make sure to include:

- an explicit and detailed statement of your goal;
- the team members involved;
- your hypothesis for improvement;
- the specific variables you want to measure;
- how data will be collected and analyzed; and
- how improvement will be assessed.

Explain any barriers that you need to overcome to achieve your goal and what strategies or processes you used to overcome them.

Suggestions for Further Reading

Kowalenko, T., S. R. Hauff, P. C. Morden, and B. Smith, B. 2012. "Development of a Data Collection Instrument for Violent Patient Encounters Against Healthcare Workers." *Western Journal of Emergency Medicine* 13 (5): 429–433.

U.S. Department of Labor, Occupational Safety and Health Administration. N.D. "Guidelines for Preventing Workplace Violence for Health Care and Social Service Workers." https://www.osha.gov/Publications/osha3148.pdf

Williams, P. M. 2001. "Techniques for Root Cause Analysis." *Baylor University Medical Center Proceedings* 14 (2): 154–157.

Wu, A. W., A. K. M. Lipshutz, and P. J. Pronovost. 2008. "Effectiveness and Efficiency of Root Cause Analysis in Medicine." *JAMA* 299 (6): 685–687.

Useful Websites

https://www.ache.org/pubs/Releases/2014/top-issues-confronting-hospitals-2013.cfm

http://www.heart.org/HEARTORG/Conditions/HighBloodPressure/AboutHighBloodPressure/Understanding-Blood-Pressure-Readings_UCM_301764_Article.jsp

http://www.ihi.org/resources/Pages/Tools/FailureModesandEffectsAnalysisTool.aspx

https://www.osha.gov/SLTC/healthcarefacilities/violence.html

http://www.patientsafety.va.gov/professionals/onthejob/rca.asp

http://www.psnet.ahrq.gov/primer.aspx?primerID=10

http://asq.org/learn-about-quality/process-analysis-tools/overview/fmea.html

https://medicine.umich.edu/sites/default/files/content/downloads/CPRs2013.pdf

CHAPTER SEVEN

WORKING WITH QUALITY DATA

Chapter Outline

Working with Measurements
Understanding Issues in Data Collection
Using Data to Understand Appropriateness of Care
The Value of Aggregated Data in Performance Improvement
The Role of Data in Managing Chronic Disease
Using Data to Monitor Variability
Publicly Reported Data
Interpreting and Making Use of Data
Quality Management in the Future
Summary
Key Terms
Quality Concepts in Action
References
Suggestions for Further Reading
Useful Websites

Key Concepts

- Understand the distinction between collecting measures for compliance and for performance improvement.
- Highlight issues involved in defining, collecting, standardizing, and interpreting accurate data for measurements.
- Recognize issues involved in managing vulnerable populations and patients with chronic disease.

- Appreciate the importance of monitoring variation from the standard.
- Realize the implications of publicly reported measures for administration and quality professionals.

Health care professionals use data to ascertain whether the care that is being delivered is "good." How does one define "good care" in an objective way? Data provide objectivity to an otherwise subjective concept. Quality care—processes, services, outcomes—is quantifiable. Staff effectiveness and efficiency and meeting patient expectations can also be quantified, as can meeting the goals for the organization. The constant stream of information that is available about the daily activities of a unit or department or practice, budget concerns, employee turnover, patient treatment plans, complaints, and errors, as well as those measures that are mandated, has to be interpreted in order to be useful. If the data reveal that improvements are necessary, then asking focused questions that gather more information can help to uncover what improvements are desirable. Then data can monitor whether the improvements are sustained or not. Information is the key to performance improvement, to the delivery of "good" care.

Data support the foundations of quality management, and quality management data provide the foundation for performance improvement. This chapter illustrates, through case studies, how to use data for improvement, and discusses how to educate administrators and physicians about the value of data in interpreting performance and prioritizing improvements. The case studies, and the tools that are included with them, are presented to suggest methods of managing common issues that exist in working with quality data in a health care setting.

Working with Measurements

There is a difference between using measures for **compliance** and for performance improvement. Hospital and health care administrators and policy makers understand why it is crucial to comply with government measures. Compliance is mandated for reimbursement programs and is used for hospital rankings. Rates of compliance are reflected in hospital care, in report cards, and in criteria for "best" hospitals. Performance improvement measures go further than compliance and are used to assess, monitor, and improve care processes.

It is the role of the quality management department to aggregate various data sources and databases to understand performance: the medical record, blood bank, reports of adverse events and incidents, laboratory information, pharmacological information, billing and claims data, infection control, patient satisfaction data, and so on. Quality management is expected to oversee compliance with the reporting of measures, educate the health care community about the importance of measures, make sense of the data that are collected, analyze it correctly, interpret the information for different specialists, and make reports that tell an effective story from the data so that it is comprehensible to leaders who can then make intelligent use of the data for performance improvement.

As the government defines methods for monitoring quality and containing costs, especially through creating increased accountability for care through Accountable Care Organizations, health care providers have to develop new methods of practice to proactively meet the government objectives.

Compliance

Physicians are required to record information in the medical record that relates to the measures. There is no way to opt out of the system and still receive payment. Data about patient care are reported to the government, and if there is not full compliance, if there are "0s" in the numerators because clinicians have not responsibly filled in the data, then the government investigates and there are financial implications. Therefore administrators have to be sure that the process is working.

In 2006, the Centers for Medicare and Medicaid Services (CMS) implemented the Physician Quality Reporting Initiative (now called Physician Quality Reporting System), which financially rewarded physicians who provided data regarding quality measures for Medicare patients (https://www.cms .gov/Medicare/Quality-Initiatives-Patient-Assessment-Instruments/PQRS/). By reporting on these quality measures, individual physicians and group practices would quantify how often they were meeting a particular quality metric. In 2015, under the Accountable Care Act, the CMS began to penalize providers who do not participate or are unsuccessful in meeting the goals (http://www.ama-assn.org/ama/pub/physician-resources/clinical-practice-improvement/clinical-quality/physician-quality-reporting-system.page).

Case Example: Using Data to Change Practice

When the New York State Department of Health felt that the cardiac information presented by the health care system in which we work was incorrect or insufficient, leaders contracted with an outside agency, a peer review organization, to review our records and ensure data validity. Using outside expertise was useful to the surgeons who did not like quality management evaluating and interfering (as they experienced it) in the way they practiced medicine. As a result of the review, a registered nurse who had responsibility for reviewing medical records, communicating with the cardiac surgeons about information, and ensuring data integrity was hired. Slowly, the physicians grew to accept data as a valid measure of performance and as a yardstick with which to evaluate their process of care for opportunities for improvement.

Performance Improvement

Using measures for performance improvement requires leaders not only oversee measures for compliance but use the measures to monitor, interpret, improve, and sustain the delivery of care. The goal of improvement is to ensure patient safety. The health care literature has stressed the importance of inculcating a culture of safety for decades (Pronovost and Sexton 2005), and the Institute for Healthcare Improvement (IHI) has structured a program for organizations to develop a culture of safety (http://www.ihi .org/resources/Pages/Changes/DevelopaCultureofSafety.aspx). Ensuring patient safety involves understanding structure, process, and outcomes; that understanding is founded on databases that monitor care and can identify where improvements are necessary. Data can show which groups of patients or patient populations can best benefit from changed or improved processes.

Case Example: Pressure Injury Performance Improvement Initiative

Skin integrity is a traditional quality indicator, and collecting data and reporting data about skin integrity has been required for decades. Pressure injuries are considered nursing-sensitive measures because, with appropriate nursing care, injuries to the skin can be minimized or prevented. Pressure injuries can result from prolonged pressure on a bed surface, as may be the case with immobilized patients. If pressure injuries are not recognized and treated early, complications can be quite serious. Effective treatment for patients who are vulnerable to pressure injuries is also very well known. For example, at-risk patients should be turned—that is, their position should be changed—at frequent regular intervals to prevent too much pressure on the skin. Therefore, daily nursing vigilance is critical. The CMS considers pressure injuries never events and will not reimburse organizations for expenses associated with this avoidable condition.

Guidelines regarding staging (levels of severity) of pressure injuries, such as the Braden Scale, have been available for many years (Bergstrom et al. 1987). The National Pressure Ulcer Advisory Panel developed the Pressure Ulcer Scale for Healing Tool as a quick, reliable tool to monitor the change in pressure ulcer status over time (http://www.npuap.org/resources /educational-and-clinical-resources/push-tool/). Although information has been available for many years about reducing the incidence or severity of pressure ulcers, hospitals across the country continue to have patients suffering with such injuries.

FIGURE 7.1. HOSPITAL-ACQUIRED PRESSURE INJURY INDEX

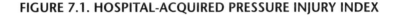

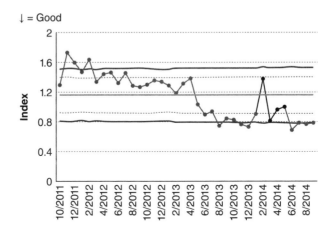

Typically nursing staff reports data on pressure injuries to unit managers who in turn report the information to quality management. In the system in which we work, quality management staff aggregates the data from hospitals and for the system and reports to leaders and back to the units through the quality communication structure. Figure 7.1 is an example of such a report. Hospital-acquired pressure injuries are tracked over a three-year period for leaders, who can see that the trend for pressure injuries has basically decreased over time.

This decrease was the result of performance improvement efforts. The first step in identifying and treating pressure injuries involves examining the skin for redness and sores, then entering this information into the medical record. Stage 1 of pressure ulcer identification is noting redness of a localized region of the skin. It became evident that there was variation in the interpretation of "redness" across units and hospitals and that we needed to establish clear and standardized definitions and training to ensure that the measure would be accurate and consistent. Although nurses were expected to examine and turn patients as a preventive approach, the process was not standardized and was varied across units and nurse leaders. There was a communication gap between clinicians and administrative staff. Specialty beds had been ordered and delivered but remained unused because the accountability and communication structure about bed assignment was unclear.

Quality management staff began a performance improvement effort. They made rounds with the unit clinicians (physicians, nurses, residents) several times a week to reach consensus on the identification of pressure injuries and define potentially risky conditions for increased observation, such as the association between an immobilized patient and pressure injuries. To spur improvement efforts, multidisciplinary teams were established that included all professionals involved in pressure ulcers, such as geriatricians, nutritionists, nurses, physicians, vascular specialists, pharmacists, plastic surgeons, and equipment managers. It was determined that the system would collaborate with a large specialty bed manufacturer, Hill-Rom, because the company had vast amounts of data that could be leveraged to better interpret our delivery of care. The company added value by defining benchmarks, understanding the population via prevalence studies, and including information about the experience of other hospitals.

Data on the prevalence of pressure ulcers were collected at every one of our institutions. Over the course of two years, the teams and quality management established a standardized definition of the different stages across the system and developed a standardized methodology to collect and record data. A standardized tool, the Braden Scale, was adopted to ensure standardization of guidelines about what to measure and how. This objective tool enabled caretakers from various units across the continuum of care to define pressure injuries statistically rather than impressionistically. The reliability of the data collection efforts was vetted through inter-rater reliability methodology. Aides were trained to observe and turn patients. Everyone had a stake in the process, and therefore there was a great deal of professional buy-in for changed practices. A regional education program on our findings was provided to professional staff.

The data collection efforts helped to focus clinician attention on identification and treatment of the problem of pressure ulcers, and their volume and severity were monitored and reported to performance improvement committees throughout the system.

These changes led to improved care. The improvements were so successful that the health system won the coveted Ernest A. Codman Award for improved pressure ulcer management. And most important, a real coalition was formed between nursing and quality management; the nurses realized the power of standardizing care, accurate reporting of data, and the accountability provided through measurements.

Understanding Issues in Data Collection

Since quality data are the foundation of compliance and performance improvement, it is important to understand how data are collected, validated, and communicated. Traditionally, the charge of quality management was to report specific measures required by external agencies. Until recently, these measures were extracted from handwritten medical records. Medical records also include **free text narratives** handwritten by physicians. These narratives provide a great deal of information, and nurses were expected to accurately extract and record information from them.

Because physicians have different styles of recording information in the charts and because the nurses had no formal training about how to collect information, the completeness and accuracy of the data were suspect. Nurses were expected to screen for inclusion and exclusion criteria, and physicians, administrators, and quality management professionals were not sure whether data collection was standardized, valid, and reliable. It was unclear whether extractors were collecting the same information in the same way. Due to lack of rigor and standardization, it was easy to reject conclusions based on these data because the data were thought to be—and sometimes were—incomplete or inaccurate.

Case Example: Standardizing Data

In an attempt to address these reservations and to standardize the process, the quality management department established an educational training program to ensure inter-rater reliability for data collection. Nurses were expected to review patient charts for compliance with specific measurements, such as those established by the CMS for **chronic disease** management. They had to screen for inclusion and exclusion criteria to ensure that the correct population was documented appropriately for the measure. The measurement was explicitly defined, with inclusion and exclusion criteria, and the nurses educated about how to extract the correct and complete information from charts.

For example, the raw severe sepsis/septic shock mortality rate is calculated as: the percentage of sepsis patient deaths out of all sepsis discharges.

$$\frac{\text{Sepsis patients with a discharge status of expired} \times 100}{\text{Number of severe sepsis/septic shock discharges}}$$

Inclusion criteria are patients diagnosed with severe sepsis or septic shock. Exclusions are patients less than 18 years old and those patients on hospice care.

Not only was education provided about how to gather information, a statistical analysis was undertaken to measure the accuracy of collection efforts. The goal was to achieve 99 percent reliability, and that goal was met. The many nurses across the system were effectively trained to collect information about a single measure in a standardized way.

Physicians also required education to understand that the data about a measure reflected information about their care practices. Education was provided, focused on explaining what the measures meant and how they might be used. When documentation was missing from the medical record, physicians were shown the consequences through database reports. They also required education about issues involved in measurements; specifically physicians needed to understand what defined the numerator and denominator of the measure. When the denominator (i.e., the population that the measure is concerned with) increases and the numerator remains stable, it only appears as if the rate is declining. The measurement is not an accurate indicator of the quality of care.

Moving from Manual to Electronic Records

The enormous amount of data required for collection and the complexity of the measurements that need to be reported to regulatory organizations, governmental agencies, and insurance companies encouraged web-based collection efforts, especially electronic health records (EHRs). EHRs were developed to encode patient information and replace the often idiosyncratic handwritten medical chart in a more accurate and standardized way.

There are problems involved in transferring information from medical records to EHRs. For example, EHRs use **binary categorical variables**, which means that caregivers have to indicate either yes or no about specific issues in the delivery of care. Free text narratives—where physicians write notes in their own words, and which are a critical part of the medical record—contain information that may not be captured in the binary checklist structure of EHRs.

Another issue in making the transfer from manual to electronic records is that many physicians require education about how to use EHRs effectively, which is to say as documents that reflect the process of care, and to recognize that electronic records do not simply duplicate paper records. Also, physicians have to be trained to enter information differently. There is a great deal of resistance, especially from older physicians who are uncomfortable with the new technology. Clinicians who are familiar with entering free text are not always happy to go through menus and alerts to fill in categorical data that would reflect what they might have previously written in narrative form.

Extracting Accurate Data from Electronic Health Records

Regardless of these issues, in order to be reimbursed, health care providers are expected to extract clinical quality measures from EHRs and submit them to the CMS. Theoretically the quality measures extracted from the EHR can be superior to those reported from administrative claims data, which are not clinically reliable, and the manual review of the medical record, which is limited in scale because it requires so much staff time. However, a study by Kern et al. (2013) has shown that when comparing manual and electronic medical records, there is variation in accuracy and statistically significant differences, what they refer to as "substantial" discrepancies, between the two. Clearly, the EHR is not a mirror of the manual medical record. Also, a review of the literature (Chan, Fowles, and Weiner 2010) revealed that there are pervasive problems with data accuracy and with the structured fields in EHRs, especially with regard to medications lists. It will take time to resolve these limitations.

Yet even as flawed as they are, EHRs are what is used to determine compliance with CMS measures, and that compliance is crucial for reimbursement and for hospital rankings about performance. Since the CMS and insurers are looking at measures, those measures need to be accurate and complete and valid. A physician will check "yes" or "no" about whether certain specific care measures were provided. EHRs then become a kind of checklist about whether a physician did his or her job properly. Compliance with measures will be a kind of quality control of the entries into EHRs. Have all the patients diagnosed with heart failure had all the measures related to this diagnosis completed in the record? Simply, are the appropriate boxes checked, and if not, why not?

When data are extracted in the aggregate, EHRs can be powerful sources of information about the scope of care and type of care. Such data can offer a snapshot of the organization and enable decision makers to make rapid and informed decisions. Diagnosis codes from EHRs can help leaders track high-risk population information.

The big problem is that software companies that design EHRs compete for customers and are reluctant to make their technology transparent. Patient information is different in different databases, and it becomes a challenge for analysts to link the information to create a central repository of data. Merging databases is not the complete answer either; duplicate records have to be recognized and removed, and typographical errors, such as incorrect Social Security numbers, make patient identification troublesome. **HIPAA** regulations have to be honored.

HIPAA

HIPAA is an acronym for the Health Insurance Portability and Accountability Act, which is a law developed by the Department of Health and Human Services to protect the privacy of information contained in a patient's medical record by keeping that information confidential and secure.

Another issue that will have to be resolved in the near future is that EHRs are not structured to collect information for both inpatient and outpatient variables. Today's information technology challenge is to integrate data from ambulatory/physician office through inpatient hospitalization, postdischarge, and outpatient care. In order for health care organizations to make a profit, patients who can be treated appropriately in the outpatient setting rather than the more expensive acute hospital care setting need to be seen outside the hospital. Therefore, data from ambulatory centers and rehabilitation services, as well as from nursing homes, must be integrated into a single care episode database. If the organization guarantees a certain outcome for a certain procedure, such as hip replacement surgery, for example, and payers pay for that procedure and outcome, which is the bundled payment model, the organization needs to monitor and measure how care is delivered.

Using Data to Understand Appropriateness of Care

Data are collected to ensure appropriateness of services and resources, as well as for comparative analysis of care practices, improvement prioritization, performance evaluation, and analysis. Understanding hospital mortality can be an integral component of evaluating the quality of care delivered by the health care organization (Lau and Litman 2011). The IHI and other organizations have focused attention on analyzing mortality in order to identify gaps in care and institute improvements. The CMS has been publicly reporting data on 30-day mortality rates (deaths that occurred within 30 days of a hospital admission) for specific conditions, such as acute myocardial infarction, heart failure, and pneumonia, since 2008. The reported measures have expanded to include other conditions and in-hospital mortality. Understanding mortality, according to the CMS, can assist hospitals in improving quality and safety (https://www .medicare.gov/hospitalcompare/Data/30-day-measures.html).

Case Example: Analyzing Mortality

Leaders at the system at which we work wanted a better understanding of which patients were dying in the hospitals and why. When quality management attempted to gather data about mortality, it was evident that few tools were available to do so. To help data collection efforts, a standardized process was developed so that each death in the multihospital system would be reviewed in the same way and in real time (within a month of death).

A team of trained nurses reviewed the medical chart of each mortality and entered information into a central database from which summary reports could be made (see Figure 7.2). If the nurses thought a further review of the death was required, the medical chart was sent to the hospital site for physician review, a second-level site review.

Figure 7.2 shows that the morality surveillance report encodes a great deal of information: monthly mortality rate for all hospitals over time; of the individual records that were reviewed, how many were referred for more detailed site-specific review; and the specific diagnosis of the patients under review. Other information was identified for patients who died: age, diagnosis, from where they were admitted (nursing facility, home, etc.). Readmissions

FIGURE 7.2. MORTALITY SURVEILLANCE TOOL SUMMARY REPORT

June 2013 – September 2014

Monthly Hospital Mortalities and Raw Mortality Rate from Hospital Billing System

Note: Excludes Hospice cases. Data through date range of current hospital billing data.

Source: Hospital Billing Data	Totals	Jun13	Jul13	Aug13	Sep13	Oct13	Nov13	Dec13	Jan14	Feb14	Mar14	Apr14	May14	Jun14	Jul14	Aug14	Sep14
All Hospital Mortalities																	
Raw Mortality Rate (%)																	

Mortality Review Tool Totals

	Totals	Jun13	Jul13	Aug13	Sep13	Oct13	Nov13	Dec13	Jan14	Feb14	Mar14	Apr14	May14	Jun14	Jul14	Aug14	Sep14
Records Reviewed																	
Referrals for Site Review																	

Distribution of Age, Top 10 ICD-9 Diagnoses and Admit Source Percentages (Jun-13 to Sep-14)

Source: Hospital Billing Data	N= (Records Reviewed)	Age Range %	N= (Records Reviewed)	Admit Source %
Top 10 Primary ICD9 DC Diagnoses				
0389: Septicemia NOS		18 to 49	Home	
51881: Acute respiratory failure		50 to 59	Other	
486: Pneumonia, organism NOS		60 to 69	Rehab	
41071: Subendo infarct, initial		70 to 79	SNF	
431: Intracerebral hemorrhage		80 to 89	Transfer	
43491: Crbl art ocl NOS w infrc		90 and Above	Unspecified	
5070: Food/vomit pneumonitis				
42823: Ac on chr syst hrt fail				
4280: CHF NOS				
5849: Acute kidney failure NOS				

Note: Top 10 Primary DX data is available through date range of current hospital billing data.

Note: Percents may not total to 100.00% due to rounding.

Admissions Related to Previous Admission

N= (Records Reviewed)	Total
Numerator (Total Related to Previous Admission)	
Denominator (Total Records Reviewed)	
Rate (%)	

Note: Numerator includes any 'Yes' marked under "Is this admission related to the previous admission?"

Deaths within 24 Hours of Admission

Jun-13 - Sep-14

N= (Records Reviewed)	Total
Numerator (Total Expired w/ in 24 hrs of Admission)	
Denominator (Total Records Reviewed)	
Rate (%)	

24 Hour, 7 and 30 Day Readmissions

Jun-13 - Sep-14	Total
24 Hours (#)	
7 Days (#)	
30 Days (#)	

N= (Records Reviewed)

Note: 24 hour readmission does not imply 7 and 30 day readmission. 7 day readmission does not imply 30 day readmission.

Skilled Nursing Subset

	Deaths within 24 hrs of Admission with Admit Source: SNF
Total #	

N= Deaths within 24 Hours of Admission

for related conditions were also counted and displayed, as were deaths that occurred within 24 hours of admission. The wealth of standardized information enabled leaders to understand the population who died and ask data-driven questions. By reviewing these reports, leaders can initiate improvements.

Analyzing End-of-Life Care

The intensive care units (ICUs) are among the most expensive in a hospital because they require vast financial, technical, and human resources. Many hospitalized patients die in ICUs because those units are where severely compromised patients generally are placed. However, although patients may be at the end of their lives—as, for example, elderly, chronically ill patients whose diseases have progressed regardless of treatment—they do not necessarily require the sophisticated interventions and technology typical of an ICU. In fact, end-of-life care is among the concerns of health care reform because our hospitals often do not treat people who are dying efficiently and humanely.

Health care organizations have attempted to better understand ICU utilization by using data to analyze appropriateness of ICU care. End of life is not solely a medical issue; social and psychological issues also require rethinking. Often families encourage physicians to place their desperately ill loved ones into the highest level of care, even though that level may not be best for caring for that patient. Therefore, social workers, geriatricians, and others need to develop skills to help family members understand alternative end-of-life care decisions. Many physicians also are not easily persuaded to allow end-of-life patients to die peacefully without useless and expensive interventions, and they too may require reeducation to ensure that their patients receive appropriate care.

Case Example: Understanding Mortality

The health system in which we work investigated mortality using data of patients admitted to the ICU and patients who were admitted for comfort care within the first 24 hours of hospital admission. Mortality had to have occurred any time within that particular hospital admission. Cross-tabulation, a tool developed by the IHI, showed four distinct populations.

COMFORT CARE

Comfort care is care given to maximize patient comfort and relieve suffering at the end of life. It does not seek to aggressively treat or cure a terminal illness, recognizing that death is a natural ending to a disease process. The focus of comfort care is quite different from ICU care; whereas comfort care is palliative and nonaggressive, ICU care uses every means possible to treat or cure illness.

In this initiative, analysts (most often trained nurses) conducted a **retrospective review** (looking back at the patient's care) of the charts of all patients who died. Patients were categorized by where they were admitted:

1. ICU care for comfort care only
2. Non-ICU (such as a medical unit) for comfort care
3. ICU for active treatment
4. Non-ICU for active treatment

It is important to note that preventing mortality is not a realistic goal for patients placed on comfort care. Therefore, those patients placed in ICU care for comfort care (1) have not been appropriately placed. The analysis suggests that those patients who died who were not admitted to an ICU for treatment (4) might have been misplaced. If their conditions were serious enough to result in death, what were the reasons that prevented them from being placed in ICU care? Were their conditions not recognized, or was there a failure to rescue when the patient's condition became critical?

Analyses such as these can generate important insights into the care of seriously ill patients who died. Patients who were admitted for comfort care only do not belong in an ICU, which is designed for active and complex treatment. Therefore, this expensive resource is being used inappropriately for these patients. Patients who were not in the ICU and admitted for comfort care only may have been better served in hospice care. Patients who were admitted for active ICU treatment and non–comfort care were not expected to die; therefore, there may be opportunities for improvement, either in the ICU care itself or in the treatment plan or communication. Those patients admitted without either ICU or comfort care were not expected to die; yet they did. Further analysis might expose reasons for their possibly preventable deaths.

Armed with this objective information, quality management is able to tell clinical leaders about the effectiveness and efficiency of care delivery. Each hospital in the system gets its own report, and system leaders receive a system-level analysis. The goal is not only to reduce mortality, a worthy enough goal for sure, but to change the culture, to educate the medical staff about their role in providing treatment and in the process of care. The categories involved in the standardized mortality collection tool and the ICU effective utilization analysis have helped health care providers to better serve their patients and to utilize resources more effectively and efficiently.

Future plans are to investigate a correlation between this analysis and the APACHE (see Chapter 5) score given to ICU patients to better quantify which patients should be in an ICU and which patients would be better served on another type of service. In the future, this combined data analysis could be used to generate palliative care consultations in real time.

The Value of Aggregated Data in Performance Improvement

Data reports are valuable for administrators so that they can ask the right questions of the right professionals. Quality reports and analyses provide the administrator with a platform from which to ask why a certain outcome is below the benchmark or what intervention has been developed by a discipline or service to reduce such quality and safety variables as mortality, sepsis, readmissions, or others. Data reveal when an entire program or service is in trouble and improvements need to be implemented.

Case Example: Improving Transplant Mortality

The transplant program at a local hospital provides an example of how introducing data analytics helped to change physician practice there and to educate clinicians to rely on data. The CMS had put the program on notice that unless improvements were made in mortality rates, Medicare reimbursements were at risk. Not only was patient safety a critical issue, but the financial implications of closing a transplant program are enormous.

The first step was to investigate what issues might be contributing to the high mortality rate and to uncover gaps in care for improvement efforts. When administrative leaders expressed their concern to physicians, the physicians responded by asserting that the mortality rates were artificially high because their denominator was so small. In other words, the doctors claimed that their high rate was due to having few patients. Obviously, if the program has four patients who undergo transplants, and two of the four have to be operated on again or have serious complications, the complication rate is 50 percent. If the program has 100 patients and two have complications, the complication rate is 2 percent. But the doctors were misinterpreting the data. The risk-adjusted methodology that was used to determine complication rates and calculate mortality took denominator size into account. Therefore, a more productive response would be to examine the management of care for the transplant patient before, during, and after surgery and to locate vulnerabilities in safety.

In order to analyze what was going wrong, it was important to understand the clinical profile of the patient population. A standardized web-based tool was developed through a collaboration between quality management and residents and fellows that encoded information about all transplant patients.

Figure 7.3 shows an example of the data collected on the input screen for a kidney transplant patient. (Liver and cardiac transplant procedures have input data screens appropriate to their patients.) Demographic and clinical details are entered in a standardized way so that data can be collected, aggregated, and reported. Fellows were trained to enter data on process and outcome variables. Using the data from this web tool, information was accumulated about this patient population in the aggregate for the first time.

FIGURE 7.3. KIDNEY TRANSPLANT DATA INPUT

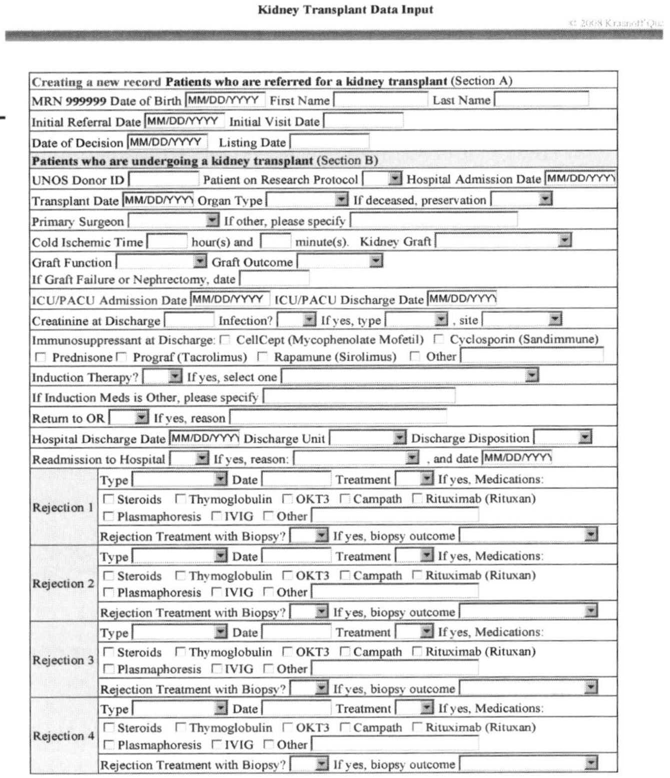

Kidney Transplant Data Input

Creating a new record **Patients who are referred for a kidney transplant** (Section A)
MRN **999999** Date of Birth MM/DD/YYYY First Name Last Name
Initial Referral Date MM/DD/YYYY Initial Visit Date
Date of Decision MM/DD/YYYY Listing Date
Patients who are undergoing a kidney transplant (Section B)
UNOS Donor ID Patient on Research Protocol Hospital Admission Date MM/DD/YYYY
Transplant Date MM/DD/YYYY Organ Type If deceased, preservation
Primary Surgeon If other, please specify
Cold Ischemic Time hour(s) and minute(s). Kidney Graft
Graft Function Graft Outcome
If Graft Failure or Nephrectomy, date
ICU/PACU Admission Date MM/DD/YYYY ICU/PACU Discharge Date MM/DD/YYYY
Creatinine at Discharge Infection? If yes, type , site
Immunosuppressant at Discharge: CellCept (Mycophenolate Mofetil) Cyclosporin (Sandimmune) Prednisone Prograf (Tacrolimus) Rapamune (Sirolimus) Other
Induction Therapy? If yes, select one
If Induction Meds is Other, please specify
Return to OR If yes, reason
Hospital Discharge Date MM/DD/YYYY Discharge Unit Discharge Disposition
Readmission to Hospital If yes, reason: , and date MM/DD/YYYY

Rejection 1	Type Date Treatment If yes, Medications:
	Steroids Thymoglobulin OKT3 Campath Rituximab (Rituxan) Plasmaphoresis IVIG Other
	Rejection Treatment with Biopsy? If yes, biopsy outcome
Rejection 2	Type Date Treatment If yes, Medications:
	Steroids Thymoglobulin OKT3 Campath Rituximab (Rituxan) Plasmaphoresis IVIG Other
	Rejection Treatment with Biopsy? If yes, biopsy outcome
Rejection 3	Type Date Treatment If yes, Medications:
	Steroids Thymoglobulin OKT3 Campath Rituximab (Rituxan) Plasmaphoresis IVIG Other
	Rejection Treatment with Biopsy? If yes, biopsy outcome
Rejection 4	Type Date Treatment If yes, Medications:
	Steroids Thymoglobulin OKT3 Campath Rituximab (Rituxan) Plasmaphoresis IVIG Other
	Rejection Treatment with Biopsy? If yes, biopsy outcome

Data Collection Elements:

1. Identifiers
2. Select demographics
3. Process variables
4. Outcome variables

Table 7.1 shows the measurements (with numerator and denominator) that were extracted from the web tool and reported to leaders. With this information, leaders can track the volume of transplants, the average length of stay, the number of patients who were readmitted to the ICU, as well as complications, adverse reactions, survival, and other data. Before the creation of this database, each case was evaluated individually, and leaders had no data that would help find commonalities in the population; therefore, no processes could be developed to improve care.

Often aggregated data reveal information that would be impossible to uncover with individual analysis. For example, analysis of the liver transplant data revealed that 82 percent of patients did not have an infection after the transplants (see Figure 7.4); but the chart reveals that 18 percent of transplant patients did have infection, a number that leaders should be aware of.

Aggregated data also revealed that the patients with the highest rate of complications were patients of one senior surgeon. This surgeon took on very

TABLE 7.1. KIDNEY TRANSPLANT TABLE OF MEASURES

	Numerator	Denominator
Total # of Transplants		
Hospital ALOS (Average Length of Stay)	Hospital LOS	Total # Transplants
ICU Readmission Rate	# ICU Readmissions	Total # Transplants
Pretransplant Nutrition Consults Rate	# Pretransplant Nutrition Consults	Total # Transplants
Unplanned OR Returns (excluding retransplant) Rate	# Unplanned OR Returns	Total # Transplants
Retransplant Rate	# Retransplants	Total # Transplants
Adverse Drug Reaction Rate	# Adverse Drug Reactions	Total # Transplants
Ventilator-Associated Pneumonia Index	# Ventilator-Associated Pneumonias	# Ventilator Days in ICU
Line-Related Bacteremias Index	# Line-Related Bacteremias	# Line Days in ICU
Other Nosocomial Infections Rate	# Other Nosocomial Infections	Total # Transplants
Organ Rejection Rate	# Organ Rejections	Total # Transplants
Hospital Readmission Rate	# Hospital Readmissions	Total # Transplants
Survival Rate	# Alive Patients (disposition <> 20)	Total # Transplants
New-Onset Diabetes	# of Patients Identified with New-Onset Diabetes	Total # Transplants

FIGURE 7.4. WOUND INFECTION RATE

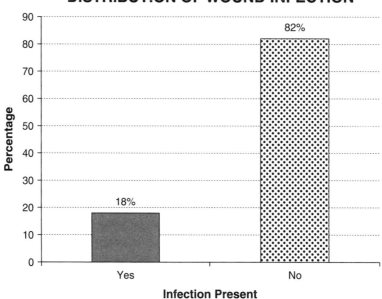

DISTRIBUTION OF WOUND INFECTION

high-risk patients, and these patients were not treated any differently from other, less high-risk patients. Once this information was revealed, different protocols were established for high-risk and low-risk patients. Also, intensivists were put in charge of high-risk patients. These changes led to a reduced complication rate.

To further improve care, checklists were instituted, based on CMS criteria. Standardized processes were developed for appropriate patient evaluation, for preparing patients for surgery, and for postoperative care. A quality council was formed with the responsibility to review the information in the database and ensure that care was efficient and effective. These and other improvements, based on data collection and analysis, caused the mortality rate to decrease and also educated physicians about the value of using aggregated data to analyze and improve the delivery of care. The transplant program has met all CMS standards and is now financially stable.

The Role of Data in Managing Chronic Disease

According to the Centers for Disease Control and Prevention:

> As a nation, we spend 86% of our health care dollars on the treatment of chronic diseases. These persistent conditions—the nation's leading causes of death and disability—leave in their wake deaths that could have been prevented, lifelong disability, compromised quality of life, and burgeoning health care costs. (http://www.cdc.gov/chronicdisease)

For these reasons, improving the care of patients with chronic disease has become a focus of health care reform. As concern about the management of chronic diseases mounts, new approaches are being developed and evaluated.

Health care professionals need to understand not only the care of hospitalized patients but also how care is delivered in the community, nursing homes, and physician offices. They also have to identify what barriers exist to better management and what interventions will be successful. Health care administrators need to understand how various interventions interact along the continuum of care and what can be done to improve care and lower readmissions. They need to analyze available information to better understand the patient population and outcomes. They need to know where to invest resources. Administrators need to work with clinicians and quality management personnel to develop better processes, such as a better discharge process or improved follow-up care after hospitalization. To do so, data analytics are necessary to establish metrics for evaluating, monitoring, and improving care.

Understanding Readmission

One of the metrics that can be useful in understanding chronic disease is readmission to the hospital within 30 days. If a patient with chronic disease has to be readmitted to the hospital within 30 days of discharge, the readmission might signal a flaw in the care of that patient. Perhaps the care was not adequate during the first admission, the patient was discharged prematurely, or the discharge instructions were inadequate or poorly understood. Not only is readmission a red flag about care, but the CMS penalizes hospitals financially for unplanned readmissions of patients with chronic diseases. Therefore, for patient safety and for organizational and financial reasons, monitoring readmission makes good sense. According to the Agency for Healthcare Research and Quality (AHRQ), "measuring readmission will create incentives to invest in interventions to improve hospital care, better assess the readiness of patients for discharge, and facilitate transitions to outpatient status" (http://www .qualitymeasures.ahrq.gov/content.aspx?id=49196).

Case Example: Heart Failure Readmissions

Heart failure (HF) or congestive heart failure is a progressively deteriorating condition where the weakened heart muscle has trouble pumping blood. The goal of HF treatment is to manage the condition with medicine, such as diuretics, and with lifestyle changes, such as diet, exercise, and weight control so that the condition does not deteriorate. HF can be managed at home unless there is a crisis, such as the onset of chest pain. When there is a crisis, most patients are admitted to a hospital for treatment. If they are treated appropriately and released with effective discharge instructions and follow-up care instructions, they should not be readmitted within 30 days. However, it is to be expected that patients who have chronic deteriorating conditions will return to the hospital in crisis multiple times.

Under the bundled payment model, in order to avoid penalties, early and accurate identification of HF is essential so that an appropriate plan of care can be developed that would avoid penalties. An analyst has to verify that the patient with a HF diagnosis matches the information on the medical record and determine whether the admission was within 30 days of a previous discharge. Once that identification has been made and information about the patient has been gathered, quality management collects, analyzes, and reports data so that leaders can better understand the care management of this patient population. When leaders of the health care system in which we work prioritized an investigation into the causes of readmission of HF patients, quality management used EHRs to collect information on admission date, discharge date, and diagnosis.

In order to know how to evaluate and how to allocate and prioritize resources, it is important to understand the scope of the problem. Figure 7.5 displays information that shows that over a two-year period, the readmission rate for the system remained around 20 percent, which is below the national average (Ross et al. 2010). The goal, of course, is for this number to be reduced.

Since HF is a progressive disease, it is not surprising that many patients who are readmitted are elderly. Figure 7.6 shows that for the same two-year

FIGURE 7.5. 30-DAY OBSERVED READMISSION RATE FOR HEART FAILURE ANALYSIS

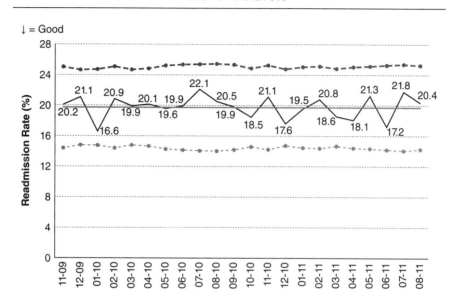

FIGURE 7.6. HEART FAILURE READMISSIONS BY AGE

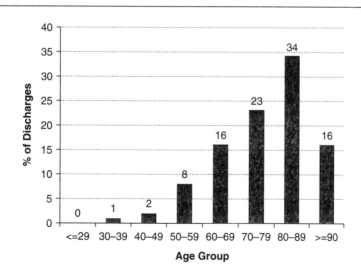

period, more than half the readmissions were of patients between 70 and 90 years old. Although this information does not seem remarkable, having data to support suppositions helps to objectify personal observations.

Data tracked where readmitted patients came from, whether from home, a skilled nursing facility, rehabilitation, or somewhere else. Data reported in Figure 7.7 show that over 70 percent of the patients who were readmitted came from home care, which is care that is monitored by RNs or other professionals, or from home, where the patient has no external services or self-care, where the patient has been instructed to follow specific care protocols.

This information may indicate that HF patients who were discharged to home might not have complied with their discharge instructions, such as to reduce their salt intake, or perhaps they did not receive adequate education while hospitalized about how to manage at home, such as instructions to call the doctor for weight gain, or perhaps they were not given adequate discharge

FIGURE 7.7. HEART FAILURE READMISSION ANALYSIS: HF DISCHARGES BY DISCHARGE DISPOSITION

	HF Discharges	%
TOTAL	**12,188**	**100%**
Home Care	4,396	36%
Home or Self-Care	4,354	35%
Skilled Nursing Facility	2,298	18%
Another Hospital	493	4%
Hospice—Home	184	1%
Left Against Medical Advice	152	1%
Hospice—Medical Facility	114	0%
Intermediate-Care Facility	58	0%
Unknown	56	0%
Rehabilitation Services	37	0%
Other Inpatient	35	0%
Psychiatric Hospital	9	0%
	1	0%
Federal Hospital	1	0%

Note: 0% indicates percentages <1%.

instructions. Therefore, their disease progressed, and they had to be readmitted to the hospital.

If improvements could be made for this population, it would significantly reduce the readmission rate. One improvement was to develop a standardized process for trained professionals to make follow-up calls to recently discharged HF patients and ask probing questions about physical and functional status. If the professional is alerted to a problem, such as weight gain, or medication issues, he or she can suggest solutions and follow-up before there is a crisis that requires hospitalization.

Another improvement involved educating HF patients about their follow-up care. Based on data reports, a tool was developed to help patients monitor whether to contact a doctor and what to look for as symptoms of the progression of the condition (see Figure 7.8).

The different zones (green, yellow, red) indicate all clear, caution, and medical alert, and explain both what patients should look for and what they should do. For example, if a patient notices swelling of the feet or legs (yellow/caution), he or she should contact a physician or nurse, who may

FIGURE 7.8. KNOW YOUR HEART FAILURE ZONES

Green Zone: All Clear	Green Zone Means:
You have:	Your symptoms are under control
o No new or worsening shortness of breath	o Continue taking your medications as ordered
o No new or worsening swelling of your feet or legs	o Continue daily weight
o No weight gain Goal Weight:	o Follow low-salt diet
o No chest pain or tightness	o Keep all physician appointments
o No decrease in your ability to maintain your activity level	
Yellow Zone: Caution	**Yellow Zone Means:**
CAUTION: CONTACT YOUR DOCTOR OR HOME HEALTH CARE NURSE	Your symptoms may mean you need an adjustment of your medications
o Weight gain of 2 or more pounds in one day OR a gain of 3 or more pounds in one week	CALL YOUR PHYSICIAN OR HOME HEALTH CARE NURSE.
o Increased swelling of feet or legs	Doctor:_____
o Increase in shortness of breath with activity	Phone #:_____
o Increase in number of pillows needed to sleep at night	Nurse:_____
o New or more frequent chest pain or tightness	Phone #:_____
o New onset of dizziness or lightheadedness after standing up	(Please notify your home health nurse if you call or visit your doctor)
Red Zone: Medical Alert	**Red Zone Means:**
MEDICAL ALERT: CONTACT YOUR DOCTOR OR HOME HEALTH CARE NURSE	**You may need to be evaluated by a doctor right away**
o **Unrelieved shortness of breath: shortness of breath at rest**	****Call your doctor right away**
o **Unrelieved chest pain**	**Doctor:_____**
o **Wheezing or chest tightness at rest**	**Phone #:_____**
o **Need to sit in chair to sleep**	**(Please notify your home health nurse if you visit the emergency room or are hospitalized.)**
o **Confusion**	
o **A fall related to dizziness or lightheadedness**	

modify the medication and thus control a potentially serious situation before it escalates. However, if a patient experiences unrelieved chest pain or dizziness or confusion (red/medical alert), he or she should get to a physician right away. Delays could cause harm. With these instructions explicitly articulated, elderly people can better manage their condition at home and thus avoid unnecessary readmissions.

In addition to the patients who are readmitted from home, data show that many patients are readmitted from skilled nursing facilities. To improve this situation, quality management and physician leaders met with nursing homes CEOs to educate them about care and establish what criteria should be used to define an acute incident from one that could be handled without hospitalization.

The reports generated from the data collected and analyzed by quality management enabled improvements to be made in the care of the chronically ill patient and a more sophisticated understanding of the causes of readmission.

Using Data to Monitor Variability

One of the primary goals of health care managers is to improve the quality of care and outcomes for groups of patients—that is, patient populations—and one of the techniques they use to do this is to monitor variation, especially unintended, even harmful variation from the recognized standard of care. Health care managers are expected to monitor performance over time and ensure that if gaps in care are identified, improvements are implemented and evaluated.

Reducing variation to create a stable process can lead to improved clinical outcomes and better organizational efficiency (Berwick 1991). Of course there must be a balance between the evidence that may be effective for a population of patients and specific patient/physician decisions about what is best for the individual. And the strength of the evidence has to be weighed as well in determining whether to follow guidelines or not. Nonetheless, recognizing variation and analyzing it is often very useful.

Control Chart

A quality tool designed to monitor variation and stability is the control chart. Variation in any process is to be expected, as normal or the result of chance. Statisticians graph variation in the shape of a bell curve, with most data points occurring 2 or 3 standard deviations (SD) away from the mean (the average or central value of all the data points). If you turn a bell curve on its side, you can establish the upper and lower control limits of a control chart. If you want a process to be in tight control, more stable, you can use 1 SD from the mean in a control chart.

CONTROL CHART

A *control chart* is a quality tool that was developed in the 1920s by quality theorist William Shewhart (see Chapter 1) to monitor variation from standards in industry. Control charts are used to monitor variation from acceptable norms. Once a norm is established, a control chart can be used to monitor whether there is excessive or unacceptable deviation from the defined standard of care.

A control chart plots performance over time, with upper and lower limits that define statistical control (i.e., allowing for normal variation in a process). If several points fall outside the limits, then the process is not in control and should be investigated. Control charts help users discover whether variations are due to common or special causes. Control charts use SDs to determine variation from the mean. Every process contains some normal variation. However, extremes of variation might signal that an investigation into the process should be conducted.

Statistical significance means that the variation is more than the normal and expected variation that exists in any process. Normal variation is the product of chance, or something random, said to be of common cause. Statistical analysis is necessary to determine whether variation in a process is significant. Statistical analysis uses mathematics to determine whether the variation is based on chance or is significant, said to be of special cause.

In statistical process control, the variation in a process is categorized as either common (general) cause variation or special (assignable) cause variation. The **common cause variation** arises from a multitude of small factors that invariably affect any process and will conform to a normal distribution (a bell-shaped curve when graphed) or a distribution that is closely related to the normal distribution. The **special cause variation** arises from specific factors that have an identifiable effect on the process. Common cause variation is inherent in the process and can be reduced only by changes to the system. Special causes often can be tracked down and fixed without extensive changes to the system.

Special cause variation is created by a nonrandom event leading to an unexpected change in the process output. The effects are intermittent and unpredictable. If special causes of variation are present, the process output is not stable over time and is not predictable. All processes must be brought into statistical control by first detecting and removing the special cause variation.

There are four rules for identifying special cause variation:

Rule 1: There is a single data point beyond the 3 SD upper or lower control limit

Rule 2: Data show a run of 8 points above or below the mean

Rule 3: Data show 2 out of 3 consecutive points beyond the 2 SD upper or lower warning limit

Rule 4: There is a run of 6+ points ascending or descending

Figure 7.9 shows a control chart that tracks the rates of *Clostridium difficile* (a serious intestinal infection) over time. Because 3 SDs is thought to indicate that the process is in control, the dotted lines mark the upper and lower levels of control. Points of data that fall outside of those lines, such as April 2007, show a spike in infection that may require investigation. Other months (August 2006, January 2007, June 2007) are above the acceptable upper limit, indicating that the process is out of the desired control limits.

Variation could signal some problem with the infection control process or a problem with data collection. Only further investigation clarifies the issue. Variation below the control limits should also be investigated. Remember that one data point can be above or below the control limit as a result of chance variation; if three or more data points are out of control, the cause of the variation in the process should be investigated.

When the control chart reveals that a process requires improvement, those improvements can be instituted with a Plan-Do-Study-Act or other quality methodology. Control charts should be presented to leaders regularly, every month so that opportunities for improvement or gaps in care are recognized in a timely way and corrected.

Variance Analysis

Variance analysis can also show that a process is not meeting the goal of an established benchmark. If the variation from a benchmark indicates poor outcomes, then leaders can look for processes that might give better results. Once a new process is implemented, the control chart will display whether improvements have resulted from the intervention. For example, if mortality is high, and higher than the benchmark, it could be for a number of reasons. Mortality could be coded differently by different coders (were hospice patients included?), which might provoke an inter-rater reliability study and educational programs. Or perhaps high-risk patients account for the high mortality. If so, perhaps the processes for high-risk populations should be examined. Until you know what to look for, you do not know what to fix.

Variability can also be usefully examined in relation to cost of services. A control chart can be used to assess cost efficiency related to some established standard. If it looks as if a process is inefficient and the costs are excessive, investigation as to causes can yield improvements.

The **Dartmouth Atlas** (http://www.dartmouthatlas.org/) has published a great deal of evidence of variability as to the cost of care around the country. Variation in costs across the country has led Congress to push for increased transparency for costs of care. Information regarding variations in costs for common procedures has alerted consumers that they should do some comparison shopping before committing their health care dollars to one hospital over another. For example, in Massachusetts a magnetic

FIGURE 7.9. CONTROL CHART OF *CLOSTRIDIUM DIFFICILE*

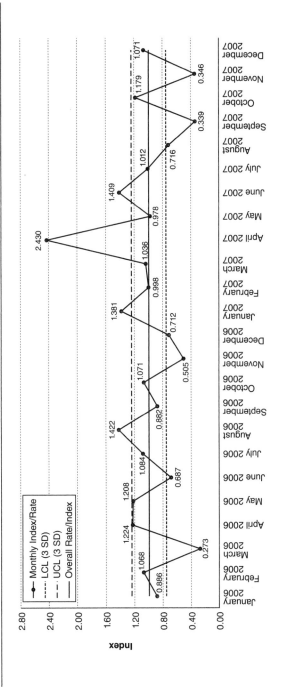

resonance imaging (MRI) test costs $382 in one Massachusetts hospital and $8, in another (http://www.masslive.com/news/index.ssf/2015/06/price _shopping_cost_of_mri_at_area_hospitals_report_finds_persistence_needed .html).

Many other states show similar cost variation. An article by Meier, McGinty, and Creswell (2013) published in *The New York Times* was titled "Hospital Billing Varies Wildly, Government Data Shows." The article cited huge differences in costs for identical procedures not only across the country but within the same geographical region.

Publicly Reported Data

To encourage greater transparency and to motivate improvements in efficien-cies and outcomes (such as pay for performance, bundled payments), the government has not only demanded that health care organizations collect data on specified variables in order to receive Medicare reimbursement; it also has published the results of the data on their website for consumers of health care to compare and evaluate organizations.

Hospital Compare

The website http://www.medicare.gov/hospitalcompare/search.html offers a wealth of highly specific information about the delivery of care offered in a par-ticular hospital. Once you specify a hospital, the site offers information about patient experiences, taken from the Hospital Consumer Assessment of Health-care Providers and Systems (HCAHPS) survey, about timely and effective care, readmissions and complications, use of medical imaging, and other informa-tion. In this way consumers really can make considered choices about which hospital will provide them with the best service.

Figure 7.10 shows several indicators (of many) related to inpatient surgi-cal infection prevention for an acute care teaching hospital. The report shows the percentile over time for specific evidence-based indicators, such as timely catheter removal postsurgery and temperature management. The figure shows the hospital score compared to the national average and also the COTH hos-pitals (members of the Council of Teaching Hospitals and Health Systems).

In addition to a numerical average, median, 75th percentile, and 90th percentile, the scores show the ratings. The web report was adapted to include emoticon faces. A smiley face indicates that the score is greater than or equal to the 75th percentile (which means that 25 percent do better on that indicator); a neutral face means that the score is greater than or equal to the median score; and a frowning face shows that the score is less than the median (indicating that the score is at the 50th percentile or lower than

FIGURE 7.10. HOSPITAL COMPARE BENCHMARK REPORT: INPATIENT CLINICAL MEASURES—INPATIENT SURGICAL INFECTION PREVENTION

1. Surgical Patients Whose Doctor Ordered Prophylaxis for Venous Thromboembolism (VTE)

Your Scores Over Time				Summary Discharge Data for Oct 11 – Sep 12					
				Average	Median	75th Percentile	90th Percentile	Your Score	Rating*
99	99	99	National	96.7	99.0	100.0	100.0	99.0	☺
Apr 11 – Mar 12	Jul 11 – Jun 12	Oct 11 – Sep 12	COTH Hospitals	98.9	99.0	100.0	100.0	99.0	☺

2. Surgical Patients Whose Received Venous Thromboembolism (VTE) Prophylaxis

Your Scores Over Time					Summary Discharge Data for Apr 12 – Mar 13					
					Average	Median	75th Percentile	90th Percentile	Your Score	Rating*
99	99	99	99	National	96.6	98.0	99.0	100.0	99.0	☺
Apr 11 – Mar 12	Jul 11 – Jun 12	Oct 11 – Sep 12	Apr 12 – Mar 13	COTH Hospitals	98.4	99.0	99.0	100.0	99.0	☺

3. Surgery Patients Whose Urinary Catheters Are Removed within 48 Hours After Surgery

Your Scores Over Time					Summary Discharge Data for Apr 12 – Mar 13					
					Average	Median	75th Percentile	90th Percentile	Your Score	Rating*
91	90	91	93	National	95.4	98.0	99.0	100.0	93.0	☹
Apr 11 – Mar 12	Jul 11 – Jun 12	Oct 11 – Sep 12	Apr 12 – Mar 13	COTH Hospitals	96.4	97.0	99.0	100.0	93.0	☹

4. Surgery Patients Who Are Under Perioperative Temperature Management After Surgery

Your Scores Over Time					Summary Discharge Data for Apr 12 – Mar 13					
					Average	Median	75th Percentile	90th Percentile	Your Score	Rating*
100	100	100	100	National	99.5	100.0	100.0	100.0	100.0	☺
Apr 11 – Mar 12	Jul 11 – Jun 12	Oct 11 – Sep 12	Apr 12 – Mar 13	COTH Hospitals	99.7	100.0	100.0	100.0	100.0	☺

*AAMC-Assigned Ratings: ☺ = greater than or equal to the 75th percentile;   ☹ = less than the median.

☺ = greater than or equal to the median, less than 75th percentile;

Inpatient Clinical Measures Notes:

National rates differ from those reported on Hospital Compare web site. Hospital Compare reports average case rates, while this report shows hospital-level rates.

Adapted from AAMC Analysis of HHS Hospital Compare Database—December 2013

comparable hospitals). Leaders can see at a glance that improvements should focus on "surgery patients whose urinary catheter are removed within 48 hours after surgery" because the score is below the national average and that compliance with temperature management is excellent.

Other indicators reveal other kinds of information. For example, a consumer can search any hospital and target the question: "Patients who reported that their room and bathroom were 'Always Clean.'" Say a search reveals that patients agreed with this statement only 56 percent of the time; why would consumers want to go to a hospital where the bathrooms are reported as not clean half the time?

Another tab on the **Hospital Compare** site indicates "timely and efficient care," which shows how often the specific hospital provides care that research shows leads to best outcomes for specific conditions (see Figure 7.11). Measures of heart attack care, for example, show that this hospital provides good care. For the variable "Average number of minutes before outpatients with chest pain or possible heart attack got an ECG (electrocardiogram),"

FIGURE 7.11. TIMELY HEART ATTACK CARE

Medicare.gov | Hospital Compare
The Official U.S. Government Site for Medicare

TIMELY HEART ATTACK CARE	ACUTE CARE HOSPITAL A	NEW YORK AVERAGE	NATIONAL AVERAGE
Average number of minutes before outpatients with chest pain or possible heart attack who needed specialized care were transferred to another hospital *A **lower** number of minutes is better*	74 minutes	75 minutes	59 minutes
Average number of minutes before outpatients with chest pain or possible heart attack got an ECG *A **lower** number of minutes is better*	6 minutes	9 minutes	7 minutes
Outpatients with chest pain or possible heart attack who got drugs to break up blood clots within 30 minutes of arrival ***Higher** percentages are better*	54%	54%	59%
Outpatients with chest pain or possible heart attack who got aspirin within 24 hours of arrival ***Higher** percentages are better*	97%	97%	96%
Heart attack patients who got drugs to break up blood clots within 30 minutes of arrival ***Higher** percentages are better*	49%	47%	55%
Heart attack patients given PCI within 90 minutes of arrival ***Higher** percentages are better*	96%	95%	96%
Heart attack patients given aspirin at discharge ***Higher** percentages are better*	95%	99%	99%
Heart attack patients given a prescription for a statin at discharge ***Higher** percentages are better*	91%	98%	98%

the lower the number of minutes, the better. Hospital A provides the ECG at 6 minutes, with the state average at 9 and the national average at 7. That is useful information to potential patients. For another measure of timely and efficient heart attack care, "Outpatients with chest pain or possible heart attack who got aspirin within 24 hours of arrival," where the higher the number, the better, show Hospital A at 97 percent, the state average at 97 percent and the national average at 96 percent

This website provides detailed, specific, and informative data for the public to understand the delivery of care at specific hospitals and compared to regional hospitals. It enables people to see where the delivery of care is superior. All administrators should be watching this website and asking serious questions when the numbers are poor.

Interpreting and Making Use of Data

Administrators take these regulatory and private organization's reports seriously, as does the public. Some health care providers believe there are too many reports available. Certainly the reports generated by the CMS Hospital Compare data are more reliable than those that are generated by political or financial interests. (For example, the Leapfrog Group requires that hospitals purchase licenses to advertise their scores. The *U.S. News & World Report* data are influenced by subscriptions and advertising.) CMS measures reflect a standardized methodology for evaluating health care quality, and they are valid, reliable, and based on evidence. Other reputable report cards, such as The Joint Commission Quality Check or the New York State Department of Health Profile Quality section (http://profiles.health.ny.gov/hospital/) are based on clinical rather than administrative data and are relatively current. The CMS and the AHRQ use risk-adjusted data to score their rates, which is important for fair comparisons.

Administrative Concerns

With so many reports out there, and with some more reliable and valid than others, it is easy to see why so many administrative leaders can become overwhelmed. It is certainly quicker and easier to reject unflattering reports as based on bad or inappropriate data than to respond with analysis and performance improvement initiatives. Administrators require education so that they understand the value of these reports. They need people who will explain to them the fine points of deciles, percentages, indexes, and benchmarks. Today's administrators have to cope with these reports in meaningful and intelligent fashions, which requires education.

If, for example, the hospital ranks low on "recommend to others," administrators should want to know why. If the rankings are not improving, they should want to know the reason as well. Analysts who drill down the data might see that obstetric patients say they were satisfied and would recommend the hospital but chronic disease patients were not satisfied and would not recommend the hospital. What is the difference in their treatment? What could be instituted to make the experience more positive for chronic disease patients? Most administrators today do not drill down. They do not have the experience or education to ask pertinent questions; nor do they have sophisticated analysts who explain numerators and denominators, percentages and sample sizes, and can explain when to look at the mean, or the median, or the mode, and why.

Future administrators and health professionals will need to use statistics and data for developing strategic plans and making resource allocations. Administrators should dissect the numbers in the reports and ask: Where does the data come from? Who can benefit from change/improvement? How much benefit and at what cost? Under what circumstances do we use the numbers? To create efficiencies and change numbers, outcomes data need to be analyzed and variables need to be identified that can explain the phenomena under investigation.

For example, let's say that turnaround time between appointments in a clinic is poor. How should this problem be addressed? What baselines should be used to measure change? Are all appointments equally time consuming, or are some issues more or less so? In order to improve, these and other questions have to be asked and answered with objective information.

Once databases are established to measure a process or explain an outcome, the analytic team can partner with the performance improvement team to define and assess improvements. Quality teams that deal with the analytics should be part of any Plan-Do-Study-Act or Six Sigma/Lean process improvement. Analysis and explanations should be in the hands of experts who can interpret and report back. These quality teams would be specialty groups to mediate between the performance improvement team and administration. One reason it is so difficult to sustain improvement is because there is no oversight on the process improvement—that is, no analysis of the data; someone actually has to react to the control charts and public reports and interpret them for administrative leaders in order to monitor what improvements are made and sustained.

Data Analytics in the Future

Clinical and business decisions are based on data. New methodologies are being developed to use the wealth of available data effectively. Health care has always used data descriptively, to understand and assess performance;

today, quality management uses data for identifying gaps in care for performance improvement opportunities. Descriptive data used for reports and databases can reveal historical information about performance, compare current performance to benchmarks, and be used to analyze problems, errors, or issues that require further investigation. These data are used for monitoring processes.

Predictive analytics, a new field of data analytics, uses large quantities of (past) data to predict future performance by detecting patterns and projecting into the future through machine learning techniques. It uses data mining techniques, decision trees, neural networks, clustering, and other new computational tools that can identify patterns and trends, determine causality, and answer why one group of patients has better outcomes to a specific treatment intervention than others, for example. With the advent of sophisticated new computer technologies and mathematical models, data are being used to explain performance—that is, to relate input, in the form of treatment and interventions, to outcomes. The future of improvement lies in these new analytic processes.

Big-data analytics is another new development in the evolution of health care data (Raghupathi and Raghupathi 2014). **Big data** refers to large and complex data sets that cannot be managed with traditional tools, not only because of the volume but also because of the diversity of data. Everything related to patient health makes up big data. By using new analytic techniques to discover associations, patterns, and trends within the data, big-data analytics has the potential to improve care, save lives, and lower costs.

Quality Management in the Future

Health care is so complex and complicated and so filled with bureaucracy and hierarchies that there is little capacity for innovation. And for most health organizations, monitoring compliance takes whatever resources are available. For example, databases can be developed to monitor compliance with immunization. But that is a far cry from actually understanding barriers to receiving vaccinations and developing a successful immunization program. A similar situation exists with other processes. For example, if an organization wants to reduce central line infections (infections associated with having a long tube that carries medication or nutrients throughout the body), which are associated with extended length of stay and mortality, a serious analysis of these infections must be accomplished. At this point in the evolution of quality management, we should be able to address why there are high rates of infection and which interventions or improvements are successful, not simply whether an antibiotic was administered or not.

However, with the pressure to comply with measures and with overwhelming cost pressure to trim budgets, quality management is often concerned solely with crisis management, not long-term care improvements. With so many measures to collect and report for payment, there is hardly time to focus on developing an ideology that might be the basis for fundamental changes, creative thinking, and innovative processes. There is little opportunity to look at the big picture, to be proactive, and actually to enact change that might lead to cultural shifts. Understanding complex processes requires time and resources, both of which hospitals have in short supply.

Quality management is itself complex. Prioritization for improvement has to be based on data. And with the many measures developed by the government, organizations have to establish a process, detailing how the data will be collected for each measure, who will collect it, who will review the data for compliance, and what kind or reports, such as control charts, will be shown to leaders for decision making. Also, leaders should know about performance—that is, whether benchmarks are being met, and if not, why not and what is being done to improve. Also, a process has to be developed to care for specific populations: Who will be in charge of oversight, how will improvements be prioritized, who will develop and implement improvements, and what measures will be used to gauge their success? In addition, the process should be evaluated for efficiency, cost, service excellence, and outcomes. It is easy to see why this amount of information is overwhelming. Most organizations are hard-pressed just to monitor compliance with the large number of measures required.

Summary

Working with quality data poses challenges for health care professionals. Among them are:

- ensuring that valid data are the basis of performance improvement decisions;
- understanding issues related to standardizing measurements and monitoring variation;
- educating health professionals to use data to monitor and sustain performance improvements;
- establishing standards for defining appropriate end-of-life care;
- developing improved processes for managing quality for vulnerable populations;
- managing patients with chronic disease effectively and efficiently; and
- using publicly reported measures to improve processes and outcomes.

Key Terms

big data, binary categorical variables, chronic disease, common cause variation, compliance, Dartmouth Atlas, free text narratives, HIPAA, Hospital Compare, predictive analytics, retrospective review, special cause variation, variance analysis

Quality Concepts in Action

Quality professionals who work with data often have to convince clinicians that the data are reliable and an accurate reflection of their care management. Mortality, for example, can be considered a quality variable. It's not meaningful to simply count how many people died over a period of time. What is meaningful is to understand the cause of each death and determine whether appropriate care was delivered. As an administrator of a hospital or health system determined to lower your mortality rate (especially if it is publicly reported as high), would you:

- try to place as many patients as possible in palliative or hospice care because that would lower the rate?
- demand that ICU directors justify each mortality in the ICU?
- honor the wishes of the patient and family in placing the patient in either the ICU or palliative care?
- use data, such as APACHE, to understand acuity levels in the ICU and direct care accordingly, with low-acuity patients on other units?

Argue the pros and cons of each of these alternatives, with special emphasis on using arguments to influence physician behavior.

References

Bergstrom, N., B. J. Braden, A. Laguzza, and V. Holman. 1987. "The Braden Scale for Predicting Pressure Sore Risk." *Nursing Research* 36: 205–210.

Berwick, D. M. 1991. "Controlling Variation in Health Care: A Consultation from Walter Shewhart." *Medical Care* 29 (12): 1212–1225.

Chan, K. S., J. B. Fowles, and J. P. Weiner. 2010. "Review: Electronic Health Records and the Reliability and Validity of Quality Measures: A Review of the Literature." *Medical Care Research & Review* 67: 503–527.

Kern, L., S. Malhotra, Y. Barron, J. Quaresimo, R. Dhopeshwarkar, M. Pichardo, A. Edwards, et al. 2013. "Accuracy of Electronically Reported 'Meaningful Use' Clinical Quality Measures." *Annals of Internal Medicine* 158: 77–83.

Lau, H., and K. C. Litman. 2011. "Saving Lives by Studying Deaths: Using Standardized Mortality Reviews to Improve Inpatient Safety." *Joint Commission Journal on Quality and Patient Safety* 37 (9): 400–408.

Meier, B., J. C. McGinty, and J. Creswell. 2013, May 8. "Hospital Billing Varies Wildly, Government Data Shows." *New York Times.*

Pronovost, P., and B. Sexton. 2005. "Assessing Safety Culture: Guidelines and Recommendations." *Quality and Safety in Health Care* 14(4) : 231-233.

Raghupathi, W., and R. Raghupathi. 2014. "Big Data Analytics in Healthcare: Promise and Potential." *Health Information Science and Systems* 2 (1): 3.

Ross, J. S., J. Chen, Z. Lin, H. Bueno, J. P. Curtis, P. S. Keenan, S. L. Normand, et al. 2010. "Recent National Trends in Readmission Rates after Heart Failure Hospitalization." *Circulation: Heart Failure* 3 (1): 97–103.

Suggestions for Further Reading

Institute for Healthcare Improvement. *Move Your Dot™: Measuring, Evaluating, and Reducing Hospital Mortality Rates (Part 1).* IHI Innovation Series white paper. Boston: Author, 2003.

Lustig, I., B. Dietrich, C. Johnson, and C. Dziekan. 2010. "The Analytics Journey." *Analytics,* pp. 11–18.

Massachusetts Health Care Quality and Cost Council and Massachusetts Division of Health Care Finance and Policy. 2009, November. *Measuring Healthcare Quality and Cost in Massachusetts.* N.P.: Commonwealth of Massachusetts, Division of Health Care Finance and Policy.

Neuhauser, D., L. Provost, and B. Bergman. 2011. "The Meaning of Variation to Healthcare Managers, Clinical and Health Services Researchers and Individual Patients." *BMJ Quality & Safety* 20 (Suppl. 1): i36–i40.

Robbins, W. A., and F. A. Jacobs. 1885. "Cost Variances in Health Care: When Should Managers Investigate?" *Healthcare Financial Management: Journal of the Healthcare Financial Management Association* 39 (9): 36–42.

Sinaiko, A. D., and M. B. Rosenthal. 2011. "Increased Price Transparency in Health Care —Challenges and Potential Effects." *New England Journal of Medicine* 364: 891–894.

Weiner, J. P., J. B. Fowles, and K. S. Chan. 2012. "New Paradigms for Measuring Clinical Performance Using Electronic Health Records." *International Journal for Quality in Health Care* 24 (3): 200–205.

Useful Websites

http://www.cdc.gov/chronicdisease/

https://www.cms.gov/Medicare/Quality-Initiatives-Patient-Assessment-Instruments/PQRS/

http://www.dartmouthatlas.org/

http://www.hhs.gov/hipaa/

http://medicaleconomics.modernmedicine.com/medical-economics/content/tags/
2013-salary-survey/ehr-holdouts-why-some-physicians-refuse-plug?page=full

www.masslive.com/news/index.ssf/2015/06/price_shopping_cost_of_mri_at_area_
hospitals_report_finds_persistence_needed.html

https://www.medicare.gov/hospitalcompare/Data/30-day-measures.html

http://www.medicare.gov/hospitalcompare/search.html

http://www.npuap.org/wp-content/uploads/2012/01/NPUAP-Pressure-Ulcer-
Stages-Categories.pdf

http://www.npuap.org/resources/educational-and-clinical-resources/push-tool/

http://www.nytimes.com/2014/12/11/opinion/dont-homogenize-health-care.html?
emc=eta1

http://profiles.health.ny.gov/hospital/

http://www.qualitymeasures.ahrq.gov/content.aspx?id=49196

CHAPTER EIGHT

WORKING WITH QUALITY AND SAFETY MEASURES

Chapter Outline

Commitment to Quality
Using Measures to Understand Care
Defining the Measure
Process Measures
Pay for Performance
Patient Satisfaction Measures
Monitoring Measures
Safety and Environment of Care Measures
Summary
Key Terms
Quality Concepts in Action
References
Suggestions for Further Reading
Useful Websites

Key Concepts

- Understand how measurements are essential for monitoring and improving care.
- Describe how measures are used by physicians, administrators, and patients.
- Recognize how measures can improve processes and identify gaps in care.
- Realize the importance of measures for P4P.

- Define how measurements can address patient satisfaction issues.
- Visualize the process of care through dashboard reports.
- Link patient safety, good clinical outcomes, and the environment of care via measurements.

In the past, good care was defined primarily through the prestige of the institution, the academic credentials of the physicians, and technological equipment, not numbers or data or measurements. Poor performance, including errors that resulted in mortality, was often considered an acceptable complication, and patients who were emotionally attached to their physicians did not rush to judgment.

Today, the push toward objectivity and quantification is creating new approaches to care—and, importantly, defining value for health services. Now, perhaps because of the fragmented nature of medical care, with the Affordable Care Act enabling consumers to select their health insurance providers and with the OpenNotes program, initiated by the Robert Johnson Foundation and expanded throughout the country, enabling patients to see what their physicians write in their notes (http://www.rwjf.org/en/how-we-work/grants/grantees/OpenNotes.html), patient loyalty has become more complex and subject to financial pressure. More consumers are focusing on quantitative data, such as measures of outcomes, cost, and satisfaction.

Reliance on numbers is certainly not new in medicine. Physicians have always relied on numbers to assess their patients' condition, from the history and physical to laboratory reports about blood panels. They trust **quantitative information** to establish whether their patient's condition is improving or not, and they communicate with nurses about quantitative analysis, rarely about the narrative progress notes. What is new is the use of quantitative information, in the form of measurements, to respond to government, insurers, and the public's mandates to ensure quality, lower costs, and increase satisfaction. Health care is being quantified to reduce variation from the standard of care, create efficiencies, reduce waste, ensure evidence-based treatment, understand outcomes, define populations, and monitor patient satisfaction.

Commitment to Quality

The goal of using measures is to develop new processes and new structures to improve care, reduce mortality and complications, and increase efficiencies, thus reducing costs. Once improvements are made, there has to be a strong structure in place to maintain the new processes, especially as staff and leaders change. The key to improvements is to reach a level of success that integrates quality and safety into the culture of the organization and create structures and processes that are not susceptible to changed management. For example, if the medical board has approved employing intensivists for postoperative intensive care unit (ICU) care, that structure is likely to remain in place, even if the personnel of the ICU change. If a new chief executive officer (CEO) prefers Six Sigma/Lean improvement methodologies to Plan-Do-Study-Act (PDSA) ones, the underlying structure of using a quality methodology to target areas for improvements does not change. Or if ICU admission criteria are in place, having been established by the medical board, that too is a structure that is unlikely to be affected by management changes.

The Future of Quality

As quality analytics become more sophisticated and data from electronic health records (EHRs) become more reliable, future health care professionals who are trained in statistics and research methods will be able to better understand how to utilize improvement methodologies such as PDSA. They will understand and develop hypotheses, collect reliable and valid variables, research clinical and quality literature for defining appropriate variables, and use measures to reveal the relationship between performance improvement and quality management.

Future CEOs will understand that they have to be involved in quality management processes to analyze and change care for improvements. It is unproductive to try to improve patient satisfaction without understanding what is involved; to improve outcomes, leaders need to understand the processes that led to those outcomes. For the organization to be successful, administrators have to be involved in overseeing the delivery of care. Gaining consensus from the clinical staff also increases commitment to the measures. With the help of quality management, senior leaders have to define which measures best define safe care. Sometimes measures can be used for marketing purposes, to establish good public relations, saying that one organization excels in safety or some surgical procedure according to some ranking.

Using Measures to Understand Care

The government, insurers, and private agencies take measurements seriously and publish data for the public. Consumers are aware that medicine is becoming a commodity like others on the marketplace. The purchasers of health services and patients are looking for value, and measurements are available for them to gauge whether their dollars are being spent productively and wisely.

For the Consumer

If you are a candidate for open heart surgery, for example, you might look to the Dartmouth Atlas (see Chapter 7) to check for comparative cost, complications, and **mortality rates** for this procedure. You might also look at the Hospital Consumer Assessment of Healthcare Providers and Systems

(HCAHPS) (see Chapter 4) and other patient satisfaction surveys to assess patient experience. You can also compare physician credentials and quality statistics. You can see whether the organization has high or low compliance with process measures for this procedure at the Hospital Compare website (https://www.medicare.gov/hospitalcompare/compare.html). Today the customer for a hip replacement, for example, can research the numbers, be selective about choosing an organization and physician, determine price, infection rate, complications, pain control, communication effectiveness, and levels of functioning after surgery, among other variables.

Since measures are available to evaluate processes, outcomes, and structures, which means that these aspects of care are quantified, customers are beginning to define the product of health care services through these numbers. In the past, physicians have asserted their effectiveness based on experience, intuition, and training, and that definition may not be consistent with the patient experience. If an endoscopy patient ends up in the hospital, the physician may say it is a normal consequence of the procedure, but the patient may not see it the same way. If the patient was at high risk for complications, why was the procedure done in the physician's office? Or if the procedure was so low risk, why did the patient end up in the hospital? Was the problem related to incompetence or inexperience, poor equipment, poor assessment, or other? When patients demand good care, physicians may change practices to accommodate their expectations. Now that care is measureable and transparent, the move will be from subjective experience of the physician to objective numbers from data.

Patients and their families are also being educated about measures, usually by the clinician. Explaining to the family, for example, that antibiotics will be given prior to surgery because evidence indicates that outcomes will be improved helps patients and their families understand what is occurring and why. This is good medicine, effective communication, and good public relations.

For the Administrator

Administrators use measures for their organizations to remain competitive in the health care marketplace. Measures reflect whether an organization's care is as good at providing efficient quality services as another is, or whether it is better or worse. Organizations have to align themselves with national quality benchmarks to be accountable to the public for the clinical and financial quality of their services. Transparency and availability of measurements lead to increased accountability because consumers can obtain quantitative information about specifics of care.

Today's health care administrators do not have to be physicians to understand effective and efficient care. Like patients and physicians, however, they do have to understand the measurements and react to the numbers, especially if improvements are necessary. Administrators need to challenge physicians to comply with the measurements because compliance is rewarded financially. Also, because the measures are publicly reported, compliance may lead to retaining and increasing market share, traditionally an administrative concern.

For example, the Centers for Medicare and Medicaid Services (CMS) tracks rates of pneumococcal vaccination because, according to evidence, outcomes are better when patients are vaccinated. However, many physicians do not believe that survival rates increase with vaccination and therefore are not interested in collecting data about this measure. Because it is a CMS requirement, however, administration and quality management insist these data be collected for compliance with the measure, and it is up to them to educate physicians about its importance to patients, the organization, and their reputations. Administrators have to use numbers to objectify the discussion. The numbers can help move from an emotional response to a rational objective one. However, this may be a tightrope for administrators to walk because annoyed physicians can always walk away with their patients and move to another health care organization.

For the Physician

Because physicians define the scope of care and understand the implications of the measures and where they have an impact, they should be involved in any discussion about measures. Today's health care environment collapses many of the old boundaries among quality, policy, and clinical care.

For measures that are dictated by the government or outside agencies, physicians are expected to document the medical record and be educated about the importance of understanding numerators and denominators. If physicians think measurements are irrelevant to their practice, they will not comply and there will be serious consequences to the organization. Quality management professionals and administrators work hard to help clinicians accept and implement measures.

Quality measures are distinct from research data, with which physicians are often more familiar and comfortable. In research, it is acceptable to take a sample. But in quality, everyone in the denominator has to be counted and documented. Often physicians do not like to have details of clinical practice dictated to them, for instance, from measures that have been formulated from evidence-based medicine. To ensure compliance with these measures, quality professionals have to convince them, via databases, that the measures are reasonable and that compliance with them will improve outcomes. It is a rare physician who eagerly participates in the quality process, but doing so is necessary today to ensure compliance and improved reimbursements.

Physicians are understandably sensitive about measures because their performance is being judged by them. If a physician's data reveal that his or her patients are high in readmissions, with long lengths of stay (LOS), and neglect to follow-up on post hospital discharge visits with the physician, indicating poor discharge instructions, then the physician will be notified of poor results and perhaps questioned about his or her practice.

Working with measurements, especially process measures, is a challenge for most clinicians because they are not trained in how to look at care from a process and population point of view. They are trained to examine specific problems and target specific outcomes for those problems. They usually are not concerned with the way care is delivered generally to a patient population or with the analysis of measures, such as for throughput.

Also, with the availability of EHRs, many clinicians think they are entering data, as requested and required for compliance with measurements, when what they are entering are simply progress notes and information about care. Information included in the medical record and the EHR has to be converted to data to be analyzed and measured. As with the example of the HEAL 10 project (see Chapter 4), physicians thought information was being communicated across the continuum of care, specifically from the physician's office to labor and delivery and back to the office in a loop, but when we analyzed the situation, information was often missing and what was documented was not being communicated effectively.

Defining the Measure

Measures enhance accountability for specific variation in care. If national or regional benchmarks are not reached, administrators and physicians need to make changes. The 2013 Institute of Medicine (IOM) report, *Best Care at Lower Cost*, recommends generating, collecting, compiling, and using data for improved care management. It encourages the development of a clinical data infrastructure to support improvements in both the delivery of care and the patient experience.

The IOM report asks three important questions about data:

1. What does the hospital need to know?
2. How will the information be captured and used?
3. How will the resultant knowledge be organized and shared?

Define the Numerator and the Denominator

Take, as an example, sepsis. Sepsis is a potentially life-threatening complication of infection. What does the hospital need to know about sepsis? What kind of data would be most useful? These are not simple questions. Should all sepsis patients be grouped together, or should mild sepsis be distinct from patients with septic shock? In other words, what is the denominator of the measure, the population of patients under scrutiny? Should the cause of sepsis be analyzed, or at what point in the treatment or procedure it occurred? Should the patients with sepsis be tracked by demographic information to see whether one group—for example, the elderly—had more sepsis than other groups, or if patients with a specific illness/procedure—for example, transplant—were more prone to infection, or even whether specific physicians accounted for more than a chance occurrence of sepsis patients? In other words, what should be the numerator of the measure, the specific patients that are of interest? Should the data be gathered by service line or otherwise? Clearly the data will be different according to what is of interest; therefore, it is important to define the reason to collect the data.

Another example is readmission. Professionals may think about how the data will be captured and used differently, depending on their orientation. Quality management might track readmission rates differently from strategic planning departments. Since the focus is different for each, and they use different data sources (medical record review, charge data), they will have different populations, or denominators, in their measures. Strategic planning may want to know how many patients are readmitted in order to track expenses, reimbursements, and resources; quality management might want to analyze which patients return and for what reason in order to make improvements and reduce the rates.

Another new challenge for quality professionals is to try to track **outpatient measures**, such as administering the right kind of antibiotic to individuals having an outpatient surgical procedure. Tracking of these measures is required by the CMS and is extremely difficult to do. How should the data be gathered? By whom? In what fashion? And then, how should the data be documented? Processes that are successful in the inpatient hospital setting may not be viable in private physician outpatient offices. Yet every office needs to standardize the way measures are collected. The problems of standardization across multiple offices becomes most challenging when physician offices are affiliated with health systems, as most of them are.

It is also important to try to eliminate politics to reduce special interests and work together toward improvements. Even seemingly straightforward measures can be complex. Committees can spend months attempting to define "falls," for example. Is it necessary to fall from a standing position, or is sliding out of a chair onto the floor considered a fall? Defining a problem has to precede attempts to improve. Even with the CMS's carefully defined inclusion and exclusion criteria for what constitutes a numerator to a measure, there is conflict. How should aspiration pneumonia be defined? Even within the same health organization, definitions are inconsistent. Pressure injuries can be interpreted differently by physicians, nurses, and nutritionists. Especially when the numbers show poor care and that improvements are necessary, people can become defensive, and the issue becomes political.

Measuring for Improvement

Leaders, especially the CEO, have to determine which of the hundreds of measures being collected should be tracked for improvements. The CEO wants to focus on those measures that meet his or her prioritization criteria and are congruent with strategic planning goals. CEOs, who are used to considering financial and operations measures, now also have to assess quality measurements in order to move the organization forward successfully.

Measures not only are required by the CMS, but data submitted are scrutinized for accuracy and completeness. Because the CMS oversees billing as well as quality, it is impossible to produce false reports of better care than what is being billed. In other words, if you have to treat someone for a fall or for a reoperation and hope to be paid for it, the CMS can cross-check the bill with your reports on falls and reoperations. Therefore, the CMS provides checks and balances for accurate reporting.

But measuring for the sake of measuring or even simply for compliance teaches us nothing about improving care. It is the analysis that accompanies the measure that makes a difference. For instance, hospitals have been tracking mortality for ages, but that's all; they have simply counted the numbers. Understanding how the numbers are derived and what they mean is not simple.

In fact, the debate over calculating mortality rates has been going on since 1863, when Florence Nightingale claimed that mortality rates were calculated differently depending on the goal of the hospital. She said that London hospitals were dangerous and supported this assertion with statistics showing that the hospitals had mortality rates above 90 percent. However, that calculation relied on dividing the total number of patients who died in a year by the number of inpatients on a single day, which is akin to dividing apples by herrings (Iezzoni 1996). When the calculation was changed to the number of patients who died in a year by the number of inpatients during that year, the rate of mortality was 10 percent. When this came to light, Nightingale criticized the data and said it was necessary to understand statistical methods when calculating quality of care (Batalden and Mohr 1999).

When the IOM reported that mortality was high, people took notice. Why? Because the IOM interpreted the high mortality and said that it was caused by avoidable errors and mistakes—that is, poor care. Only then did the health care community sit up and take notice. Sometimes it takes an external agency to tell you that your numbers signify a problem. If overall mortality is 2.3 percent, that seems low, especially across a large health system. But if, on closer analysis, mortality of a certain disease is 20 percent (once the denominator changes, the percentage changes), that may shock the health system into further analysis and improvement efforts.

Measures are not only changing the way we think about the delivery of care but also about how improvements are made. The PDSA methodology is becoming more sophisticated because measures now are incorporated. For example, in the Planning phase, national benchmarks can be used to focus improvement goals; in the Do stage, the culture has changed so that data collection is accepted as critical to the process, and quality improvement data, patient satisfaction data, and CMS measures are integrated into the improvement efforts. The Study phase focuses on ensuring that the denominators being studied are well defined. In the Act phase, process measures are monitored to ensure that benchmarks and deciles are being reached.

Process Measures

It is not sufficient to have a good Joint Commission (TJC) survey score or even to be above the benchmark on a process measure. To excel, administrators need to understand the details of the process, the patient population, the expectations about treatment and outcomes, and the different issues involved at different levels of care. They should also be involved in engaging all staff members in understanding the measures.

Process measures, based on medical evidence, specify the best way to deliver care for particular diagnoses or procedures, and they reflect how efficiently clinical and organizational processes are implemented. Analysis of process measures can be useful in identifying bottlenecks or delays in care and services. The CMS publishes information about process measures on its Hospital Compare website (https://www.medicare.gov/hospitalcompare/search.html). Compliance with these evidence-based measures means the organization will be in the top decile in the nation. Although a direct link between compliance with process measures and improved outcomes cannot be guaranteed, as the measures get better—that is, more carefully defined—better outcomes may indeed be the result.

Quality management helps organizations comply with established measures and uses any gap between actual and ideal compliance rates to develop improvements via PDSA or other improvement methodology. In order to develop improvements, however, the process related to the measure has to be clearly and minutely understood. The goal is to understand the process in order to improve the measure and meet expectations—that is, to achieve the benchmark or leadership expectations.

To evaluate any process adequately, the analytic team associated with the quality management department needs to assess deviance, variation, and interpret data results. The analysts can also develop and monitor control charts for compliance with the measure and note whether the peaks and valleys are due to special cause variations or simply chance occurrences (see Chapter 7).

Case Example: Medication Measures

For example, medication is the most frequent intervention in medical care, and the medication delivery system is highly complex. Many disciplines are involved, and often the process is fragmented, especially because often there is no single authority overseeing the process from beginning to end. To deliver the correct medication to the correct patient at the correct time involves the physician correctly diagnosing the patient's condition and prescribing the correct medication at the correct dosage and the correct method of delivery (intravenous or oral). The prescription has to be communicated correctly to the pharmacy. The pharmacist has to fill the order correctly and label it correctly for the right patient. The correctly labeled correct medication has to be delivered to the correct patient in a timely way, and then it must be administered correctly.

Errors can occur at any time during this complex process (see Figure 8.1). Because errors are almost inevitable, processes have to be developed to ensure patient safety, and those processes are measured (Dlugacz 2011).

Collecting medication measures helps to reduce errors and identify gaps in the process. In the health care system in which we work, several measurements are used to monitor medication safety and reported to leaders on a regular basis. For example, we collect carefully defined data on **adverse drug reactions** (harm or injury as a result of medication) rates, medication error rate, and medication near-miss rate (see Figure 8.2).

By monitoring these measures, analyzing the data, and reporting them, leaders know when improvements are necessary.

Figure 8.3 is an example of an executive summary that tracks and compares medication errors, near misses, and suspected drug reaction reported rates at several system hospitals. The chart reveals that Hospital I is doing better

FIGURE 8.1. HOSPITAL MEDICATION ADMINISTRATION PROCESS

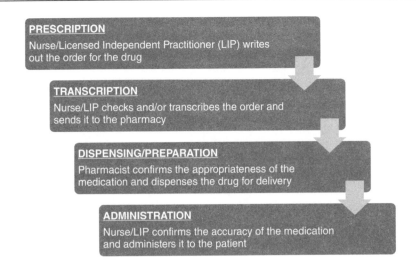

FIGURE 8.2. MEDICATION ERROR MEASURES

Drug Name/Category: (e.g.) Lipitor/Statin	
Adverse Drug Reaction Rate	# of patients with suspected adverse drug reaction(s)
	Total discharges (excluding Psychiatry/Chemical Dependency, Newborns)
Reported Medication Error Rate	# of medication errors reported
	Total discharges (excluding Psychiatry/Chemical Dependency, Newborns)
Medication Near-Miss Rate	# of events that were corrected or reported prior to administration
	Patient care days (excluding Psychiatry/Chemical Dependency, Rehabilitation, Hospice, Newborns)

than the benchmark for medication errors whereas the others are performing at average or lower than the benchmark. When leaders see this, they might suggest that the successful hospital explain its excellent rate and that others learn from that hospital's processes.

NEAR MISS

The term *near miss* refers to an error that *almost* occurred. The classic example is of two airplanes that almost collide because they inadvertently come too close to each other. Since a near miss is something that might happen if not prevented, it is important to identify what in the process is vulnerable to error and then correct it before it actually occurs. Near misses occur often in health care and are usually corrected with no consequence to the patient.

For example, a nurse realizes at the last minute that the medication she is about to administer is for the patient in the next bed and quickly corrects the problem. Or a diabetic patient receives the incorrect meal and a family member tells the nurse, who contacts nutrition services for the correct one.

It is important to bring near misses to consciousness and to identify them as gaps in care that could lead to patient harm. Therefore, the system in which we work collects data on near misses and reports them to make staff aware of potential problems. The idea is that if a mistake could happen once (even if corrected), it could happen again and perhaps not be corrected. Then harm could come to the patient. By collecting data and reporting information about near misses, patient safety is increased and processes can be improved. It is only natural that professionals do not want to admit to mistakes, but discovering areas where near misses occur is so important that many organizations have developed an anonymous form for reporting.

FIGURE 8.3. EXECUTIVE SUMMARY MEDICATION MEASURES

MEDICATION MEASURES	HOSPITAL A	HOSPITAL B	HOSPITAL C	HOSPITAL D	HOSPITAL E	HOSPITAL F	HOSPITAL G	HOSPITAL H	HOSPITAL I	HOSPITAL J
Medication Error Reported Rate										
Benchmark Range: (7.86–1.47)	0.61	2.38	1.49	1.37	0.68	0.61	2.15	0.89	12.44	0.99
Near-Miss Reported Rate										
Benchmark Range: (19.07–1.45)	11.72	1.97	0.92	3.15	1.4	1.98	0.72	7.18	0.86	26.26
Suspected Drug Reaction Reported Rate										
Benchmark Range: (3.62–1.56)	2.03	1.36	1.9	0.95	1.56	1.49	2.47	1.61	3.13	2.58

▦ = Green = Hospital/System performed BETTER than the benchmark*

▥ = Yellow = Hospital/System performed within AVERAGE

▨ = Red = Hospital/System performed WORSE than the benchmark*

*Benchmark: Developed using the system's previous year's performance

FIGURE 8.4. MEDICATION SAFETY ALERT

MEDICATION SAFETY ALERT	
Don't hold onto dangerous habits: *SPELL IT OUT*	
DON'T USE	INSTEAD
(U)	Write "unit"
(μg)	Write "microgram"
(q.d.)	Write "daily"
q.o.d.	Write "every other day"
q.i.d.	Write "four times daily"
x.0 or .x	Write "X mg" Write "0.X mg"
(MS)	Write "morphine sulfate" Write "magnesium sulfate"

Errors that occur in the medication administration process can lead to risks to patient safety. TJC has identified various abbreviations, acronyms, and other commonly used shortcuts in handwritten medication orders that should be avoided. A list of not-to-be-used abbreviations was distributed to all clinicians across the United States (see Figure 8.4). For example, the symbol U could be confused with a 0 (zero), leading to dangerous overdoses.

Those systems that have fully adopted computerized provider order entry technology for prescribing and ordering mediation have significantly reduced the incidence of medication errors (Radley et al. 2013).

Complying with Process Measures

Understanding process measures is quite complicated. However, without understanding the process, there is no way to improve compliance with the measure. Measures should not be collected simply because the government expects it; the issue is to understand how the process works so that risk points for compliance with the measure can be identified. Only once the process is understood and analyzed can a protocol for improvement be developed, education can be provided if necessary, changes to the process can be suggested, barriers to success can be identified, and risk assessments can be performed.

Measures are not simple. Meeting the criteria of a measure—let's say, for Hospital Compare—means that there is a good process in place. Also, there has to be responsibility or accountability for the measure. Who will provide oversight? Sometimes an entire program needs to be developed to ensure compliance with the measure. Even something as seemingly simple as giving aspirin is a process: Prescribe, order, dispense, administer.

All patients who present at the hospital with chest pain are supposed to receive aspirin. Again, if compliance with this measure is not meeting the benchmark, the process has to be analyzed. Another measure is that all sepsis patients should receive antibiotics immediately upon diagnosis. Compliance with the measure involves correctly and quickly diagnosing sepsis in the patient, and the diagnosis may be difficult because the symptoms can be masked. People make quick decisions. The laboratory results have to come in quickly, perhaps radiological studies as well. To develop efficient processes, you have to understand the processes and eliminate obstacles and risk points so that compliance with the measure is maximized.

Although health organizations can develop their own measurements, many measures are dictated by the government to develop national benchmarks and enforce data collection objectivity. For example, the CMS collects and publishes data on measures related to the effective use of medication, such as antibiotic administration prior to surgery. This measure was developed because evidence shows that giving an antibiotic prior to surgery reduces infections and therefore improves outcomes. It is also cost effective since LOS may be reduced and fewer resources, such as the ICU, may be used.

If the compliance rate with the measure is not what it should be, a multidisciplinary team needs to analyze where in the complex process of antibiotic delivery the problem occurs. The problem could be in the emergency department (ED) or in the perioperative phase of the surgery. Perhaps different clinicians have different prescribing strategies, or there is a barrier to dispensing in the pharmacy or perhaps there is an issue with the nurses delivering the medication at the appropriate time. And even once the process problem is identified, there should be an investigation into whether the process is standardized or idiosyncratic to individual EDs or operating rooms (ORs) or pharmacies or nurses.

For example, if a health system wanted to improve compliance with the evidence-based process measure of administering antibiotic prior to surgery, two approaches could be taken. Nurses could be assigned the task of reminding the team that the antibiotic should be administered and also be held accountable for monitoring compliance. Another and superior approach would be to define how antibiotic administration fits into the entire process of preparing a patient for surgery. Once defined, adjustments to the process could be made so that antibiotic administration would be delivered on a routine basis. Accountability for ensuring compliance could be assigned to a team member.

Data about compliance would be reported regularly to leaders. The more process-oriented intervention for improvement would internalize the measure as part of the normal work flow; compliance would be accepted as routine. Without real change, any improvements in compliance are short-lived.

Process measures with benchmarks that are received from the government create consistency across the country. With the transparent rating of variables, organizations can compare themselves and strive to attain the highest percentiles. This kind of competition may improve the quality of care, but for there to be a real cultural change in the delivery of care, measurements have to be used for improvements.

Once an organization uses measures appropriately for improvement, analysts can begin to make hypotheses based on the data findings and pursue strategies to improve processes. For example, using measures, quality analysts and clinicians in the health system in which we work hypothesized that reoperation, caused by bleeders not closed, leads to sternal wound infection. This **hypothesis**—that bleeding leads to infection—could be studied. Analysis of data supported the hypothesis, and new processes were developed for improved intraoperative and postoperative care. Educational efforts improved competency. Until processes are analyzed via measures, it is not clear which processes need improvements and change.

Case Example: Mammography Rate

Quality management provides the health system in which we work with the definition of every measure—that is, the explicit definition of the numerator and denominator as well as an explanation of how the measure is calculated. The population involved in the measure is defined, through the inclusion and exclusion criteria. For example, for mammography screening, the numerator is defined as those women of a specific age (40–69) who have had a mammogram in the past year; the denominator is the number of women of those ages who are part of our patient population (see Figure 8.5). The numerators can be changed depending on what specific population is of interest. If a professional is interested in tracking the mammography rate of patients with a history of breast cancer, the definition of the measure would be changed so that the numerator would be those women with a history of breast cancer, of a specified age, who have had a mammogram in the past year, and the denominator would be all women with a history of breast cancer of a specified age.

Inclusion and exclusion criteria are also defined. Perhaps a researcher wants to exclude from the definition of the measure women who have had a complete mastectomy. These definitions and inclusion and exclusion criteria depend on the goals of the data collection. The measure might be defined differently if leaders were interested in the effectiveness of and compliance with the referral process or in identifying and screening an at-risk population.

FIGURE 8.5. MAMMOGRAPHY RATE

$$\frac{\text{Numerator}}{\text{Denominator}} = \frac{\text{\# of women (ages 40–69) who have had mammography in the past 12 months}}{\text{\# of women (ages 40–69)}} \times 100$$

Inclusion Criteria	Women ages 40–69 years
Exclusion Criteria	Women who have had a complete mastectomy (may occur on the same or separate dates)

Understanding Variables

To understand certain phenomena, it is often useful to study how one variable can predict, explain, or influence another. A variable is an item, factor, or condition that varies—that is, can change its value. Researchers can manipulate variables (the **independent variable**s) to observe the effect on another variable (the **dependent variable**).

For example, to develop a hypothesis (i.e., an idea or theory to be tested) such as if a patient falls, that patient will have a prolonged LOS, two variables are involved: falls and LOS. The hypothesis suggests that falls may predict LOS. Falls, then, is the independent (or predictor) variable that may have an impact on LOS, the dependent variable. The dependent variable is measured to learn the effect or impact of the independent variable (see Figure 8.6). The independent variable causes a change in the dependent variable. Therefore, it is the dependent variable that is measured for change.

Many variables that are required by the regulatory agencies are dependent, such as mortality rates, infection rates, aspirin administration to heart attack patients. The CMS is concerned with analyzing variables that have an impact on care. If an organization is in compliance and understands the characteristics of a patient population, such as its heart failure patients, it can begin to ask questions, or develop hypotheses to better understand care, such as: What impact does LOS have on heart failure patients? or What is the relationship between readmission and mortality? It is questions like these, based on measures, that lead to improved care.

Making Compliance Meaningful

If an organization is in compliance with quality process measures, an intelligent next question for a manager or leader to ask is how compliance relates

FIGURE 8.6. INDEPENDENT VARIABLES

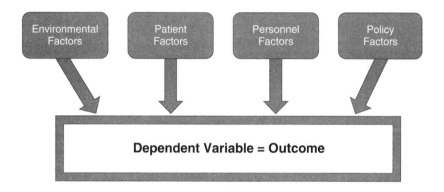

INDEPENDENT VARIABLES

Environmental Factors

Patient Factors

Personnel Factors

Policy Factors

Dependent Variable = Outcome

Independent variables PREDICT dependent variables

to improved care. Compliance should only be the first step toward defining relationships for improvement. Is the compliance tied to any research hypothesis that might advance the understanding of medical care? Understanding, for example, the expectations defined in measures associated with myocardial infarction (i.e., heart attack care) might lead to new questions about cause and effect and also enable predictions about outcomes.

Once there is compliance with measures, especially process measures by disease, improvement efforts using PDSA methodology can be instituted. Is there any relationship between zero infection and LOS or between zero infection and fewer complications? These are important and interesting questions that can be asked only once the measures are understood and compliance is reached. If you are an organization in compliance with infection control measures, for example, is mortality lower? It is important for leaders to make compliance meaningful.

For example, the American Heart Association developed a program, *Get with the Guidelines* (https://www.heart.org/HEARTORG/HealthcareResearch/ GetWithTheGuidelines/Get-With-The-Guidelines-Stroke_UCM_306098_Sub HomePage.jsp), to encourage data reporting of predetermined metrics with the goal of improving care for heart failure and stroke patients by following the latest evidence. This initiative is a collaborative effort among the American Heart Association, the American Stroke Association, and TJC to establish objective criteria for designating certain organizations as Comprehensive Stroke Centers.

In order to be so designated, organizations are expected to meet highly specific **performance measures** in treating stroke patients; the measures were developed by experts and supported by the latest available scientific information. Among the goals of the program is to properly assess the patient early in the process to prevent deterioration. Using metrics such as the ones established by these national professional organizations helps leaders see the value of early intervention and gain a better understanding of outcomes. Measures should be used for more than compliance; they should be used to improve patient care.

Case Example: Reducing Central Line Infections

Regulatory agencies have developed and promoted guidelines regarding how to place a central line (an intravenous line inserted into a large vein) with minimal risk of infections. The guidelines from the Centers for Disease Control and Prevention (http://www.cdc.gov/HAI/bsi/bsi.html) suggest proper insertion practices (e.g., perform hand hygiene before insertion, use maximal sterile barrier precautions) and proper maintenance practices (e.g., access catheters only with sterile devices, perform dressing changes using clean or sterile gloves). The guidelines also suggest that facilities provide recurring education sessions on central line insertion, handling, and maintenance, and collect and evaluate data about compliance with these and other guidelines as an initial step in promoting patient safety. Analysis of any barriers to compliance with these straightforward and nontechnologically sophisticated measures should help to reveal structural and process issues that may require investigation and improvements.

It is important to define accountability and explicitly state the roles and responsibilities of the nurse on the floor, the physician who places the line, what communication channels are available and efficient, and what interventions lead to reduced infections. Once improved processes and procedures are implemented, data on central line blood stream infections (BSIs) can be reported to leaders who can then assess whether the improvements have made an impact on safety.

The control chart in Figure 8.7 shows that the infection rate declined over time in the non-ICU area. To move an organization to zero infection rate takes time. Usually new processes have to be implemented after problems have been identified via data. Once the new processes have been developed, it takes time to ensure that the changes can be maintained.

Analytic reports help to promote vigilance since they can be used to communicate information in real time to leaders. Figure 8.7 shows that improvements initiated in 2012 had a positive impact. Reports are powerful tools to convince clinicians to review and change their process of care. Measures provide a status report about progress in improvement efforts.

FIGURE 8.7. NON-ICU CENTRAL LINE–ASSOCIATED BSI CONTROL CHART

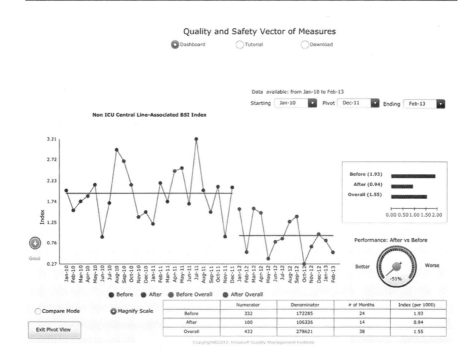

If necessary, new hypotheses might be needed to figure out what kind of change is necessary. Reviewing the measures allows leaders to evaluate whether the changed process had the desired impact.

Pay for Performance

Meeting specific clinical quality or performance measures is the foundation for pay for performance (P4P) or **value-based purchasing**, a payment model that provides financial incentives (and disincentives) to health care providers and organizations for improving quality and efficiency. P4P provides an alternative to the current fee-for-service reimbursement model, which rewards providers for volume of patients and the number and complexity of services. The concern is that fee for service might encourage *more* care, which may not necessarily result in *better* care; it is hoped that P4P would eliminate unnecessary tests and procedures.

P4P Measures

Two IOM reports, *Preventing Medication Errors* (2006) and *Rewarding Provider Performance: Aligning Incentives in Medicare* (2007), suggest that P4P initiatives might be useful in improving quality and efficiency. If health care providers meet or exceed the performance measure, the organization will be rewarded with a financial bonus. If they fail to meet the measure, organizations may be penalized. For example, Medicare will not reimburse organizations for hospital-acquired pressure ulcers or other never events. Presumably this lack of reimbursement will encourage hospitals to improve care.

The P4P measures include process measures—that is, activities that promote healthy outcomes, such as administering aspirin to patients with heart attacks or providing smoking cessation counseling to pneumonia patients. **Outcome measures**, which are associated with the effectiveness of care, are also included. Outcome measures reflect the consequences or results of processes, systems, or phenomena. But outcome measures are controversial because outcomes often are a result of the patient's social factors, such as diet or exercise, which might be unrelated to provider services.

For example, an outcome measure would be following guidelines for controlling glucose levels for diabetic patients; diet and exercise have an impact on glucose, and once a patient leaves the hospital, the provider cannot control the behavior. Therefore, professional medical organizations have suggested that it is unfair to penalize physicians for patient activities that are out of their control.

Patient experience or **satisfaction measures**, such as the quality and effectiveness of communication between patient and providers or the cleanliness of the rooms in the inpatient setting, are also included in P4P. Finally, **structure measures**, such as innovative technology or equipment, are also involved, and organizations are rewarded for innovative treatment modalities or for the integration of health information technology. Private sector initiatives of physician groups or insurers are also exploring whether P4P improves quality and reduces costs.

It should be noted that studies of the long-term (more than five years) effectiveness of P4P initiatives do not support its success ("Health Policy Brief" 2012). There is also concern that providers of care to underserved populations, who may have language barriers and other socioeconomic issues that would prevent optimal care, will score poorly on the measures and would not be able to support their organizations if they lose even a small portion of their reimbursement fees.

Patient Satisfaction Measures

Some health professionals are critical of the view that patient satisfaction measures reveal information about quality of care. Patients are not trained in medical care, the critics say, and are in no position to assess the quality of care delivered. But even if the surveys are imperfect and patients are untrained, research shows that the patient satisfaction surveys are robust indicators of health care quality and improved outcomes and should be taken very seriously (Manary et al. 2013).

Interpreting Patient Satisfaction Scores

It is important to realize that the interpretation of measurements is not static; different perspectives lead to different kinds of assessments and different types of analytics. Numbers by themselves, removed from an analytic context, are not meaningful. If Hospital Compare shows that patient satisfaction is a certain percentage, the clinician may feel satisfied with the number or look at a run chart to see whether satisfaction is going up or down. However, the administrator may view the same number differently. The administrator wants to improve patient satisfaction because doing so may increase market share and profits to the organization. The administrator may compare the percentile number to that of other organizations in the region because it is important to be in the top decile. Measures are tied to physician and hospital compensation.

Quality management professionals may see the number from yet another point of view, as something that should be investigated in order to improve. They may want to drill down to see where in the process patients felt dissatisfied, what the specific issues were, what procedure or treatment was involved, what the disease population was, and the kind of patient involved: everyone or only a subset? In other words, quality management might want to know what factors are contributing to the measure/results. Quality management would develop methodologies to analyze problems and recommend improvements. Depending on your point of view, the number or measure leads to different responses.

If patient satisfaction is generally lower in the northeastern part of the country than other regions, clinicians may believe that it is because patients in the Northeast are more sophisticated and thus more demanding. Perhaps their expectations are higher, and thus their satisfaction is lower. Clinicians who interpret the measure in this way may not believe change is necessary; it is what it is. Administrators may also accept this point of view but seek to make this population happier by adopting hotellike services to improve satisfaction.

Understand the Process

In order to get a handle on how to work with the patient satisfaction measure, there are several basic issues to address. The first step is to define the product: What does patient satisfaction mean, and who gets to decide: the clinician, the patient, the administrator?

What are the role of hotel services, such as cleanliness, friendliness of staff, good food, in patient satisfaction? For many years, administrators thought hotel services would increase satisfaction, and they attempted to introduce services into health organizations that were similar to what is offered at four-star hotels. But these attempts, although certainly pleasant improvements, were not successful in raising satisfaction rates.

Among the reasons for the lack of success was the false assumption that "patients" comprise a homogenous group. Hotel services are the same across hotels and locales. Different patients experience the health care delivery system in different ways. Does the measure control for the differences among inpatients, outpatients, and nursing home patients? Even in the inpatient setting, an obstetrical patient who has a normal, uncomplicated delivery may experience her care quite differently from an elderly patient with heart failure who falls and breaks a hip. In other words, to understand the measure and to institute improvements, one has to look into the details.

Refine the Process

To understand the patient satisfaction measure, different measures for different experiences and different patient populations should be developed. A general measure is simply too broad to offer useful information. Once distinctions are defined and understood, improvements in the appropriate areas can be instituted. Just introducing hotel services across the board does not target specific issues that need to be addressed.

Perhaps it is outcomes that have the greatest impact on the patient satisfaction measure. Perhaps surgical patients who have a short LOS, no complications, and good outcomes are more satisfied than patients with the same surgery who do have complications and poorer outcomes. Does outcome impact satisfaction? One has to do analysis in order to answer that question.

Effective communication is among the most robust indicators of satisfaction. For example, when protocols were developed for pneumonia patients to better understand certain sequelae of their disease process, such as the likelihood of depression, the patients had better outcomes and were more satisfied. It is not clear whether the increase in satisfaction was generated from the information or simply from the communicative interaction. More investigation is necessary. Certainly if outcome is the salient factor, that is quite different from friendliness of staff or annoying noise.

Not only is it necessary to carefully define the product—in this example, patient satisfaction—but it is also important to address different product lines—that is, the context in which the services are delivered. Pediatric care is different from surgery, which is different from medical. The level of care may also influence satisfaction. Patients in the ICU are not as satisfied and happy with their experience as patients who come in for medical treatment whose outcomes are good and go home quickly. Satisfaction may be dependent on context-specific experience.

In order to understand the measure, hospital environment may also play a part. For example, when organizations introduced private rooms for labor and delivery, obstetrical patients and families were more satisfied with their hospital experience than before these improvements were introduced.

In addition to defining the issue and the patient population and understanding the scope and level of care, it is also important to understand the mode of production—that is, how the care is delivered. A patient in a typical ICU, according to the Dartmouth Atlas survey, sees multiple clinicians (http://www.dartmouthatlas.org/). Are those patients happier than those who see a single physician?

And finally, it is important to understand the labor force. What kind of people are doing the work? If nurse practitioners talk to patients about their disease and help them to understand their discharge instructions, is that more likely to satisfy patients than when a physician hands them a sheet of paper with a list of instructions as they leave the hospital? All these factors require analysis in order to interpret the survey scores.

Define Expectations

Satisfaction may be related to expectations; different patient groups may have different expectations. Customers who want to purchase a car, for example, not only look for the best price, but also want to be confident that their needs are foremost to the salesperson and not his or her commission. Customers want to trust him or her to be honest and take care of their interests. If people have trouble trusting a car salesperson, imagine how difficult it might be for patients to trust their medical care. Patients, unlike car consumers, are vulnerable, often frightened, sick, and at the mercy of the system. Many patients who interact with health organizations are also cynical about how they will be treated. The fact that patients are asked for their insurance number and credit card before anyone asks what has brought them to a hospital or doctor's office certainly does not inspire trust in care.

To understand the product of patient satisfaction, professionals need to understand the patient/consumer expectations, cultural and social barriers to satisfaction, and exactly what variables are involved in and are basic to a good experience. An overarching measure, such as patient satisfaction, can and should be broken down into other, more specific measures, such as effective communication, comprehensible discharge instructions, friendliness of staff, and so on. Only through this kind of careful analysis of the process can improvements be effective.

The patient experience is also dependent on the doctor-patient relationship. In the past, physicians were trained to focus on the problem rather than the individual. Today, physicians are being trained to focus on the entire patient, and residents are taught empathy, role playing, the value of narratives, and listening skills. As patient satisfaction measures are taken more seriously by administrative and clinical leaders, improvements in these important areas may be forthcoming.

Monitoring Measures

Regardless of whether the measure is about patient satisfaction, mortality, sepsis, medication errors, ICU care, or any other indicator, leaders require reports to help them understand the relationship between measures and the delivery of care. **Dashboards**—reports in the form of tables or charts of quality measures—are tools that help leaders understand measures for decisions about improvement opportunities. Unsurprisingly, dashboards have evolved and changed over time, becoming more sophisticated as health care information technology has changed. For example, in 2004, the health care system in which we work reported very different measures than we do today.

Dashboards in the Past

Figure 8.8 shows a hospital's quarterly report on specific measures for 2004. Results were color coded to easily show whether the results were above (green), below (red), or meeting (yellow) the CMS benchmarks for those indicators. The chart shows that this particular hospital did very well—it exceeded the CMS benchmark of 10 percent for prescribing aspirin at discharge for heart attack patients.

However, the hospital did below the benchmark at administering aspirin at arrival, as the CMS requires. Hospital leaders can look at this dashboard and quickly ascertain where opportunities for improvement exist, establish accountability for improvement efforts, and initiate new programs where necessary. Without this dashboard of aggregated data, over time and in comparison with established benchmarks, it would be most difficult to determine which indicators need to be improved.

At the system level, the dashboard aggregated the information from all the hospitals and reported results in a slightly different format. Figure 8.9 shows the system dashboard that compares individual hospitals. The colors alert leaders about which hospitals were doing well and which were not, and on what indicators. The color-coded circle shows the overall picture, and the individual table has color-coded stars that indicate better, worse, or the same as the CMS benchmark.

This example shows indicators for outcomes measures and patient safety. Viewers can see that only one hospital, Hospital A, is successful in exceeding the CMS benchmark for unplanned 30-day readmission rate. Leaders know from this dashboard that improvements are necessary for the other hospitals. Likewise with the surgical site infection (SSI) rate. Only one hospital, Hospital I, exceeded the CMS benchmark.

FIGURE 8.8. PUBLIC REPORTING SCORES

	2004 Q2	2004 Q3	2004 Q4
AMI ACEI or ARB for LVSD	100 N=2	100 N=5	100 N=4
AMI Adult smoking cessation advice/ counseling		0 N=1	80 N=5
AMI Aspirin at arrival	84 N=44	95 N=39	94 N=47
AMI Aspirin prescribed at discharge	100 N=12	100 N=10	100 N=12
AMI Beta blocker at arrival	96 N=28	95 N=19	95 N=20
AMI Beta blocker prescribed at discharge	100 N=13	100 N=12	
CAP Adult smoking cessation advice/ counseling		60 N=5	
CAP Blood culture before first antibiotic		87 N=52	
CAP Initial antibiotic received within 4 hours of hospital arrival	69 N=97	82 N=57	86 N=105
CAP Oxygenation assessment	100 N=98	100 N=66	99 N=122
CAP Pneumococcal vaccination	48 N=67	72 N=46	76 N=84
HF ACEI or ARB for LVSD	76 N=21	96 N=24	82 N=17
HF Adult smoking cessation advice/counseling		78 N=9	57 N=7
HF Discharge instructions		11 N=44	13 N=62
HF LVF assessment	97 N=86	84 N=62	88 N=77

Trends of Performance

⬜ = Green = Percent Indicators above the CMS 10% Benchmark

⬛ = Yellow = Percent Indicators between the CMS 10% and 50% Benchmarks

⬛ = Red = Percent Indicators below the CMS 50% Benchmark

⬜ = Green = Hospital Performed above the CMS 10% Benchmark

⬛ = Yellow = Hospital Performed between the CMS 10% and 50% Benchmarks

⬛ = Red = Hospital Performed below the CMS 50% Benchmark

Dashboards Today

Today the dashboard at the health system in which we work looks different and measures different indicators. Also, it is web-based and interactive, enabling end users to drill down to data that are of interest to them, offering more detail than on the overall dashboard.

FIGURE 8.9. EXECUTIVE SUMMARY

Outcomes	HOSPITAL A	HOSPITAL B	HOSPITAL C	HOSPITAL D	HOSPITAL E	HOSPITAL F	HOSPITAL G	HOSPITAL H	HOSPITAL I	HOSPITAL J
Autopsy Request Rate Benchmark Range: (72.69–25.66)	87.16	0.51	30.60	6.28	14.50	23.68	36.48	87.96	4.99	52.98
Excess Days per PT Benchmark Range: (0.46–1.71)	1.94	2.67	2.16	1.88	1.75	1.55	1.79	0.70	1.94	0.26
Unplan 30 Day Readm Rate Benchmark Range: (4.62–7.12)	3.60	7.65	7.74	8.58	7.75	7.60	9.09	11.59	4.70	5.14
Unplan Return OR Rate Benchmark Range: (0.78–1.28)	1.93	1.73	0.83	1.60	2.07	2.30	1.62	1.60	0.76	1.14

Patient Safety	HOSPITAL A	HOSPITAL B	HOSPITAL C	HOSPITAL D	HOSPITAL E	HOSPITAL F	HOSPITAL G	HOSPITAL H	HOSPITAL I	HOSPITAL J
Nosocomial Press.Ulcer Rate Benchmark Range: (0.74–1.33)	0.95	1.19	0.97	1.13	1.03	1.32	1.20	0.99	1.65	1.22
PT Fall Index Benchmark Range: (2.80–3.10)	2.97	3.09	3.75	4.09	2.91	2.75	2.26	3.92	5.17	2.81
PT Med/Surg Restraint Index Benchmark Range: (5.10–31.80)	13.09	52.30	32.58	51.97	4.54	15.50	26.69	53.72	29.54	13.74
SSI Rate Benchmark Range: (0.95–1.31)	1.39	1.26	1.19	1.48	1.59	1.89	1.69	1.80	0.79	0.96

☐☐☐ = Green = Hospital/System performed BETTER than the benchmark

☐ = Yellow = Hospital/System performed within average

☐☐ = Red = Hospital/System performed WORSE than the benchmark

The dashboard shown on Figure 8.10 reports indicators that reflect leadership priorities. For the year 2012, for example, leaders focused on mortality, readmission, and infection (BSI and sepsis). These specific indicators are a subset of the more than 60 indicators that are calculated and available.

The dashboard shows at a glance whether the goal is being met. The risk-adjusted year-to-date mortality rate as of December was 1.16, which is higher than the threshold (an internally defined baseline), the goal, and a stretch goal. Since the desired direction is down and the current rate is higher than system leaders desire, the labels are in red, indicating that the system hospitals are not meeting the goal. This high-level chart provides leaders with information about progress or the lack thereof.

The complex statistics and analytics that underlie the dashboard are invisible to the user, who sees a flexible web tool that reveals specific information about variables. Today's dashboard reflects quality measurements that are

FIGURE 8.10. RISK-ADJUSTED MORTALITY INDEX

Quality and Safety Vector of Measures

⦿ Dashboard   ◯ Tutorial   ◯ Download

⦿ Overview   ◯ Performance Details

YTD as of	Indicator Name	YTD	Threshold	Goal	Stretch Goal	Desired Direction
Dec 2012	Risk Adjusted Mortality Index	1.16	◉ 1.09	◉ 1.06	◉ 1.00	
Nov 2012	Risk Adjusted Readmission Index	1.08	● 1.00	● 0.98	● 0.96	⬊
Nov 2012	Risk Adjusted HF Readmission Index	1.01	● 1.00	● 1.00	● 0.97	⬊
Dec 2012	ICU Central Line-Associated BSI Index	0.90	◉ 1.27	◉ 1.23	◉ 1.20	⬊
Dec 2012	Non ICU Central Line-Associated BSI Index	0.99	● 1.80	● 1.75	● 1.71	⬊
Dec 2012	Abx Within 180 Minutes of Sepsis Identification Rate	75.65	◉ 75.00	● 80.00	● 90.00	⬈

Green = ◉   Red = ●

accessible and easily available to all stakeholders, from the governing body to the bedside worker, who can look at and analyze the data according to their priorities and interests by clicking on the performance details circle. The tool allows users to drill down and fine-tune the analysis of the measure, which increases accountability for improving problems.

Performance Details

From the main overall overview of the indicators page (Figure 8.10), a user can click on "performance detail" for a specific variable, such as non-ICU central line–associated BSI index, and a control chart showing month-by-month details of this infection can be accessed (see Figure 8.11).

Clicking on the "pivot" view (Figure 8.12) enables the user to do a comparison between two time periods, here 2012 and 2013–2014, for this specific variable. Figure 8.12 shows the trends for the year by month along with the average. If an intervention was introduced at the end of 2012, for example, this graph shows whether it was effective at lowering the incidence of this infection.

With the interactive dashboard, users have easy access to both general and highly specific information. Therefore, the dashboard has proved invaluable for understanding the delivery of care for everyone from the high-level system leaders to the specific end user, perhaps the infection control specialist at the individual hospital. With available dashboard reports, no one can say they had no idea, for example, that the infection rate at their hospital was increasing. Awareness of the measures, communicated via the dashboard throughout the organization, leads to monitoring and improvements.

FIGURE 8.11. NON-ICU CENTRAL LINE–ASSOCIATED BSI INDEX

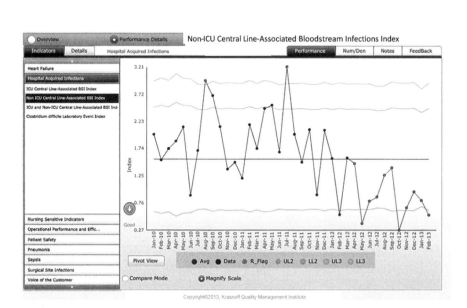

The dashboard is the end product of sophisticated and complex analysis that requires expertise, skill, and resources. The data have to be valid and reliable. Numerators and denominators have to be checked for missing values and updated regularly as circumstances change. The data need to be "cleaned" for missing or mistaken entries.

Measurements are not static. Denominators change as population characteristics change or become better understood. Circumstances change as well. Winter months may have an increase in pneumonia patients, perhaps especially elderly or unvaccinated patients; analysts watch these fluctuations and build them into the dashboards and control charts. The point of dashboards is to reflect care on an ongoing basis; viewers cannot compare months or see trends if the data are not cleaned and updated regularly.

The goal of producing and communicating measurements is to act on them in order to improve. Therefore. the right measure is required in order to have an impact. Although many measures are dictated from external sources, measures usually have to be developed within a hospital or health care organization as well.

FIGURE 8.12. NON-ICU CENTRAL LINE–ASSOCIATED BSI INDEX PIVOT VIEW

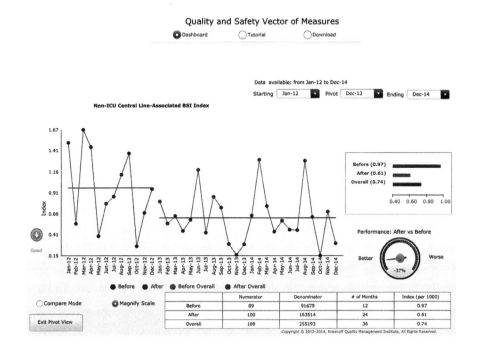

Safety and Environment of Care Measures

Many quality and safety measures are developed and monitored as part of the normal oversight of care, but some safety measures are really more administrative issues than clinical ones; for example, consider measures associated with the environment of care, equipment, and hazardous waste management. Administrators need to be aware of and supervise these safety measures in order to ensure a safe environment. It is a tremendous responsibility: ensuring that contractors for new construction build in such a way to maximize safety, ensuring that the fire safety is always in perfect working order, ensuring that safety officers interact with clinicians to understand the relevance of the environment to care.

The only way to ensure safety and prevent injuries is via measures. TJC and the Occupational Safety and Health Administration insist that safety be integrated into the oversight of care and not left up to safety officers or treated as an ancillary service.

Case Example: Monitoring Safety

For many years, the system in which we work has been measuring variables related to safety and reporting them to performance improvement committees. Among the measurements are variables related to: fire drills, such as success rates at meeting drill criteria; hazardous waste incidents; sharps injury rates; radiation safety; security; and others. These measures are reported quarterly (see Figure 8.13).

Along with the measures, detailed narratives about these safety measures are provided, articulating what happened and what was done to correct or improve any issues. In each of these monitored categories, the number of incidents is given; that number is compared to the same quarter for the previous year; explanations for these incidents are also included. For example, a narrative for occupational safety incidents might read:

> There were 38 occupational safety related injuries during the 1st quarter, a slight increase when compared to the previous quarter (which was 35) and more than the previous-year quarterly average (32). The leading cause of injury was Patient Handling (10), and the leading type of injury was Contusion/Bruise (13). Rehabilitation Unit was the department with the most claims during this reporting period (4). Regional risk management, XYZ Insurance Company, and the Ergonomic and Safety Committees continue efforts to reduce employee injuries.

Another example from emergency management plan activation:

> There was 1 incident requiring activation of the HEICS (Hospital Emergency Incident Command System) during the 3rd quarter. A worker used gasoline as a tar solvent while installing a skylight in the ED construction area. This work was directly upwind from the main intake heating and ventilation duct for the east part of the ED, and fumes were ventilated into the ED. HEICS was activated at level 2. Patients were evacuated. Ventilation fans were installed. There were no adverse patient outcomes. Opportunities for improvement were identified and are in process of implementation.

This impressive specificity of detail about one variable is repeated for each and every variable. Therefore, a filter system is necessary so that reports to senior leaders and the board of trustees are not simply compendiums of overwhelming information.

A special high-level committee, the Joint Conference Professional Affairs Committee for Safety and Environment of Care, chaired by a member of the board of trustees and comprised of other board members, senior quality professionals, safety experts, and clinicians, met monthly; reports to the committee were compiled monthly, and minutes and agendas were distributed.

This structure enabled concurrent ongoing oversight of the environment and a multidisciplinary approach to solving problems and implementing improvements. For example, a patient undergoing a magnetic resonance

FIGURE 8.13. SAFETY SERVICES QUARTERLY REPORT

Campus: Hospital A

Quarter: First

	ENVIRONMENT OF CARE PERFORMANCE INDICATORS	PREVIOUS YEAR PERFORMANCE	THIS QUARTER PERFORMANCE
1	**Fire/Life Safety** Drills	25 Drills Failure Rate = 6.6%	6 Drills Failure Rate = 2.3%
2	**Fire/Life Safety** Incidents	65	17
3	**Hazardous Materials** Incidents	16	3
4	**Emergency Management** Plan Activation	4 Plan Activations (2 Internal/2 External)	2 Plan Activations (1 Internal/1 External)
5	**Environment of Care** Knowledge/Awareness	89.5%	97%
6	**Safety Management** Sharps Injuries	161	30
7	**Security Management** Incidents	504	134
8	**Equipment Management** Incidents	4	1
9	**Utility Systems Management** Incidents	8	3
10	**Radiation Safety** Incidents	7	2
11	**Occupational Safety & Health** Incidents	694	163
12	**Occupational Safety** Lost Time (Days)	2,565	729

imaging (MRI) test complained of a burning sensation. Investigation revealed that her tattooed eyeliner was causing the problem. As a response, the questionnaire for patients undergoing such tests was updated to include this kind of information in order to avoid similar problems in the future. The reports of measures and the communication structures that we developed is more proactive than reactive. Therefore, many problems that are considered clinical but tied into the environment, such as infections, falls, and pressure injuries, can be concurrently reviewed.

More than a decade ago, the chair of the Joint Conference Professional Affairs Committee for Safety and Environment of Care reminded clinicians on the committee how important it was to take the environment seriously. He commented that when he was a pilot in World War II, checklists were used for every take-off and landing and for other complex procedures. He said pilots are often asked why they use checklists and health care practitioners are reluctant to do so. He responded that it's because the pilot gets on the plane as well as the passengers.

Linking Environmental and Clinical Variables

Although perhaps not immediately obvious, distinctions between clinical and environmental variables can be blurred, and a savvy administrator needs to understand how the environment of care has an impact on clinical processes and outcomes. When TJC surveyors examine a hospital for accreditation, they even examine whether the ice machine on patient floors have been cleaned appropriately; every aspect of the environment is examined because of the influence on safe patient care.

For example, it is important to monitor and measure whether the ORs are safe, and that safety has to be checked continuously. Not only do ORs have to be sterile; the equipment has to be mounted and secured properly. For hospital turnover to be efficient, bed cleaning processes need to be speedy and effective. Administrators need to know how to prioritize resources. If infection rates are an issue, then the environment of care has to be constantly monitored for sterility and other safe practices.

Another example: Until quite recently, patients who contracted the infection MRSA (methicillin-resistant *Staphylococcus aureus*) were in rooms with two or three patients. It was not until the infection rates went up that analysis of the problem revealed how contagious the infection could be. Now patients with MRSA are placed in private rooms, a relatively simple and commonsense approach that was instituted because leaders became aware of the rising infection rate.

Monitoring the environment is in no way a new activity. Florence Nightingale understood the crucial relationship between the environment and infection and wrote about it over 100 years ago. She recognized that unless the environment was sterile and well ventilated, patient care would be compromised. In other words, the environment changes as clinical information is updated. An administrative leader does not want to wait for an incident to occur before examining the environment of care for safety gaps. Monitoring measures on an ongoing basis enables administration to target and prioritize vulnerable areas.

In addition, employee satisfaction and injuries are dependent in large part on the safety of the environment. Employees may be unable to work due to workplace injuries. Being proactive about safety can help to avoid potential problems. For example, employees can be allergic to latex and their health can be affected; once this is recognized, new policies to be latex free can be established. Fewer allergies result in greater productivity, and less waste, for the workforce.

Summary

Measurements are critical to understanding the delivery of care and for improvements. However, there are many issues involved in collecting appropriate data, reporting information on dashboards, and meeting required benchmarks for defined measures. Among these are:

- understanding how patients (consumers) use measurements to evaluate health care services;
- using process measures as indicators of effective and efficient care;
- monitoring safety and avoiding errors through measuring good processes and identifying gaps in care;
- using dashboards to communicate effectively about the delivery of care;
- interpreting measures, such as patient satisfaction, by carefully analyzing the details of how care is delivered to specific populations; and
- linking the environment of care to improved clinical outcomes and greater efficiency.

Key Terms

adverse drug reactions, dashboards, dependent variable, hypothesis, independent variable, mortality rates, outcome measures, outpatient measures, performance measures, quantitative information, satisfaction measures, structure measures, value-based purchasing

Quality Concepts in Action

Research shows that poor communication results in adverse events and patient harm. Health care organizations are in the midst of changing channels of communication, moving away from handwritten progress notes to EHRs, moving away from hierarchies and silos to multidisciplinary teams, objectifying care processes and outcomes with database reports and dashboards. They are being subject to penalties and rewards based on Hospital Compare and the Hospital Consumer Assessment of Healthcare Providers and Systems (HCAHPS). As a senior administrator working in this changing environment, how would you encourage acceptance of these new modes of communication? Would you:

- attempt to convince the CEO to introduce educational programs to senior staff about the advantages of new communication styles and techniques?
- collaborate with quality management analysts to produce data reports and dashboards that would serve as the bases for information forums for unit managers and department heads?
- introduce clinical guidelines or care pathways so that multidisciplinary information is communicated?
- establish a formal communication and accountability structure with monthly reports and multidisciplinary meetings?

Explain the advantages and disadvantages of each of these possibilities, and articulate a formal plan (with time lines) for success.

References

Batalden, P. B., and J. J. Mohr. 1999. "An Invitation from Florence Nightingale: Come Learn About Improving Health Care." In *Joint Commission on Accreditation of Healthcare Organizations,* Florence Nightingale: Measuring Hospital Care Outcomes, pp. 11–16. Oakbrook Terrace, IL: Author.

Dlugacz, Y. D. 2011. "Medication Safety Improvement." In P. L. Spath, ed., *Error Reduction in Health Care: A System's Approach to Improving Patient Safety,* 2nd ed., pp. 335–368. San Francisco: Jossey-Bass.

"Health Policy Brief: Pay-for-Performance." 2012, October 11. *Health Affairs.*

Iezzoni, L. I. 1996. "100 Apples Divided by 15 Red Herrings: A Cautionary Tale from the Mid-19th Century on Comparing Hospital Mortality Rates." *Annals of Internal Medicine* 124 (12): 1079–1085.

Institute of Medicine of the National Academies. 2006. *Preventing Medication Errors: Quality Chasm Series.* Washington, DC National Academies Press.

Institute of Medicine of the National Academies. 2007. *Rewarding Provider Performance: Aligning Incentives in Medicare. Pathways to Quality Health Care Series.* Washington, DC: National Academies Press.

Institute of Medicine of the National Academies. 2013. *Best Care at Lower Cost: The Path to Continuously Learning Health Care in America.* Washington, DC: National Academies Press.

Manary, M. P., W. Boulding, R. Staelin, and S. W. Glickman. 2013. "The Patient Experience and Health Outcomes." *New England Journal of Medicine* 368: 201–203.

Radley, D. C., M. R. Wasserman, L. E. W. Olsho, S. J. Shoemaker, M. D. Spranca, and B. Bradshaw. 2013. "Reduction in Medication Errors in Hospitals Due to Adoption of Computerized Provider Order Entry Systems." *Journal of the American Medical Informatics Association* 20 (3): 470–476.

Suggestions for Further Reading

Committee on Quality of Health Care in America, Institute of Medicine. 2001. *Crossing the Quality Chasm: A New Health System for the 21st Century.* Washington, DC: National Academies Press.

Picardi, C. A., and K. D. Masick. 2013. *Research Methods: Designing and Conducting Research with a Real-World Focus.* Thousand Oaks, CA: Sage.

Useful Websites

http://www.cdc.gov/HAI/bsi/bsi.html

http://www.cdc.gov/HAI/pdfs/bsi/checklist-for-CLABSI.pdf

http://www.dartmouthatlas.org/

https://www.heart.org/HEARTORG/HealthcareResearch/GetWithTheGuidelines/Get-With-The-Guidelines-Stroke_UCM_306098_SubHomePage.jsp

https://www.medicare.gov/hospitalcompare/compare.html

http://www.rwjf.org/en/how-we-work/grants/grantees/OpenNotes.html

CHAPTER NINE

TRANSLATING INFORMATION INTO ACTION

Chapter Outline

Key Concepts

- Understand how quality data are used for performance improvement.
- Determine effective methods for managing throughput and alleviating bottlenecks.
- Define appropriate levels of care for end-of-life patients.

- Recognize the clinical, financial, and quality issues related to mortality.
- Analyze issues related to readmission.
- Communicate the value of measures throughout the organization.

Among the most important questions for leaders and managers to address is when to use data and for what purpose. Should data be used for decision making, to monitor processes, to ensure compliance, for improvement? Is the investment in data collection and analysis activities worthwhile? Are patients healthier and safer because of the data collection and analysis? Data also underline transparency, and is this a good thing? Is the public sufficiently educated to interpret information about services and quality accurately? What is the end result of collecting, analyzing, interpreting, and reporting quality measures and measures related to staffing, resource consumption, efficiency, and the patient experience?

Of course one wants the answers to all these questions to be: yes, the data are used for improvements and considered decision making, to ensure patient safety, and to monitor processes. In reality, however, managers have to create the time and space to consider the importance of measures and of translating the measures into meaningful change. If they are expected to review the data reports and act on them, as opposed to file them or pass them along, they should see the benefit to them or to the patients, departments, and staff that they manage. Realistically, most managers are juggling so many issues and concerns that they have little opportunity to evaluate why they are collecting data; they do it because they are supposed to do it. Unless the data reports drive leaders to actually look at processes and proactively develop improvements, they will not be able to see the big picture and will spend their days reacting to crises and putting out fires one at a time.

It is important for managers and leaders to determine which data they want to collect; therefore, they need to understand issues related to efficiency, appropriateness of care, and patient satisfaction. Using a series of examples, this chapter discusses how to implement improvements based on data that have been collected and analyzed and illustrates how quality data can be applied for performance improvement in various diverse scenarios.

Maximizing Efficiency

Among the purposes of collecting data and developing and reporting analytics is to evaluate care and take proactive steps to prevent a crisis from occurring, if possible. Today data analytics are forced on organizations from the top down, from the government to governance, from senior leaders to middle managers, to the caregivers on the floor. However, information should also simultaneously move from the bedside to the top management, reverse the flow as it were so that information is not a club to batter managers with poor results but becomes a tool for improvement. And with even more information coming via electronic health records, bedside workers and managers need to be prepared to use analytics to better perform their responsibilities.

For example, if an administrator is responsible for care and services at a 700-bed hospital, with 40 unit/department managers, how is information organized for effectiveness, and how should that information be used? Often a graph or control chart shows senior executives some data or information, but then no interpretation or action is taken. Health care executives would do well to model themselves on Jack Welch, who insisted that every employee in GE (General Electric) adopt a new mode of thinking about services and improvements or they would be replaced—not just the managers but the line workers as well. The core of the issue is that there should be an expectation that everyone makes meaningful use of data.

Throughput

Many managers prioritize efficient throughput, a term that has been borrowed from the telecommunications industry to refer to the flow of service. Understanding waiting time and patient flow is essential because it has to do with timely access to care, one of the foci of the 2001 Committee on Quality of Health Care in America and Institute of Medicine report, *Crossing the Quality Chasm: A New Health System for the 21st Century*, to improve the delivery of safe and efficient health care services. In the health care context, throughput means moving patients, and the information that accompanies them, through the health care system efficiently.

A patient enters the health care system at point 1 in time. Once in the system, the patient moves from one level of care to another, point 2, and then hopefully via a smooth and efficient discharge back to home or the community, point 3 (see Figure 9.1). At any of these three points in time, the system can break down and the efficiency of the flow can be interrupted.

Throughput is important because bottlenecks in the system that have developed over the years can create problems for patients who are being transitioned from one point to another in the health care organization or from the organization into the community, impairing patient care and safety.

To deal with issues of efficient throughput, computers manage the flow of patients, especially from the emergency department (ED) to the floor because communication between managers is often inefficient, creating bottlenecks. Computers theoretically take the burden away from head nurses. But the question needs to be asked: Who is managing the process? The people behind the computers who have access to the facts and the numbers—the data—or the

FIGURE 9.1. THROUGHPUT

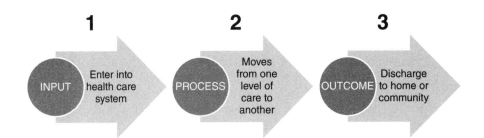

manager on the floor or in the ED? Also, evidence is still not clear regarding whether introducing computers to improve throughput has actually improved throughput.

Bottlenecks

The more complex the system, with multiple processes, the more likely there are to be bottlenecks at some point, resulting in delays or extended wait times. Managers have to not only identify where in the process the constraint or bottleneck exists—that is, the weakest point in the process—but to develop plans to fix the problem. More resources can be applied (more staff), resources can be shifted around, or some other solution can be found. The point is that the focus of improvement efforts is on the process bottlenecks. If the constraints are removed or reduced, process flow will improve.

It is not effective or efficient care to delay treatment due to nonclinical issues. For example, if an inpatient requires radiological tests, and the information is documented and communicated effectively, the patient has to be transferred from the bed, transported to the radiology unit, and back again. If turnaround time in radiology is delayed, then the patient has to wait, sometimes in a hallway. Likewise, if communication and coordination among the unit and radiology and transport are not effective, then the patient may not be ready, or be ready and waiting for a time, delaying treatment. There are many opportunities for throughput to break down: The physician has to order the test; the nurse has to implement the order and communicate with radiology; radiology has to collect the patient; and the whole system has to be efficiently reversed. Then information from radiology—the test results—has to be communicated to the physician. Some organizations have hired people, so-called navigators, to help smooth these kinds of transitions. It would be more effective to analyze the bottlenecks for cause and repair the faulty processes.

Theory of Constraints

Awareness of the importance of bottlenecks and the difficulty in managing them has given rise to many theories, including the theory of constraints (TOC) and practical solutions, such as Six Sigma. In order to manage throughput effectively, bottlenecks to seamless process flow have to be identified. The TOC, developed for manufacturing, posits that organizational **silos**—an organization working with separate, unintegrated parts—will have barriers to success, improvement, and change. The TOC calls this a core constraint (Breen, Burton-Houle, and Aron 2002).

To improve a system or process, the barriers to a holistic approach need to be identified and removed. The TOC can be applied to strategic planning, understanding processes, defining services, and improving quality and value as well as to employee and patient satisfaction. The goal of the TOC is ongoing improvement, and there is no improvement without the willingness to change. The TOC stresses reducing variability in processes and creating measurements to track and monitor improvements in processes and services. Regardless of what the theory is called, the principle is quite similar to traditional tenets of quality management.

In quality management terms, a root cause analysis is conducted to determine where and why a process is stalled or blocked, and then improvement efforts are implemented. In health care, we talk about the consequences of working in independent silos and attempt to bridge the spaces in between, enlisting multidisciplinary teams to work together to enhance communication between different disciplines and create buy-in for improvements. Various solutions have been attempted, including hiring consultants trained in GE, Six Sigma specialists, human engineering, and others. The fact is that health care is organized in such a complex fashion that bottlenecks, constraints, inefficiencies and variability are almost inevitable.

Traditional silos, a mind-set that keeps departments or sectors independent and cut off from others and prevents them from sharing information, need to be overcome in order to enhance throughput; eliminating the silo mentality may require a cultural and organizational transformation. Certainly it is easier to do one's job in the confines of a silo. Taking responsibility for ensuring that information gets moved to the next silo is a challenge.

For example, if a physician recommends a consultation with a specialist, the patient might or might not make the appointment; and if the patient makes the appointment and actually keeps it, it is not always ensured that the referring physician gets the information back from the specialist, closing the loop. Implementing EHRs will resolve some of these issues, but unless the silo culture is changed, communication gaps will result in problems, delays, and adverse outcomes.

Improvement should not just be a project but internalized as part of daily routine. The Institute for Healthcare Improvement stresses the importance of a collaborative approach, encouraging organizations to change perspective from the silo mind-set, which believes that "others" cause problems, to more systemic or holistic points of view in which each person understands that the entire system has to work together to improve (http://www.ihi.org/resources/Pages/ImprovementStories/BetterPatientFlowMeansBreakingDowntheSilos.aspx).

Queueing Theory

It is important to think about how to manage throughput and patient flow because health care processes can be riddled with delays, and those delays may have an impact on patient care and satisfaction and on organizational and financial efficiency. Health care is in many ways unpredictable and variable, which makes the mechanics of efficient throughput difficult to manage. Patient needs are unpredictable and can interrupt normal routines; demands on clinicians' time are also variable, as are medical services.

Queueing theory, which is a mathematical model of queues (waiting in line) developed in the early 20th century, has been applied to issues involved in balancing services and demand. It has been used to understand and improve traffic flow and to provide timelier customer service. Based on a complex mathematical model, queueing theory accounts for customer demand, rates of service, waiting time, and variation in demand and service capacity. Cost considerations are also factored into the equation.

In health care, queueing theory offers insight into how to manage the steps in the flow of events, from arrival, through services, taking into account how many people are involved, how many processes are involved, how many places patients have to access, and how many providers are available. The model is useful for understanding issues such as supply and demand (ED beds, staffing), priority queues such as for transplant (organ allocation), and scheduling appointments (Gupta 2013).

When the system works well, patients flow through each phase of the process easily and without delay. But when the process becomes disrupted or blocked, patients can accumulate and experience delays. Queueing is obviously minimized when patient flow is good and maximized when it is not. Patients can experience delays at many points, as when tests, treatments, and discharge are not well coordinated or when clinicians are busy and overscheduled. If the queue becomes large, patients may deteriorate and may still need to be served by staff, creating extra work.

Hospital care is organized around specialized departments and services (radiology, surgery) and various types of units (ED, telemetry, floor units) and ancillary departments (admissions, housekeeping, transportation). A patient who enters the health care system via the ED may experience delays moving from one stage to another, such as waiting for tests, empty beds, specialized consultations, or discharge. Queues are affected by poor synchronization of services, inadequate communication among departments, and processes that may be inefficient. Queueing theory has been used to help manage ambulance deployment, critical care services, and bed and staff planning. Demand and service capacity cannot be exactly predicted because they all have variation. Therefore, there will always be wait times. Using performance measures to track patient flow leads to improvements. The measures help to quantify acceptable wait time from delays that are unacceptable and can help in planning for services.

The manager has to find the balance between providing appropriate services and keeping waiting times short. In contrast to waiting in lines for many other types of services, health services may not serve people according to how long they have been waiting but, in the ED, for example, by how acute is their emergency. Even if someone has been waiting for care in the ED for some time, if a patient with more urgent needs comes in later, he or she may be seen earlier. In private physician practices, increased demand may require that a patient be seen days later than desired. Again, collecting information and analyzing daily and aggregate data about how patients move through the health system is necessary to minimize queues and maximize quality care.

Case Example: Managing Throughput

When physicians at a local specialized hospital needed help in managing efficiency and throughput, quality analysts developed an interactive web-based tool to create databases that would help the physicians track the patient from entry through recovery. In addition to identifying bottlenecks, the tool also tracked time by type of surgery and by physicians performing the surgery so that hospital leaders could understand how care was delivered in the organization.

Figure 9.2 shows the data from which reports can be tailored. The patient is identified by name and age; the operating room (OR) is identified, as is the scheduled OR time. Throughput is chronicled from the time the patient arrived and registered, how much time elapsed in the ambulatory surgical unit (ASU), the time the patient was in holding and getting ready for surgery, the time the patient entered and left the OR, the time the patient entered and left the post acute care unit (PACU), and so on until discharge. The reason for the delay, if there is one, is coded. Caregivers and administrators have the capacity via the web tool to run specialized reports from these data. The time period can be specified from daily to monthly, the type of surgery can be specified and the particular measure, in this case wait time for the OR, can also be specified.

With this tool, physicians and administrators can see at a glance how many cases were performed each day, how many per surgical procedure, and how much time patients spent in the OR and in recovery and waiting for discharge.

FIGURE 9.2. AMBULATORY SURGERY LOG TRACKING

| PATIENT NAME | AGE | OR ROOM # | OR TIME | REGISTRATION | | ASU | HOLDING | | OR | |
				PATIENT ARRIVED	TIME REGISTERED	TIME IN TO ASU	TIME IN HOLDING	READY FOR SURGERY	TIME IN TO OR	TIME OUT OF OR
A	49	12	08:30: AM	06:36: AM	07:01: AM	07:03: AM	07:37: AM	07:37: AM	08:28: AM	09:35: AM
B	81	16	09:30: AM	07:23: AM	07:58: AM	08:00: AM	08:34: AM	08:41: AM	09:19: AM	09:54: AM
C	77	17	09:30: AM	07:18: AM	07:49: AM	07:53: AM	08:43: AM	09:15: AM	09:38: AM	10:28: AM
D	55	15	09:30: AM	08:37: AM	08:57: AM	09:00: AM	09:14: AM	09:27: AM	09:43: AM	10:26: AM
E	66	12a	09:30: AM	08:12: AM	08:31: AM	08:33: AM	08:55: AM	09:11: AM	09:29: AM	10:07: AM
F	52	10	10:00: AM	08:54: AM	09:52: AM	09:55: AM	10:07: AM	10:40: AM	11:01: AM	11:27: AM
G	27	4	10:15: AM	08:24: AM	08:33: AM	08:35: AM	09:11: AM	09:11: AM	10:24: AM	11:37: AM
H	41	15	10:15: AM	08:34: AM	08:50: AM	08:53: AM	09:40: AM	10:02: AM	10:52: AM	12:29: PM

| PATIENT NAME | AGE | OR ROOM # | OR TIME | PACU | | ASU | | DELAY DESCRIPTION |
				TIME IN TO PACU	TIME OUT OF PACU	TIME BACK TO ASU	TIME DISCHARGED	
A	49	12	08:30: AM	09:35: AM	11:40: AM	11:41: AM	12:47: PM	ADD ON CASE
B	81	16	09:30: AM			09:54: AM	10:25: AM	NO DELAY
C	77	17	09:30: AM			10:29: AM	11:18: AM	TRANSPORT PERSONNEL LATE OR UNAVAILABLE
D	55	15	09:30: AM	10:26: AM	12:40: PM	12:42: PM	01:28: PM	SURGEON LATE
E	66	12a	09:30: AM			10:05: AM	11:25: AM	NO DELAY
F	52	10	10:00: AM	11:29: AM	12:06: PM	12:08: PM	01:03: PM	SURGEON LATE
G	27	4	10:15: AM	11:37: AM	01:53: PM	01:55: PM	03:21: PM	ROOM NOT CLEAN
H	41	15	10:15: AM	12:29: PM	02:12: PM	02:14: PM	03:00: PM	PT HAS MULTIPLE QUESTIONS TO BE ANSWERED

These data offer invaluable information about efficiency and effectiveness of services. Technology, data, and, most important, leadership commitment result in improved care and efficiency.

Determining Appropriate Levels of Care

Efficiency involves more than moving patients across the continuum of care. Using hospital resources efficiently requires understanding the appropriate levels of care for patients with different needs. Clinical information, in the form of data, about chronic illness, sepsis, and readmissions gives us a better understanding about advanced illness, end of life, and mortality, and helps administrators and providers understand the importance of placing patients in the appropriate level of care, such as **palliative** and **hospice** services.

END-OF-LIFE TERMINOLOGY

End-of-life care refers to the care a patient receives in the last months of life, not only the medical care but also the social and emotional support that would improve quality of life.

Hospice care is care that focuses on managing symptoms in patients who are expected to live for no more than six months. Hospice care stresses providing comfort and quality of life to someone who is dying and provides an alternative to aggressive treatment, which is costly, often painful, and frequently unproductive and futile.

Palliative care is specialized medical care for people with serious illnesses. This type of care is focused on providing patients with relief from the symptoms, pain, and stresses of a serious illness—whatever the diagnosis or prognosis. The goal is to improve quality of life for both the patient and the family. Palliative care is provided by a team of doctors, nurses, and other specialists who work with the patient's other doctors to provide an extra layer of support. Unlike hospice care, palliative care is appropriate at any age and at any stage in a serious illness and can be provided together with traditional medical treatment and interventions.

End-of-Life Care/Advanced Illness

Specific criteria have been developed for palliative and hospice care for inpatients and outpatients, and those criteria must be met in order for the organization to receive reimbursement for treatment. For example, if an end-of-life patient's pain and symptoms cannot be managed at home, short-term hospital admission is available and appropriate. Or if the patient needs a higher level of nursing skill than is available in the home care setting, hospital admission is necessary. An interdisciplinary group, including a physician and a hospice medical director, makes this determination.

Having clear definitions and criteria means that end-of-life issues are no longer subjective or fuzzy. On the contrary. From a quality management point of view, placing patients in the appropriate level of care improves performance. With the data available that help to define advanced illness and with criteria established for appropriate levels of care, much of the subjectivity, as well as the emotional distress of trying to make end-of-life decisions, is reduced. Health professionals have moved from a focus on the disease and its treatment to a focus on patients and their needs and how they would be best served. That is patient-centered, rather than treatment-centered, care.

By using data, analysis has evolved from noting the volume of mortalities to a more nuanced understanding of why people die, which people die, and what treatment options and levels of care are most appropriate at end of life. The result of the analysis is performance improvement, delivering appropriate care at the appropriate level to the appropriate patient. Without appropriate data, there would be no way to define these concepts. Not only is this good medicine, but it is the only way to remain financially viable.

Improving end-of-life care would go a long way to achieving the quality and value objectives that are basic to health care reform. Palliative care programs and hospice care are designed to deliver patient- and family-centered care that improves such quality outcomes as pain management, communication, satisfaction, and reduced costs.

The Reform Mandate

The basic goal of health care reform is to improve the quality of care while lowering costs. With the aging of the patient population, many of whom have chronic illnesses and multiple health issues, the financial burden is enormous and growing. Interestingly, even with so much money spent, there is little evidence that the quality of care is especially good. Studies have shown that despite spending more per capita on health care than any other nation, seriously ill patients in the United States receive poor medical care and little social support (Thorpe and Howard 2006, http://www.commonwealthfund.org/publications/issue-briefs/2015/oct/us-health-care-from-a-global-perspective).

Determining appropriate end-of-life care is not simple, especially because it is not uncommon for patients and physicians to have different treatment goals. When surveyed, patients reported that at the end of life, they want pain control, symptom management, to avoid treatments that would prolong dying, to have a sense of control, and to relieve the burden on loved ones (Singer, Martin, and Kelner 1999). The health care reform legislation originally included mandating physician-patient discussions about the value of interventions versus hospice for end-of-life care. However, inflamed by politicians and others who mistakenly claimed that these discussions would be "death panels," encouraging the elderly sick to go into hospice rather than have expensive treatments, the provision was deleted from the Accountable Care Act.

Nonetheless, health care policy leaders are aware that palliative and hospice care are necessary for effective and efficient patient-centered quality care. Many states have taken steps to improve end-of-life care because the quality of care is so poor and the cost of poor care is so high. As an example, New York State passed end-of-life legislation, the Palliative Care Information Act, effective 2011, which ensures that patients are fully informed of the options available to them when they are faced with a terminal illness or condition so that they are empowered to make choices consistent with their goals for care and their wishes and beliefs, and can optimize their quality of life.

Understanding Mortality

Issues surrounding end of life and advanced illness focus attention on appropriateness of care because many seriously ill patients require sophisticated services and expensive resources. But not everyone does, and not always. Therefore, it is important for administrative and clinical leaders to understand how to best manage advanced disease and end-of-life care.

Although it might seem that everyone understands what the terms *end of life* or *advanced illness* means, the definitions are not straightforward. According to the American Hospital Association (AHA) (2012), advanced illness management is vital to support today's care and business models. The AHA defines advanced illness as "occurring when one or more conditions become serious enough that general health and functioning decline, and treatments begin to lose their impact. This is a process that continues to the end-of-life." Nonetheless, studies show that managing advanced illness leads to improved quality of life; higher patient and family satisfaction; and decreased utilization of medical services, fewer hospital admissions, and reduced costs. It pays to manage well.

The AHA defines four phases involved in advanced illness (see Figure 9.3): In Phase 1, patients are healthy or have reversible illnesses. They can discuss advanced directives and have conversations about their wishes or, if they are unable to make decisions, appropriate legal documentation can be provided. Palliative care may be introduced to better quality of life. In Phase 2, patients

FIGURE 9.3. ADVANCED ILLNESS

PHASE 1	PHASE 2	PHASE 3	PHASE 4
Patients are healthy or have reversible illnesses.	Patients are still involved in active curative treatment but may be suffering from chronic conditions.	Patients have advanced disease with frequent complications.	Patients are eligible for hospice care with the prognosis of six months or less to live.

Curative -> Palliative are still involved in active curative treatment but may be suffering from chronic conditions. In Phase 3, patients have advanced disease with frequent complications. Treatment may also incorporate palliative care. And finally, in Phase 4, patients are eligible for hospice care, which means they have a prognosis of six months or less to live. As patients move through these phases, the delivery of care changes: Treatment is more palliative than curative and, in the final phase, incorporates psychosocial factors and comprehensive support to the family through the bereavement process.

The Centers for Medicare and Medicaid Services (CMS) encourages organizations to reduce mortality rates, but doing so requires having patients in Phases 1 and 2, rather than in Phases 3 and 4, when dying is inevitable. From a quality management point of view, risk-adjusted mortality data can and should be used to help define end of life (in the AHA scheme, Phases 3 and 4). Understanding the definition helps to separate mortality as a clinical issue from mortality that occurs as a natural progression of illness.

The purpose of analyzing mortality data is to provide patients at the end of life with appropriate care. Often patients who are very sick come to hospitals to die, usually from nursing homes. They do not require intensive services yet may be placed in intensive care units (ICUs). Some patients who are expected to recover die unexpectedly. Their mortality may need to be analyzed further to understand causation. Mortality is not a single unified category but should be considered a complex one that requires careful definitions.

The health care reform payment model requires a hospital culture that is focused on improving processes and efficiencies, with a better understanding of patient characteristics and disease management across the continuum, with improved understanding of different levels of care for appropriate treatment, with attention to end-of-life issues, and that is affiliated and collaborates with community health care organizations.

Financial Implications

End-of-life care is not only concerned with protecting patients from excessive pain and suffering and futile interventions; it is also of great financial consequence to health care organizations. Quality data play an important role in understanding end-of-life care issues and monitoring efficiencies. A focus on mortality forces organizations to examine their patient populations in order to reduce hospitalizations by providing preventive care and community services as much as possible. With better management, especially of palliative care patients, hospital resources can be expended more appropriately.

Ideally, understanding the characteristics of the patient population would help define the appropriate level of care for each patient (in hospital or community) and help the administration realize the levels of care required to best serve the patient population. Hospitals should work with nursing homes to provide services (such as medication administration) in order to keep patients, especially palliative ones, in the community. Prevention efforts would also reduce hospitalizations for patients who are not acute and can be treated without inpatient services. Hospitals must begin to develop partnerships with assisted living facilities, pharmacies, and community urgent care centers. In the health care reform environment, the hospital is no longer the sole locus of care.

Under the old payment systems, the more services and expensive treatments provided to patients, the greater the payment to the hospital. Many end-of-life patients have multiple specialists caring for them and expensive interventions. However, there is no evidence that intense interventions and specialized treatment lead to lower mortality rates (http://www .dartmouthatlas.org/data/topic/topic.aspx?cat=18).

Under the reformed payment system, with bundled payments, shared risk for disease management, and value-based purchasing programs, unnecessary and expensive treatments result in reduced payment to health organizations. Since 2014, the CMS has used mortality rates to determine hospital payments under the Affordable Care Act value-based purchasing program. Since mortality is now evaluated as an outcome measure on which payment is based, with either rewards or penalties, better disease management and more careful assessment of the value of interventions, especially at the end of life, are encouraged.

Financial considerations should highlight the appropriateness of services rendered. If comfort care is what is most appropriate and desired by the patient/family, then unwanted treatments and procedures may be an overutilization or inappropriate utilization of services. At the end of life especially, traditional treatment involves all kinds of last-ditch efforts and various specialized consultations. But is that valuable for the patient, and is it organizationally and economically sound? Financial administrators need to be able to assess the value of care for end-of-life patients. For example, for an end-stage patient with a chronic disease, is dialysis appropriate, or is there too much risk involved for potentially little return? Answers to these difficult and complex questions depend on objective quality data.

The new bundled payment program involves shared risk. If the risk of mortality is high and ICU care due to complications from treatments or procedures is expensive, how does a professional evaluate whether to recommend treatment? Proper utilization returns the best reimbursement, which means that administrators as well as clinicians need to be educated about alternatives and to work together to define criteria for levels of care. With better management and more sophisticated analytics that can predict outcomes as much as possible, questions about what processes to improve and which patients are at the end of life need to be addressed.

It should be noted that many health care leaders have reservations about using mortality rates as an index for quality care. The pressure for low rates and thus higher payments may result in hospitals focusing on their coding practices, which has nothing to do with improving quality of care. Or due to pressure to have lower reported mortality rates, physicians may be reluctant to treat high-risk patients, or they may recommend that palliative care patients be treated in the community or in hospice. Since palliative care can be associated with treatments and curative therapy, even though there is an expectation of death, mortality may not reveal quality of care. Moreover, in many hospitals, patients have to elect hospice care rather than traditional care on their first day of admission. Due to financial and regulatory pressure, physicians may not recommend inpatient care for high-risk patients. Forcing early referral to hospice may not serve all patients well.

Mortality Data

Since mortality measures are becoming critical to financial well-being, it is an ongoing discussion whether end-of-life patients should be included in mortality measures, since by definition they are going to die. Typically hospice patients are considered as being on a separate level of care and are excluded from mortality calculations. However. palliative care patients represent a kind of gray area and are usually included in mortality calculations.

Physicians who have reservations about using mortality as an index of quality care say that using an all-cause 30-day mortality posthospital discharge is somewhat arbitrary; the thinking is that this time period assumes a causal relation between hospitalization and outcome that may or may not be the case. Also, using mortality as a measure assumes that following the specific standardized recommendations from the CMS will have an impact on short-term mortality; some physicians find this too simplistic. The underlying assumption behind using mortality as an outcome measure is the notion that hospital-related deaths are preventable, which is also an unproved assumption.

From a quality management point of view, risk-adjusted 30-day mortality rates have to be reliably measured and reported to leaders in order to meet expectations and receive maximum reimbursement. Processes have to be analyzed in order to understand the causes of mortality. People can die for many reasons: inappropriate interventions, too many interventions, mishap, or to the natural process of the disease. Health care organizations need to understand the characteristics of patients who die. It is important to understand why people die and why they die at one time and not at another, later time.

Therefore, unit managers have to investigate why people on their unit die. They need to assess whether the protocols are adequate to prevent harm, to determine whether (re)education of staff is necessary to maximize safety, and to evaluate whether the delivery of care is appropriate. Using multidisciplinary teams to analyze mortality can provide an understanding of the cause of death and about the appropriate level of care for expired patients. With the help of data analytics to address these issues, improvements can be embedded into the culture.

Also, from a quality management perspective, processes of care have to be analyzed across the entire continuum of care, from the community to the hospital and back into the community. Transitions need to be smooth, communication must be effective, and high-risk points have to be identified for improvements. Mortality as an outcome measure should lead to analysis of processes that may result in unnecessary mortality and to improvements. When cardiac surgery mortality rates were high in the hospital system in which we work, analysis showed that better postoperative ICU care and close observation by intensivists, as well as improved sterile procedures and better medication management, reduced mortality. In other words, investigating causes of mortality should lead to improved processes.

Improving ICU Care

Mortality is best understood by collecting and analyzing objective information about patients who die. The **APACHE** system is a tool that analyzes ICU patients, including their risk of dying. APACHE is an acronym for Acute Physiology, Age, and Chronic Health Evaluation; APACHE provides data on each patient's clinical characteristics, demographics, severity of illness (acuity), appropriate levels of care, and patient outcomes (see Chapter 5).

If a patient is at low risk for dying and also requires low-risk monitoring, an administrator may well ask why that patient is placed in the ICU. If a patient has a high risk of dying (due to the progression of a disease process) but requires low monitoring (few services), perhaps that patient would be better served on a palliative care unit. If a patient was at low risk for dying and died, further investigation might be valuable to understand causation. By stratifying and objectifying mortality risk and need of services, leaders gain useful information about levels of care and can better evaluate resource allocation.

Case Example: Introducing APACHE

When leaders in the hospital system in which we work wanted to ensure that the ICUs were being used effectively and efficiently, quality management and clinical leaders introduced the APACHE system. Every ICU—critical care, medical, surgical, cardiothoracic, neonatal—in the system receives its own APACHE report on a monthly basis as part of the Quality and Safety Vector of Measures Dashboard. Figure 9.4 shows an excerpt from a yearly report of the medical ICU (MICU) at one of the system's hospitals. Because this ICU is medical, the primary admitting diagnoses involve sepsis. In the critical care unit, the top admitting diagnoses are different and may involve heart issues, such as acute myocardial infarction, congestive heart failure, unstable angina,

FIGURE 9.4. APACHE REPORTS

APACHE IV Monthly Report for MICU
May 2014 –May 2015

	Total	May-14	Jun-14	Jul-14	Aug-14	Sep-14	Oct-14	Nov-14	Dec-14	Jan-15	Feb-15	Mar-15	Apr-15	May-15
Number of ICU Patient Encounters	1,193	105	81	83	94	98	102	85	89	93	83	92	90	98
Number of ICU Stays	1,267	113	86	89	97	103	106	93	100	100	85	99	96	100
ICU Stays with APACHE IV Predictions	1,231	113	84	82	95	99	102	92	98	97	82	97	93	97
Average Age of ICU Patients	68	67	68	68	70	68	68	70	71	68	69	68	66	68
Average APACHE Score	76.18	77.5	72.2	78.3	75.5	80.4	76.7	80.0	70.1	78.7	78.2	78.6	75.5	68.5

	Total	May-14	Jun-14	Jul-14	Aug-14	Sep-14	Oct-14	Nov-14	Dec-14	Jan-15	Feb-15	Mar-15	Apr-15	May-15
72 Hour ICU Readmissions	27	3	2	3	2	2	1	3	3	1	1	1	3	2

Note: In-hospital readmissions are given new APACHE IV predictions for the ICU only. External readmissions are given new APACHE IV predictions for the ICU & Hospital.

Top 5 APACHE IVa Admitting Diagnoses (N = 1,267 ICU Stays)	Number	Percent
Sepsis, pulmonary	257	20%
Sepsis, renal/UTI (including bladder)	125	9%
Cardiac arrest (with or without respiratory arrest; for respiratory arrest see Respirato	75	5%
Sepsis, GI	63	4%
Bleeding, upper GI	56	4%

ICU Raw Mortality Rate & Actual to Predicted ICU Mortality Ratio   N = 1,231 ICU Stays

	Total	May-14	Jun-14	Jul-14	Aug-14	Sep-14	Oct-14	Nov-14	Dec-14	Jan-15	Feb-15	Mar-15	Apr-15	May-15
Raw ICU Mortality Rate %	16.4	14.2	14.0	16.9	17.5	17.5	19.8	20.4	14.0	19.0	21.2	18.2	13.5	8.0
Actual to Predicted Mortality Ratio	0.70	0.65	0.80	0.51	0.66	0.82	0.80	0.80	0.80	0.76	0.84	0.76	0.56	0.37

ICU Ventilator Days: Actual Average & Actual to Predicted Vent. Day Ratio   N = 686 ICU Stays

	Total	May-14	Jun-14	Jul-14	Aug-14	Sep-14	Oct-14	Nov-14	Dec-14	Jan-15	Feb-15	Mar-15	Apr-15	May-15
Actual Average Vent. Days	4.3	4.5	4.3	4.4	4.4	5.1	3.9	3.3	4.1	5.2	4.3	4.2	5.1	3.3
Average Predicted Vent. Days	4.2	4.1	4.4	4.4	3.9	4.3	4.0	4.2	4.3	4.2	4.4	4.0	4.0	4.1
Actual to Predicted Vent. Ratio	1.03	1.02	1.05	1.00	1.12	1.18	0.98	0.79	0.95	1.23	0.96	1.05	1.29	0.80

ICU Stays by Risk Level of Predicted Hospital Mortality
Low Risk: <10% Hospital Mortality   Medium Risk: 10-50% Hospital Mortality   High Risk: >50% Hospital Mortality

	Total	May-14	Jun-14	Jul-14	Aug-14	Sep-14	Oct-14	Nov-14	Dec-14	Jan-15	Feb-15	Mar-15	Apr-15	May-15
Low Predicted Risk ICU Stays	332	26	22	19	27	26	31	20	27	24	21	19	33	37
Medium Predicted Risk ICU Stays	537	51	46	36	38	42	38	43	47	39	36	48	33	40
High Predicted Risk ICU Stays	267	23	11	21	27	24	26	21	11	26	23	19	19	16

Low Risk Monitor: <10% Predicted Hospital Mortality & No ICU Intervention   N = 1,136 ICU Stays

	Total	May-14	Jun-14	Jul-14	Aug-14	Sep-14	Oct-14	Nov-14	Dec-14	Jan-15	Feb-15	Mar-15	Apr-15	May-15
Low Risk Monitor ICU Stays	199	14	14	11	16	18	17	16	12	16	11	11	20	23
Low Risk Monitor ICU Stays %	17.5	14.0	17.7	14.5	17.4	19.6	17.9	19.0	14.1	18.0	13.8	12.8	23.5	24.7

Low Risk Mortality: Actual Low Risk Mortalities & Raw Mortality Rate   N = Low Risk ICU 332 Stays

	Total	May-14	Jun-14	Jul-14	Aug-14	Sep-14	Oct-14	Nov-14	Dec-14	Jan-15	Feb-15	Mar-15	Apr-15	May-15
Low Risk Hospital Deaths	8	0	0	0	0	0	4	2	0	0	0	1	0	1

Note: "Low Risk" indicates < 10% predicted hospital mortality. "Low Risk Monitor" indicates < 10% predicted hospital mortality and no active ICU intervention.

and heart rhythm disturbances. In a cardiothoracic ICU, the top diagnoses involve coronary artery bypass grafts and valve replacement issues.

Every month, the chief of the clinical care units in each system hospital receives APACHE data detailing the average age of the patient, the top five admitting diagnoses, mortality rates, ventilator days, and patient risk levels. Even this small excerpt from the larger report contains much valuable information. In addition to the top five admitting diagnoses, the number of patients who were readmitted to the ICU within 72 hours is tracked. Mortality rates are stratified into predicted levels of risk: low, medium, and high.

It took time for physicians to accept APACHE scores as valid. Many physicians were in the habit of placing patients in the ICU because they knew they would be monitored carefully, not because of any established admission criteria. In order to ensure that the ICUs were being properly utilized, we needed not only admission and discharge criteria to standardize care but also to compare the services delivered in our ICUs with those offered in the rest of the region and across the nation.

When this improvement effort began, the ICU was an "open" unit, which means that physicians controlled who were admitted to the unit and were in charge of the treatment rather than dedicated intensivists. No gatekeepers ensured appropriateness of admission, nor was there any consistency of criteria throughout the multihospital system.

The quality management department enlisted physicians and chairs of departments to define appropriate admission criteria and to act as champions for the change so as to encourage physician buy-in. The multidisciplinary team, chaired by a newly hired intensivist, recommended that the APACHE tool be used to gather consistent data across the system. Although the APACHE system is expensive and complex to interpret, understanding ICU utilization and creating efficiencies in resource utilization would reduce costs to the health system and provide a return on investment in terms of decreased length of stay (LOS), appropriate use of beds, and improved patient flow into and out of the ICU.

Administration agreed to implement APACHE. As a result of the data analysis, explicit admission criteria were established that reduced ICU utilization. The health system established step-down units to provide appropriate care to patients with low acuity. APACHE data showed physicians that many of the patients who died in fact were defined as low acuity and needed very little intervention and certainly not the kind of intervention appropriate to ICU care. Leaders began questioning the appropriateness, effectiveness, and efficiency of keeping low-acuity patients in the ICU. Over time, many became convinced that not all dying patients should be subject to ICU interventions. The team also considered other issues, such as whether intensivists should oversee care and report to the primary physicians or were they not needed (i.e., should the ICUs be open or closed).

Other improvements were made because data enabled leaders and physicians to better understand and define issues in the ICU population. For example, data revealed that patients who were on ventilators to help them breathe were self-extubating (i.e., attempting to remove their breathing tubes themselves). Patients who self-extubate can injure themselves. If patients are removing the tubes themselves, it might be a sign that they are not being monitored closely enough by the staff who are supposed to recognize when patients are ready to be weaned from ventilators.

Weaning patients from ventilators in a timely and safe fashion depends not only on an explicit protocol but also on a team working together to assess and monitor each patient's status. Respiratory therapists, intensivists, and staff from nursing, pulmonary medicine, and other areas need to communicate and agree on a plan for each patient on a ventilator.

Quality management staff worked with ICU nurses on developing standardized weaning protocols and collected data to assess improvements. The end result was that data inspired new practices that resulted in better and more efficient and cost-effective care. Quality data led to process improvement, structural changes, and greater efficiencies.

Another improvement related to APACHE data is relatively recent and reflects how new information can be incorporated effectively into patient care. It used to be thought that critical care patients who have undergone an intervention should remain immobilized for several days. New research shows that, on the contrary, the earlier the mobilization of the patient, the better the outcomes. APACHE scores are being used to identify the population (based on age, score, etc.) who should be targeted for early mobilization.

Analyzing Readmission

Mortality is only one of the outcomes measures that the CMS is analyzing and connecting to reimbursement. Unplanned readmission is now considered as an outcomes indicator, one that indicates failure to provide appropriate care during the first admission or is a sign of poor discharge instructions or follow-up care. This perspective—considering readmission as an outcome—is a relatively new point of view. For many years, hospitals received payment for readmission; indeed, administrators saw readmission as a source of revenue. Clinicians accepted readmission as a normal manifestation of chronic disease. Few clinicians involved patients in their own care in order to prevent readmission.

However, once unplanned readmission became defined as "waste" and the government began to penalize organizations financially, administrators began to prioritize reducing unplanned readmission. Just as occurred with mortality, tracking readmission data moved from the clinical domain to the administrative one. The paradigm shift in payment systems caused a paradigm shift in the interpretation of how care is delivered.

Case Example: Readmission

When leaders at the health system in which we work realized that the system's readmission data was higher than the national average, they prioritized a task force to spearhead an improvement effort. Leadership support is critical for any improvement effort since resources (funds, staff time) have to be allocated. As with any improvement effort, the first step is to ask questions to get a sense of the problem.

The overarching question is: Can readmissions be prevented? To answer this question, more specific questions have to be asked in order to understand who is being readmitted and why. What disease conditions account for readmission? Were readmissions primarily from patients with chronic disease in advanced illness or some other factor? Were there demographic factors or psychosocial factors that contributed to readmission? Until these and other specific questions are answered, the causes of readmission will remain opaque.

Our data analysis indicated that many readmissions involved patients with chronic disease. To target improvements, we decided to focus on patients who had the diagnosis of congestive heart failure, chronic obstructive pulmonary disease, pneumonia, and stroke. The goal was to define the patient population that was being readmitted, to understand the cause of their readmission, especially whether it was from the same diagnosis as previous admissions, and to understand and evaluate whether the delivery of care was good. Good care includes not only treatment but also effective discharge instructions, patient/family education, and follow-up visits.

With further analysis, we realized that patients with chronic disease who were being readmitted were really patients with advanced illness who were at end of life. They needed appropriate support services, including emotional support, but not necessarily hospital resources. Again, data led to better understanding of the process of care, and both patients and the organization reaped the benefits.

Using Data for Improvements

The two examples of performance improvement activities discussed in this section show how quality data can be used to transform and improve care and increase organizational efficiency. It should be noted that it is not always clear cut or obvious that an improvement opportunity exists. Not all professionals agree on what is a cause for concern. Busy clinicians who are asked to attend meetings and discuss opportunities and methodologies to decrease or eliminate a problem should agree that there is in fact a problem.

But what data define a problem, and who in the health care organization determines whether it is a problem? What is the role of administrators, who are concerned with margins, efficiency, malpractice, and good care, in determining whether a problem exists? Should everyone wait for regulatory agencies and/or payers to determine that a problem exists? Or should there be a proactive approach, with data and good analytics and administrative and clinical support to define an opportunity for improvement.

Case Example: Joint Replacement Surgery

According to the National Institute of Health, more than 1 million people in the United States have hip or knee replacement surgery annually (http://www.niams.nih.gov/Health_info/Joint_Replacement/default.asp). Clearly, improving the care of these patients should be a priority. Joint replacement surgery is not without risks. Among the surgical risks of joint replacement is what is called venous thromboembolism (VTE). VTEs cause blood clots in a deep vein, usually in the thigh or calf. An especially risky complication of VTE is that the blood clot can lead to a pulmonary embolism, a blood clot in the lung, which is often fatal. When our system collected data about our patients undergoing hip and knee replacement surgery, clinicians, administrators, and leaders agreed that improvement opportunities existed to reduce VTEs in the health system's program.

To investigate VTEs, a multidisciplinary team was established, including the director of anesthesiology, chief of general surgery, chief of medicine, hematologists, orthopedic physicians, surgical nurses, leaders of quality management, and social workers. From this team, a subcommittee was formed to better define patient risk factors for developing VTEs. Criteria for risk reflected established guidelines from professional associations. Improved screening procedures were developed, and the team created new order sheets to standardize prevention practices. All involved staff members were educated about risk for VTEs. Now team members assess patients postoperatively, and the committee meets quarterly to review medical innovations in the published literature.

Data were used to monitor the effect of the changes; data revealed that the changes resulted in a significant reduction of VTEs during the first year of the improvement initiative, and that success has continued. Rates of pulmonary embolisms also fell. LOS was decreased, which resulted in lowering costs to the hospital; and patient satisfaction increased because outcomes were improved. Examining processes, standardizing practice, monitoring outcomes with quality data, and using a multidisciplinary approach resulted in success.

Case Example: Bariatric Surgery

Yet another example of quality in action involved the initiative to improve bariatric surgery (i.e., surgery related to obesity) at the health system in which we work when we first began performing this surgery a decade ago. As with any new procedure, the more quantification that can be made of an experience, the more performance is understood and the more improvements can be generated.

Among the objectives of this initiative was to better protect the safety of this complex surgical population. Not only are obese patients complex physically, they are also complex socially and psychologically. Reviews of mortality after bariatric surgery led to concern that outcomes were not as expected. Also, there was a great deal of variation in mortality rates by hospital within the system. We realized that many special circumstances existed for a procedure that was relatively new at the time. For example, special equipment, such as computed tomography (CT) scanners, had to be available to handle obese patients.

Because of the body mass of obese patients undergoing bariatric surgery, complications, such as blood loss after surgery, did not have the same physical analogs as for nonobese patients; paleness or tenderness was different as well. Also, surgeons not specially trained in bariatric surgery were not always competent to recognize problems following surgery. In addition, some patients were not psychologically suited for this surgery and were not being screened appropriately.

Quality management concluded that physician competency for this complex surgery should be reviewed and evaluated, and protocols for care and appropriateness of the procedure also needed to be reviewed. It was clear that a standard of care needed to be articulated explicitly. But again, recommendations for improvements are not always straightforward. Bariatric surgery is highly lucrative for the hospital, with a very positive impact on financial margins. If administration or quality management intervenes, disrupts ongoing ways of doing things, and attempts to make changes, it may have a negative impact on margins. But if administration does not intervene, effectively letting things go the way they are, will that eventually result in poor margins? Administrators and policy makers must be actively involved in prioritization, understanding the process of care, supporting change, and communicating effectively with everyone involved.

A multidisciplinary task force established a consistent methodology for identifying, selecting, and assessing appropriate patients for the procedure. Because good outcomes were also dependent on the patient complying with dietary protocols after surgery, the improvement team was comprised not only of surgeons, anesthesiologists, pulmonologists, and physicians but also of psychologists, nutritionists, social workers, and quality management. The team researched the available literature on the topic and came to consensus on what constituted safe patient care. Eventually guidelines were developed for physician credentialing, patient assessment, patient counseling, institutional requirements, and staff education. The guidelines were based on evidence-based practice and were standardized and measureable, from the presurgical physician office visit to one-year postoperative follow-up.

A preoperative checklist was developed to ensure that the patient had necessary consultations, including nutritional, behavioral, educational, medical, and surgical (see Figure 9.5). Quality management created a database in collaboration with the improvement task force to monitor relevant indicators for ongoing review (see Table 9.1).

These data reports improved accountability and communication about assessments, infection rates, LOS, return to the OR, and other measures. The data provide an excellent teaching tool for the risks and benefits of this procedure. Weight management services were included for all patients, and patients and their families were offered education.

FIGURE 9.5. BARIATRIC PREOPERATIVE CHECKLIST

REQUIREMENTS	DATE DONE	INITIAL	RESULTS IN CHART	COMMENTS
Medical Evaluation				
Nutritional Consult				
Behavioral Consult				
Fitness Consult				
Surgical Consult				
Support Group Attendance				
Letter to Insurance				
Educational Material				
Thyroid Function Panel				
Pre-op Testing:				
Urine				
CBC				
PT/PTT				
Type & Screen				
Chemical Profile				
Chemistry Profile				
EKG				
Gallbladder Ultrasound (unless S/P Cholecystectomy)				
Upper GI Series				
PFTs				
Pre-op ABG				
Chest X-rays				
ECHO				
MUGA				
Stress Test				
Pre-op Anesthesiology Evaluation				
Pre-op General Medicine Evaluation				
Pre-op Pulmonary Consult (if indicated)				
Pre-op Cardiology Consult (if indicated)				
Pre-op GI Consult (if indicated)				
Pre-op Vascular Evaluation (if indicated)				
Informed Consent				
Smoking Status:				
Never Smoked				
Smoked in past, not currently				
Date stopped:				
Previous usage:				
____ per day X ____ years				
Current smoking:				
____ per day X ____ years				

TABLE 9.1. BARIATRIC TABLE OF MEASURES

Indicators	2013	2014	2015
Pre-op nutrition assessment completed (%)			
Post-op psychiatric assessment completed (%)			
Post-op wound infection (%)			
SICU/SCU LOS			
Hospital LOS			
Return to OR within 30 days, excluding infection			
Post-op blood products			
Return to OR for bleeding			
Mortality			

Note: SICU = surgical intensive care unit; SCU = special care unit

The initiative resulted in improved patient care and efficient organizational processes, which resulted in decreased costs. Complications were reduced, and LOS decreased. Because of appropriate screening, rates of readmission and reoperation were low. Follow-up counseling and support were available to patients and families. Facilities and equipment were upgraded to ensure appropriateness for this group of patients, with special operating rooms, CT scanners, beds, and wheelchairs now being utilized.

Patient-Centered Care

Performance improvement has the goal of providing patients with improved care, better safety, and greater satisfaction. Today, the focus is shifting from the physician to the patient to make decisions about treatment, and patient-centric outcomes are being evaluated. Patients are evaluating the value of an intervention and are defining outcomes.

SF-36

A good example of this shift of focus is the use of the SF-36 (http://www.sf-36 .org/tools/sf36.shtml). The SF-36 is a short-form survey of 36 questions that reveals the patient's health profile and uses **quality of life** (physical and mental) **indicators** to rank patient outcomes. The goal is to be able to evaluate the relative merit of different interventions using standardized measurements across different disease processes and populations and to evaluate how patients manage in their communities after hospitalization. Physicians have used the SF-36 to better understand care involved in many disease conditions, such as arthritis, depression, cardiovascular disease, joint replacement, sleep disorders, transplant, and many more.

Case Example: Quality of Life

The hospital system in which we work has been doing a pilot study using the SF-36 to analyze the delivery of care for patients who have had joint replacement surgery. Patients are surveyed about their physical and mental status at three points of time: at the presurgical office visit, three month after surgery, and then one year later (see Figure 9.6).

This survey tool has greatly increased our understanding of how specific interventions affect outcomes and what those outcomes mean to patients. The analysis for the pilot study showed that patients evaluated their care with positive outcomes over time: less pain, more mobility, and better quality of life even a year after the surgery. Specifically, the physical components that make up the survey target general health, physical functioning, and bodily pain; the mental components ask about social functioning, vitality, and emotional and mental health.

After the surveys are entered into a database, analysts score the results. The highest score that can be achieved is 70. A score of 50 for each of the mental and physical components is considered an adequate, normal quality of life. Therefore, as the physical component gets closer to 50, a patient is getting closer to a normal quality of life. Since the average age of the patients in the pilot study was 68, a score of 45 indicates that patients have reached the quality of life that an average person in that age group is expected to have.

An interesting aspect of this study is that it was initiated by one physician, and its success and usefulness came to the attention of senior leaders after

FIGURE 9.6. SF-36 PHYSICAL AND MENTAL HEALTH COMPONENT ANALYSIS BY TIME POINT

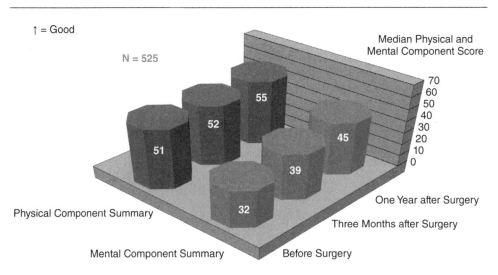

several years. Generally ideas are generated from the top and enacted by the rank and file. In this case, it was the reverse. Leaders have decided to expand this project to other areas of orthopedics and eventually to other disciplines and service lines in order to develop patient-centered benchmarks and standards of care.

Delivering the Message

Information has to be translated into action for data to make any real difference in the delivery of care. The analyzed data and the successes of the performance improvement task forces have to be communicated, in meaningful ways, to the rest of the organization. Information in the hands of just a few people cannot be useful. All employees should understand the issues involved in readmission, for example, or the importance of a sterile environment. Not only do caregivers require information; the people involved in patient education and discharge instructions need to recognize the critical importance of delivering information effectively to patients and families.

Data and Nursing Staff

The nurses in the health care system in which we work are educated in interpreting the dashboard reports, understanding the data as presented, and understanding the implications of the data for performance. They are also expected to discuss the data with the staff and with the nurses at meetings so as to determine how to improve care.

They use the analyzed data to identify their patient population; to better understand the patients on their unit; and to define their population by age, gender, treatment, illness, procedures, mobility, infection, and so on. They also track social status, discharge status, health literacy, education, and psychological status. Once they have a clear picture of their patients, they have to review the dashboard of measures to assess and monitor their delivery of care.

Those in senior positions are encouraged to help translate the data, to establish benchmarks, and to support improvement efforts via data. For example, one head nurse in our system challenges her staff at weekly meetings with actual goals: For example, she may say "Let's lower the unplanned readmission rates by 5 percent or have 100 percent compliance with discharge planning measures." Then, at the next meeting, the group discusses whether the goals have been met and why or why not. The nurses conduct a root cause analysis as to why readmission occurred and identify whether there were problems with the discharge process. This kind of effort is how information is best used.

Nurses are also encouraged to improve communication skills, participate in huddles (frequent brief meetings of caregiving staff), and participate in multidisciplinary rounds that discuss data that affect patient outcomes. For example, nursing-sensitive measures, such as pressure injuries and falls, require improvement. The more analytics are used, the more interventions can be evaluated for effectiveness and success. The measures help to identify gaps in the processes of care and failures in treatment and help to define where improvement efforts should be targeted.

Data and Medical Directors

Quality information gets reported to the chief medical officer (CMO) and chief nursing officer (CNO) who are responsible for communicating the data to medical directors and department chairs. The medical directors and department chairs are expected to communicate the information to their department, nursing directors, and staff.

Ideally, variables that identify the characteristics of the patient population being addressed (the denominator of the measure) are more clearly defined because of the data. Outcomes data (the numerator) should focus attention on interventions. The CMO, who often is in charge of quality management, communicates not only through staff meetings but via the quality performance improvement structure. Today, more and more time in medical and nursing meetings is being spent on understanding and interpreting quality data.

Multidisciplinary Teams

It is only natural that specialists are interested and expert in their specialties; but for effective communication and for patient-centered care, it is important that the different disciplines involved with a patient communicate effectively with each other and with the patient. Interpreting data analytics brings different disciplines together.

Think about a patient with infection or data that reveals the infection rate in a population or a unit is on the rise. Many different specialties need to work together on assessing the problem and improving performance: infection control, physicians, nurses, quality management, environment, housekeeping, laboratory, perhaps radiology, nutrition, pulmonologists, respiratory therapists, social workers, and so on.

Each specialty has to share a common language around disease and patient care, and often that common language is data. Also, different areas in the hospital where the patient may be exposed to sepsis need to be understood, and the team should include members from, for example, the ICU, the ED, the OR, and hospice. In order to gather the relevant data, everyone needs to be involved.

For example, if a transplant patient dies unexpectedly, a root cause analysis might show that the patient had come to the operating room with an infection, such as MRSA (methicillin-resistant *Staphylococcus aureus*), which compromised her surgical outcome. Further review might reveal that the MRSA was community acquired and that the social worker who works with patients in the community failed to inform the nurse; therefore, the information about the infection was not made part of the patient's record. Once the problem is defined, communication can be improved. If patients are coming into the hospital with infections, then surgeons need to be sure to review the notes from the community resources.

Adverse events require multidisciplinary input to understand root causes and to ensure improved processes. New processes also should enlist the input of any relevant stakeholders. The way health care organizations work today, it is no longer possible to be an independent and isolated practitioner. Care is too complex and too interdependent. Voluntary physicians, who used to be somewhat removed from hospital or organizational activities, today must participate in data collection activities and be integrated into the performance improvement of the organization. In fact, the new generation of physicians is being trained in quality, performance improvement (a Continuing Medical Education requirement), patient populations, processes, and the use of quality data. And because the medical record requires information, many physicians have scribes to enter data to ensure compliance and record completeness.

Working with Measures

Before a measure can be developed, input has to be gathered from every discipline that would have an effect on the patient. Therefore, every measure is multidisciplinary in conception. All the disciplines involved in formulating the measure, defining the numerator and denominator, need to participate so that they understand the value of the data.

Even those measures that are dictated by the government and regulatory agencies have to be addressed by multidisciplinary teams. The data collection process has to be standardized and reliable. The physicians who deal with the measures, the nurses who implement the measures, and the data collectors who enter the data all have to work together and communicate effectively for the measure to be valuable for more than compliance. For example, many disciplines are involved in collecting and analyzing whether pneumonia patients receive an antibiotic in a timely manner: radiology, laboratory, pharmacy, pulmonary, infection control, respiratory therapy. The nature of work in the hospital is multidisciplinary.

Multidisciplinary teams help to create measures, implement the measures, and communicate the results of the analytics about the measures. They need to understand the characteristics of each measure and why it is important. They need to understand how the measures affect performance and patient outcomes. Infection has to be understood not only by clinicians but also by the people who clean the operating rooms, those staff members who are involved with sterilization procedures, housekeeping, and others. Everyone is involved in the measure. Measures are not abstract notions; they should be used to understand and improve the delivery of care.

The silo organization of most health care organizations erects barriers to effective communication and to genuine multidisciplinary patient-centered care. Once a patient leaves "our" service and goes to "yours"—which is to say, as the patient travels throughout the continuum of care—who is in charge? Internal cultural barriers are much harder to redo or fix than external processes are. When something is perceived as normal or routine, it does not even appear to be a problem. For example, many caregivers assume that delays are simply part of the way things happen. For effective and permanent change to occur, there has to be a concerted effort by leaders to investigate entrenched processes and support new and better ones.

For those involved in health care administration, it is part of the job to understand the importance of measures and the multidisciplinary nature of using the measures for improvement. Administrators need to have a handle on the population involved in each measure, which disciplines should be involved in improvement efforts, how effectively information about care is being communicated vertically and horizontally across the organization, who is collecting data and implementing the measure, and how patient outcomes are affected by the measure. Processes need to be developed to incorporate measures into daily care.

Summary

Data should be analyzed and used for improving clinical and organizational performance. Professionals and staff involved in health care organizations should be familiar with the role of data in defining and interpreting the delivery of care. Data should be used to:

- assist leaders in improving the efficient movement of patients through the continuum of care;
- understand barriers to effective throughput;
- determine effective levels of care for patients with advanced illness and at the end of life;
- evaluate resource utilization and the financial and clinical issues surrounding mortality; and
- improve patient safety through careful monitoring of variables such as readmission, mortality, quality of life, and patient satisfaction.

Key Terms

APACHE, hospice, palliative, quality of life indicators, silos

Quality Concepts in Action

As a quality management professional, you want to help your organization understand the reasons for high readmission rates and help to develop processes to improve. However, the CEO and the CMO do not think lowering readmission rates should be a priority. Members of the board of trustees who may be able to influence the CEO are not sufficiently educated about quality and safety variables to realize how important it is to lower readmission rates. To help board members better understand the implications of readmission, would you:

- provide statistics and data analytics directly to the quality committee of the board and meet with them to interpret the data and explain the issues?
- attempt to meet privately with members and the chair of the board in order to provide informal education, and then expect the chair to reinforce the education to the rest of the board?
- meet with the senior executives and explain how readmission could be a proxy for evaluating clinical care and patient safety?
- meet with the chief financial officer to explain the financial implications of lowering readmission rates and hope that he or she can convince other members of the C suite to support lowering readmission efforts?
- work with the CNO to improve processes, such as discharge instructions, and hope that he or she can influence the delivery of care and improve the rates?

Discuss the value of each of these alternatives and what barriers you might foresee to success.

References

American Hospital Association, Committee on Performance Improvement. 2012. *Advanced Illness Management Strategies: Engaging the Community and a Ready, Willing and Able Workforce.* Chicago: American Hospital Association. http://www.aha.org/about/org/aim-strategies-part2.shtml

Breen, A. M., T. Burton-Houle, and D. C. Aron. 2002. "Applying the Theory of Constraints in Health Care: Part 1—The Philosophy." *Quality Management in Health Care* 10 (3): 541–547.

Committee on Quality of Health Care in America, Institute of Medicine. 2001. *Crossing the Quality Chasm: A New Health System for the 21st Century.* Washington, DC: National Academies Press.

Gupta, D. 2013. "Queueing Models for Healthcare Operations." In B. T. Denton, ed., *Handbook of Healthcare Operations Management: Methods and Applications*, pp. 19–44. New York: Springer Science+Business Media.

Singer, P. A., D. K. Martin, and M. Kelner. 1999. "Quality End-of-Life Care Patients' Perspectives." *JAMA* 281 (2): 163–168.

Thorpe, K. E., and D. H. Howard. 2006. "The Rise in Spending among Medicare Beneficiaries: The Role of Chronic Disease Prevalence and Changes in Treatment Intensity." *Health Affairs* 25 (5): w378–w388.

Suggestions for Further Reading

Fletcher, D. S., and J. T. Panke. 2012. "Opportunities and Challenges for Palliative Care Professionals in the Age of Health Reform." *Journal of Hospice and Palliative Nursing* 14 (7): 452–459.

Kupfer, J. M. 2013. "The Morality of Using Mortality as a Financial Incentive: Unintended Consequences and Implications for Acute Hospital Care." *JAMA* 309 (21): 2213–2214.

Massachusetts Expert Panel on End of Life Care, Report and Recommendations. 2010, October. "Patient Centered Care and Human Mortality: The Urgency of Health System Reforms to Ensure Respect for Patients' Wishes and Accountability for Excellence in Care." http://molst-ma.org/sites/molst-ma.org/files/2010ExpPanRep.pdf

McCarthy, D., D. Radley, and S. Hayes. 2014. "Aiming Higher: Results from a Scorecard on State Health System Performance." Commonwealth Fund. http://www.commonwealthfund.org/publications/fund-reports/2015/dec/aiming-whigher-2015

Meier, D. E., and R. Umbdenstock. 2011. "Palliative Care and Health Delivery Reform." *Hospital Health Network* 85 (2): 60.

Morrison, R. S., J. Dietrich, J., S. Ladwig, S., T. Quill, J. Sacco, J. Tangeman, and D. E. Meier. 2011. "Palliative Care Consultation Teams Cut Hospital Costs for Medicaid Beneficiaries." *Health Affairs* 30 (3): 454–463.

Murray, T. H., and B. Jennings. 2005. "The Quest to Reform End-of-Life Care: Rethinking Assumptions and Setting New Directions." In B. Jennings, G. E. Kaebnick, and T. H. Murray, eds., *Improving End-of-Life Care: Why Has It Been So Difficult? Hastings Center Report Special Report* 35 (6): S52–S57.

Palvannan, R. K., and K. L. Teow, 2012. "Queueing for Healthcare." *Journal of Medical Systems* 36: 541–547.

Turner-Bowker, D. M., P. J. Bartley, and J. E. Ware, Jr., 2002. *SF-36® Health Survey & "SF" Bibliography: Third Edition (1988–2000)*. Lincoln, RI: QualityMetric Incorporated.

Zhang, B., S. Block, A. Wright, C. Earle, M. Nilsson, H. Huskamp, M. Maciejewski, et al. 2009. "Health Care Costs in the Last Week of Life: Associations with End-of-Life Conversations." *Archives of Internal Medicine* 169: 480–488.

Useful Websites

http://www.ahrq.gov/downloads/pub/advances2/vol3/advances-dingley_14.pdf

http://www.commonwealthfund.org/publications/issue-briefs/2015/oct/us-health-care-from-a-global-perspective

http://www.dartmouthatlas.org/keyissues/issue.aspx?con=2944

http://www.health.ny.gov/professionals/patients/patient_rights/palliative_care/information_act

http://www.ihi.org/resources/Pages/ImprovementStories/BetterPatientFlowMeans BreakingDowntheSilos.aspx

http://www.ihi.org/resources/Pages/ImprovementStories/SepsisCareEntersNewEra .aspx

http://www.ihi.org/resources/Pages/OtherWebsites/Survivingsepsiscampaign.aspx

http://www.niams.nih.gov/Health_info/Joint_Replacement/default.asp

http://www.sf-36.org/tools/sf36.shtml

http://advancedcarecoalition.org/

CHAPTER TEN

PREPARING FOR THE FUTURE

Chapter Outline

The New Quality Management
The Business of Health Care
Measurements Are the Nuts and Bolts of Quality
Getting Everyone on Board
Challenges for the Future
Summary
Key Terms
Quality Concepts in Action
Suggestions for Further Reading
Useful Websites

Key Concepts

- Quality measures are linked to financial success.
- Quality management professionals should be integrated into senior leadership (C suite).
- Cultural change is required for sustained performance improvement.
- Communication must be effective for an organization to improve quality and safety.
- Oversight and accountability have to be carefully defined for successful processes.
- A quality work ethic should be integrated into data collecting, team building, and patient safety efforts.
- Measurements should reflect the values of the organization.

This book has been about preparing for the future, which is to say managing the changed health care environment successfully—clinically, administratively, and financially. This chapter reviews some of the important concepts that were discussed in previous chapters.

The New Quality Management

Health care reform has moved quality and efficiency measures into the national spotlight. Clinical measures have become performance measures that are used by insurers to influence improvements in care. Financial incentives for health care organizations are closely associated to quality measures, such as readmission, mortality, and the patient experience. Therefore, organizations need to develop tools and procedures with which to monitor quality, report on **quality metrics**, improve quality, reduce costs, and eliminate waste. To accomplish these goals, quality management professionals will become integrated into the C suite, the top leaders, and quality management programs will be designed to align with the organization's strategic planning policies.

In previous decades, quality management focused on compliance with regulations, and staff who were trained in those regulations could be quality managers. This is not the case in today's health care environment, which actually measures quality with specific variables and looks for gaps or variation in order to improve. Today, also, clinical staff must be more conversant with quality measures because metrics that evaluate the delivery of care are changing, and patient outcomes and satisfaction are being publicly reported.

The New Role of Administrators

Administrators need to understand quality metrics and analytics as well in order to provide the leadership necessary for clinical and financial success—that is, to meet quality goals by attaching quality metrics to financial variables. Poor quality, as reflected by measurements, has a financial impact on the organization. Improved quality and good quality can transform an organization for success. Because private insurers, government insurance companies, and health care systems are using quality measurements, and those measures are becoming the basis for reimbursement and financial penalties, administrators need to be familiar with the measures—that is, they need to be familiar with quality data and its implications about care and efficiency.

For example, because hospitals are no longer reimbursed for hospital-acquired infections, administrators need to take an active role in ensuring prevention. They need to understand infection, not only the reported rates, but the underlying causes of infection, the types of infection, **preventive strategies** to reduce and control infection, and the staff members involved in preventing infections. And administrators need to ensure that health care employees all work together to eliminate infections.

If administrative leaders are unhappy with the rates of infection because of financial and other implications, they need to communicate the importance of sterile conditions not just to the top infection control physicians but to the people who do the cleaning, the people who push the mops. When people understand their role in preventing infection and that someone recognizes the importance of their contribution to the "product," work is more satisfying and holistic rather than an isolated piece of action. With everyone from the physician to the cleaning staff working together to prevent infection, really functioning as a team, infection rates go down. If a barrier to **effective communication** is a language issue or a communication style, managers have to develop solutions to improve.

In addition to understanding quality analytics, administrators need to understand the principles underlying performance improvement. It is not enough to ask why certain measures are not meeting benchmarks; it is necessary to make improvements and to devote resources to those improvements. To recognize that resources will provide a return on investment, then, administrators need to introduce change via the Plan-Do-Study-Act (PDSA) or other quality improvement strategies. Change has to be led from and supported by the top for it to be effective and sustainable. Change has to be based on quality.

The Business of Health Care

These ideas are not rocket science, and no magic bullet exists that will accomplish this **cultural shift** quickly. Principles of effective teamwork and communication to staff and employees about expectations for excellence and change have to be underlined by the C suite. Obviously, people need to communicate; physicians need to share information; medical staff needs to work together; patients have to understand their treatment and hospital experience. We all know this. Yet communication is a major issue in every adverse event, error, and incident. The question then becomes this: How do you build in effective communication so that it is embedded in a changed culture, so that it is ingrained as normal? Effective health care administrators need to answer that question. In other words, what actions should be taken to make more effective communication happen? (http://www.ahrq.gov/downloads/pub/advances2/vol3/advances-dingley_14.pdf).

Health care is a business like many others, and poor quality has enormous repercussions for organizations. For example, the defects in cars that led to the recalls plaguing General Motors (GM) were known to the GM quality control people but were not communicated to the senior leaders.

One wonders what in the culture prevented such important information from being communicated? The financial consequences for GM will be far reaching (http://www.ibtimes.com/quality-crisis-gm-worst-year-recalls-2004-1588125). The same unfortunate conditions seem to have permeated Veterans Affairs hospitals, with information stalled and not communicated; the result is that no one was able to oversee what was going on in the different silos, no one was accountable, and care became substandard (http://www.modernhealthcare.com/article/20140507/NEWS/305079939).

Improve the Product

In 2014, as a result of the negative health care reports, President Obama appointed a businessman, the former chief executive of Procter & Gamble, to lead the Department of Veterans Affairs. Why a businessman and not a physician? The president knows that health care is a business, one that needs to provide customers with effective and efficient services, at a reasonable cost, and meet expectations about the "product." Meeting patient expectations should be integrated into the strategic plan and the performance improvement plan of the health care organization. Patient-centered care changes not only the way we do business but the very character of the organization. Today's executives are challenged to figure out how to sell health care services in a competitive marketplace. The new economics of health care require new attitudes and behaviors of medical and administrative leaders.

When a crisis occurs, we know very well what to do. Our multidisciplinary teams come together to do a root cause analysis of what went wrong. Everyone participates as part of the team. Ideally, this multidisciplinary effectiveness should occur when conditions are normal and the process of care is smooth. Since quality and financial data are linked in today's reform environment, administrators need to understand everything—process, outcomes, finance, measurements—and further support effective improvement implementation strategies.

Improvement is a tall order and takes many years. But with all the changes in health care, there is no choice other than to embrace quality management at every level of the organization and across the continuum of care and to make the director of quality management part of the senior leadership team. Since reimbursement is reduced for readmissions, never events, pressure injuries, falls, and infection, the specifics of medical care has to become an administrative concern. Administrators and medical staff have to work together toward a single goal of safe, quality, and efficient care. In previous decades, the concerns of administrators were separate from those of clinicians; today that is no longer the case.

A new **work ethic** has to develop, one based on PDSA and principles of W. Edwards Deming, who was able to transform floundering Japanese industries into some of the most effective and productive in the world. The new work ethic must include leaders in the trenches alongside frontline workers so that they understand each other's concerns and recognize the barriers to success.

Measures of Success

Today's business professionals, individuals involved in health care administration and policy, and those who hope to have a management position in health care organizations need to recognize the **value** of data and statistical analysis in understanding the process of care. They also need to be able to use improvement methodologies, such as PDSA, with its emphasis on data, planning, and continuous monitoring of improvements, and be able to correlate quality data to financial margins. **Oversight** involves watching the measures, monitoring improvements, and prioritizing and developing better organizational and clinical processes. In the new health care environment, health care managers have all of these responsibilities.

INTERNALIZE QUALITY

When I was a hospitalized patient, I saw the people who cleaned the room, took out the garbage, delivered the food; the nurses checked me for infection and vital signs. I realized then that if a manager wanted to know if everyone was doing their work properly, he or she need only ask a patient who observes the daily activities of the staff. More than just the clinical staff has to have the work ethic of doing things. An effective manager will attempt to rally the entire workforce to quality management methods and a commitment to change. I know hospital leaders who have put cameras in the operating rooms to enforce handwashing or time-outs. That kind of oversight is not an internalized commitment to quality and, in fact, has proved not to be effective in the long run. Appropriate care has to be internalized.

Transparency

We know what we should be doing. We know how to do it. We have the training and the skills to do it properly. We know what is expected and we understand the penalties of not doing it. Yet, remarkably, we do not do it! We are not committed to safe patient care in an internalized and consistent way. Changing a culture takes years—and, perhaps unfortunately, a financial incentive.

Quality management ethics are actually embedded in the principles of PDSA, statistical analysis, effective communication, and teamwork. Improvement opportunities should motivate the collection of accurate, valid, and transparent data. Often information that reveals gaps in care is hidden because departments, services, and clinicians want to look good. But faking the data does not lead to improvements and does not show an honest baseline from which improvement efforts can be launched.

In addition, covering up poor data usually results in expenses in the form of readmissions, complications, or malpractice claims. In the long run, it does not pay to hide from problems; it pays, literally, to fix problems before serious damage occurs. The new quality administrator wants to inculcate a quality work ethic into data collecting, team building, and patient safety efforts. Communication and teamwork have to be effective at every level of the organization, from the bedside up to management. Multidisciplinary teams foster the destruction of silos and hierarchies; roles, responsibilities, and expectations are clarified and defined. Hospitals have constant pressure from the government and other external agencies to make changes, but until those changes are internalized by every member of the institution, they will be superficial and temporary. Real change requires commitment from top leaders, middle management, and frontline workers. Real change has to be constantly monitored and reinforced.

Case Example: Improving a Hospital in Trouble

The following example illustrates how principles and tools of quality management can take a health care organization from the brink of ruin to success. Several years ago, a hospital that was on the verge of bankruptcy and had very poor accreditation scores asked the quality institute at the hospital system in which we work for help. It was clear to hospital leaders that their financial, organizational, and clinical structures were not working and needed to be rethought and revised.

Hospital leaders recognized that the first step was to create an effective quality management and accountability structure, which was critical for improvements. Administration also needed help in convincing the medical staff to work in teams and to meet policy requirements. Once improvement strategies were developed, leaders realized that they would need help with implementation and sustainability. They wanted to standardize care across each discipline and department, not have independent silos, and to develop methods to prioritize improvements.

The board of trustees of this health organization hoped to create a culture of quality that would be internally driven by senior leaders. To facilitate this goal, the chief executive officer (CEO) chose a cheerleader for quality, an expert in finance who understood the link between quality management and successful financial margins. Our consultants organized medical board meetings and educated physicians about the role of quality in improving clinical processes and patient satisfaction. Our staff also met with the nurses in various disciplines to listen to their concerns. We educated the staff on regulatory requirements as the foundation of quality but stressed that meeting requirements was only the starting point to an effective quality structure.

Roles and responsibilities in the quality structure were defined for the C suite, the physicians and nurses, the ambulatory physicians and administrators. We also explained the importance of evaluating processes using data and measurements and taught them how to interpret statistical reports. We explained benchmarks and control charts. When problem areas were identified with their dialysis process, for example, we were able to collect data and suggest improvements. We built accountability and communication structures.

Another important aspect of this project was showing leaders that improvements could be made without large outlays of capital. We showed them how much could be accomplished using effective communication and improving coordination of activities.

For example, if the roof leaked and it was no one's responsibility to report it, or it wasn't clear who was in charge of maintenance, and the information was not passed along, then the roof remained leaky. No one was in charge. No one was accountable. Once an accountability structure was defined and put in place, staff members knew who was in charge and the damage could be easily fixed. Or if the laundry contract was not being fulfilled and material was not cleaned in a timely manner, leaders came to realize that the issue was more about communication than about finance. With someone in charge and a structure in place, the contract could be monitored and fulfilled.

Over many months, our team designed new structures and processes and trained and educated staff and leaders about the changes. After a year of this, hospital employees began to identify gaps in care and take steps to improve. After two years, every discipline gave a presentation explaining a performance improvement project with implementation and data regarding success. In this example, although the CEO had a vision of improvement, he wasn't sure (and wasn't trained) in how to accomplish his goal. By becoming more familiar with tenets of quality, he was able to transform the organization successfully.

The leaders supported a proactive approach to care and encouraged new programs. The next accreditation survey of the hospital was highly successful and showed the results of changed practice. The organization began to win awards; it built a new infection control program; it became a recognized stroke center; mortality and morbidity associated with dialysis improved; it developed improved criteria for intensive care unit admission. In short, it became a quality organization.

Measurements Are the Nuts and Bolts of Quality

Once the C suite accepts that quality management should be a part of the strategic planning process and work in collaboration with the finance department to develop new and improved processes, organizations can begin to change, moving from a focus on regulatory compliance to become authentic and successful quality organizations. There is no lack of information available; the issue is what to do with the information, how to use it for better processes, and not simply be overwhelmed (see Figure 10.1).

FIGURE 10.1. DATA OVERLOAD

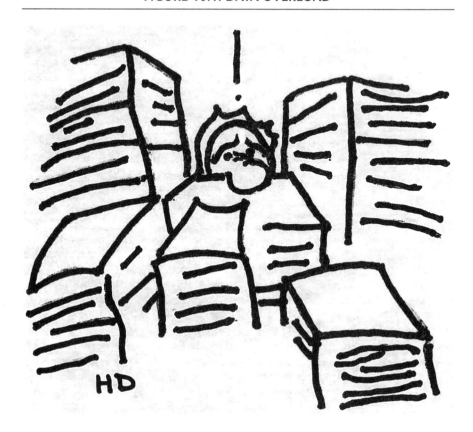

Know What the Data Mean

Measurements should be designed to help users understand which processes are more successful and efficient than others. For example, nurses, who are responsible for collecting data on required measures, such as pressure injuries, should understand why they are collecting the information and be familiar with basic statistics in order to have some sense of the meaning of the data they are collecting. If they understand the impact of numerators and denominators, the importance of sample size, the relevance of the benchmarks, and the organizational goals, then they can make intelligent decisions about improvements and help others to understand how and why to manage care. Collecting data is a rote activity; understanding the purpose of the data collection helps to move the organization forward.

It is not enough, for example, to meet one or two indicators for pneumonia to say that pneumonia patients are being treated successfully and effectively.

Nurses should be educated about all the indicators involved with caring for pneumonia patients and be able to interpret those measures in order to understand the population. Meeting indicators is a baseline only, not an indication of quality care.

Make the Data Useful

Quality management departments can interpret measures or collaborate with research groups to explain why pneumonia patients need antibiotics. If you analyze the population (the denominator) into who gets antibiotics and who does not, and why or why not, you have information that might improve care and create better processes. Does everyone require antibiotics? Do all pneumonia patients require antibiotics at the same time in the progression of the disease? Are there markers to indicate when and which patients do better than others? A look at the data can reveal answers to these questions.

This kind of analysis will be increasingly embedded into quality management. With electronic health records enabling easier and more voluminous data gathering, and with information being logged into databases, the quality manager will need to understand statistical analysis and methodology. Quality management is entirely different today than it was in the past. In an ironic way, we need to go back in time to Florence Nightingale and W. Edwards Deming, who both used statistics to analyze problems and processes for improvement. Nurses who work with data will be able to better care for populations and be more efficient in delivering that care.

Measures Reflect Values

Measures have made a difference over time. Because New York State reports cardiac mortality and other data, improvements have been generated and sustained in hospitals throughout the state; because reimbursement is compromised for never events and nursing-sensitive measures, rates of pressure injuries and falls are declining. Identifying which measures have value to an organization is critical to help with improvement efforts. Just as people value different things, organizations do as well. If someone is buying a car, one person might value safety features above all others; another gas mileage and other financial concerns; another a terrific sound system, phone connections, navigation, and so on. None of these values is intrinsically superior to the others; people value what they value and are often willing to pay more for it.

If the organization is committed to being in the top decile in cardiac care, it will put its improvement efforts into that area; if it wants to focus on customer satisfaction or the patient experience, there will be a different focus. If administration wants to improve financial margins, there will be a still different focus. Improvement efforts and resources will be dedicated to different projects, depending on the value to the organizational leaders. Data collection, analysis, and reports reflect the organization's values. Of course, improvement efforts are subject to financial resources, which also have to be taken into account. An organization may want to enlarge its bariatric surgery program but find that the equipment required and the physician credentialing requirements may prohibit such expansion. There is always a check and balance and risk/benefit analysis between quality and financial concerns.

Today's administrators realize that the financial bottom line is affected by mortality rates, unplanned readmission rates, falls, and other measures where, if criteria are not met, financial consequences occur. Data show how services provided result in value to the organization. Measures are not independent entities but are interconnected. Measures that reflect, for example, self-extubations and pneumonia patients have an impact on sepsis ratings. The interrelationship of measurements can be reflected on dashboards, and leaders can be educated about how to read dashboards effectively.

Getting Everyone on Board

With health care reimbursement associated with quality and outcomes data, quality management can no longer be an isolated department but has to be integrally involved in every department and discipline in the assessment of care delivery. Nurses not only must use data to be more efficient and to understand disease populations, but they must monitor data to think about improvement opportunities. In this way, quality management will penetrate the front line, and all staff members will be accountable for patient safety. Data will not be solely for reporting but used for improving care.

Case Example: Improving Transplant Services

An example of change can be seen in a transplant service at a local hospital. Before quality professionals were called in for consultation, when a postsurgical mortality occurred, only surgeons and fellows attended meetings to analyze and interpret the possible reasons for the mortality. In time and with the influence of quality management, more specialists were included to look at the process of care: anesthesiologists, nephrologists, nurses. Meeting together to discuss the process of care, silos began to break down and the surgeons realized that many professionals were involved in the delivery of care and that everyone should be involved in making decisions. Over more time, intensivists were included in mortality conferences because complications often arose in intensive care units. When appropriateness of patient choice for transplant was considered, social workers, psychologists, and others were also brought into the discussion.

From the original five surgeons in the transplant group, there are now 40 people who are involved in meetings and discussions about improving care. Now there is a genuine multidisciplinary team involved in ensuring good patient outcomes.

Changing Behavior

Changing physician behavior is very difficult. Issues of compliance with regulations, expectations of insurance companies, or reminders on the medical record have not made much impact. In our health system, presenting risk-adjusted measurements reflecting the physician's patient population over time makes an impact. Physicians want to deliver good care; objective proof that others deliver better care can change behavior, especially when leaders support the use of dashboards that reflect care.

Transparency of data has also helped to change behavior; when an organization is in the top decile for specific treatments or procedures, leaders and physicians feel rewarded. However, using data and measurements to change behavior requires education by quality experts so that clinicians can understand how specific variables capture aspects of the delivery of care.

If mortality is high, for example, and leaders support improvement efforts, physicians, together with others, have to analyze root causes and change processes to improve outcomes. And even mortality rates do not always immediately generate concern and change. Often physicians believe that some mortality is expected and acceptable; there is sometimes a distinction between what physicians perceive as good outcomes and what data reveal about outcomes. If two people die out of 100 procedures, the physician has a 98 percent success rate. But a 2 percent mortality rate might not be acceptable to leaders or the government. For example, if risk-adjusted mortality for transplants is above the benchmark, the Centers for Medicare and Medicaid Services investigates and the program may be at risk. Closing a program is a costly consequence, and the threat may be an impetus for changing practice. If a program is threatened with closure, processes begin to change.

The move toward pay for performance (P4P) and bundled payments places risk directly on the physicians. If they don't deliver care in the top percentile or if there is unplanned readmission or mortality above the benchmark, then reimbursement will be affected. Certain powerful data markers, such as mortality, readmission, or financial issues, might provoke change. We put a value on such measures, and they carry the stigma of bad care. But other data, such as overuse of radiological scans, may not, perhaps because the consequences do not seem immediate. But as administrators begin to realize the powerful link between quality care and financial success, they will pressure their employees to improve. Physicians are becoming aware that a strong quality infrastructure and data monitoring of processes may help them avoid poor ratings or other negative consequences.

For real improvement, leaders have to have a clearly defined mission and vision: What are they looking to provide? What do they hope to accomplish? And they need to find a way to improve without intruding on the financial viability of the organization. The mission and vision should be developed by a cabinet of top clinical, administrative, and quality leaders. Once the vision is explicit, dashboards of data can help with prioritization of short-term and long-term goals. These statements are not simply rhetoric to decorate official documents, but they define the relationship between the organization and the patients. They help to establish priorities and dictate what measures are required to attain the goals.

Case Example: Understanding Complex Processes

A hospital had a problem with sepsis and wanted mortality rates improved. Leaders incorrectly perceived sepsis as a single entity when, in fact, it is a highly complex reflection of multiple aspects of care. Sepsis that results from complications from open heart surgery or from pneumonia or from pressure injuries has distinct and different sources and requires distinct analysis and improvements.

This same organization also wanted to improve its financial picture. Our consultants explained that complex patients undergoing transplants, cardiac surgery, and bariatric surgery (all highly remunerative to the hospital) were the most likely candidates for sepsis and death and that to improve sepsis mortality, the process of care in these three complicated procedures required analysis. Teaching administrators that sepsis cannot be treated as if it were a single problem requires exposing them to various quality management processes: data collection, gap analysis, root cause analysis, PDSA, defining populations, detailing processes, and reporting and communicating information about processes and outcomes.

Challenges for the Future

Simply introducing P4P, bundled payments, or other changes in reimbursements is insufficient for change to be integrated into the delivery of care and sustained. For change to become internalized, it has to be constantly monitored with measurements; accountability for improved processes has to be clearly defined. Change often works in the short term, but once the new processes become routine, it is easy for people to revert to older routines. There are countless incidences of changes resulting in desired outcomes but, over time, the changed practices revert right back to the original problematic ones.

New Strategies

Managers therefore have to develop strategies not only for improvements but for sustainability. Usually both negative and positive reinforcements should be used. And punishing or rewarding with money may not be the answer. A culture of quality, a patient-centered culture, is not designed simply for financial gain.

Leaders and managers have to be psychologically and socially aware of how their staff functions and which dynamics might lead to sustained change.

It is interesting to observe that people do not always abide by their own guidelines; in fact, they often ignore them. Policies can state, for example, that a catheter should not be left in a patient for more than three days, and the electronic health record can even flag it; yet catheters are often left in longer, and infection may then occur. The manager of the unit has to discover why policies are not followed, what barriers need to be addressed, what issues need to be reinforced. Paper policies only go so far. People have to be on top of change. The same is true of any industry. The supervisor is on the floor watching production, identifying bottlenecks in the process, introducing improvements, and then monitoring their implementation. The role of the manager is to provide oversight, and that cannot be done effectively from behind a desk.

The key to success is to reduce variation from the standard of care and to reduce unexpected and unwanted developments in the care process. Routines are useful for standardization, as are checklists and other aids, but unless leaders are committed to standardization in an active and real way, sustained change will be difficult. What has worked most successfully for the system in which we work has been when people in senior leadership positions have been very visible, walking on the units, speaking to the frontline workers, and encouraging good work. This kind of hands-on involvement gets increasingly more difficult as systems get larger and larger, as is the trend.

Break Down the Silos

Since today's challenges are so numerous and complex, it is important for managers and administrators to develop ways to manage all the pieces and to unify them into a whole; managers need to assign accountability so that someone is responsible. All too often incidents occur because one professional believed another was responsible and in fact no one took responsibility for whatever gap in care existed. The manager or director has to be on top of that. All the talk about communication has to be actualized, put into existence in a real way, which means not just memos and meetings but huddles, conversations, and team meetings. The continuum needs to be managed, which means someone has to have oversight of the entire process. Organizations have tried to introduce patient navigators to accompany patients through the process or care episode, but having one navigator per patient is financially not viable, and navigators become overwhelmed with their caseloads and inefficient at their tasks.

With proper oversight and managerial commitment, data can be used profitably to identify variance and flaws and develop improvements with multidisciplinary input. The silo mentality, which might have worked effectively for many years, no longer does so; on the contrary, lack of communication often leads to incidents and adverse events. Silos are certainly at variance with concepts of patient-centered care. If the chair of medicine, for example, has seven units to manage and gets reports and data from each unit, how does he or she analyze and interpret all that data so that it becomes useful for improvements?

Managers and chairs of departments have to work together to deal with issues involved in moving patients through the continuum and to establish priorities for resources and changes. Hospitals set up with distinct departments encourage a model of care where it is difficult to reconcile independent silos and there are multiple barriers to effective communication. Leaders enjoy controlling their own fiefdoms; that's just human nature. Therefore, it is the senior leaders, led by the chief executive, who need to wrestle with these issues. It is not enough to write a mission statement saying the organization desires to provide patient-centered care. When silos exist and there is poor communication between them, processes will remain fragmented and safety will be impaired.

Employees need to be educated about the continuum of care, throughput, and the role of quality in order to support accountability and performance improvements. Data have to be made meaningful to everyone involved in the process of care, not recorded and filed in someone's drawer. There is always room for improvement. There are always defects in the process and variation in care. The many meetings that managers are involved with have to lead to improvements, or they are a waste of time. The goal is to identify defects and improve their cause. It is clear that having even a good and articulated process in place isn't the answer. Organizations have had all kinds of safeguards and verification techniques to avoid wrong-site surgery, and yet it still occurs. Quality has to be internalized for it to be effective.

Unless accountability is clear and based on data, and unless there is a commitment to reduce variability and promote communication, processes will be very difficult to change and improve. Using quality management principles, tools, and techniques can make change happen.

Summary

The tenets of quality management should be integrated into every level of the organization for cultural change to occur and be sustained. Data and measurements should be the foundation of performance improvement activities. In order to meet the challenges of the health care reform environment, organizations should:

- encourage administrators, clinicians, and finance staff to use quality data to evaluate the delivery of care, target efficiencies and waste, and comply with government goals;

- involve all staff members in the commitment to quality processes and patient safety;
- establish effective communication strategies across the organization and between the clinician and the patient;
- institute processes to break down traditional silos; and
- require all staff members to rely on measurements to evaluate care and monitor improvements.

Key Terms

cultural shift, effective communication, oversight, preventive strategies, quality metrics, value, work ethic

Quality Concepts in Action

As a quality manager, it is your responsibility to educate your organization about benchmarks—what they are, what they mean, and how they should be used. P4P is based on benchmarks. The Centers for Medicare and Medicaid Services dictates benchmarks. Insurers target benchmarks. Many organizations have established internal benchmarks. What data and processes would you use to explain that:

- benchmarks are goals to be achieved;
- benchmarks are used for comparison among organizations;
- benchmarks are data based; and
- benchmarks should be used for performance improvements?

What barriers to do imagine you might encounter, and how would you overcome them?

Suggestions for Further Reading

Berwick, D. M., A. B. Godfrey, and J. Roessner. 2002. *Curing Health Care*. San Francisco: Jossey-Bass.

Glickman, S. W., K. A. Baggett, C. G. Krubert, E. D. Peterson, and K. A. Schulman. 2007. "Promoting Quality: The Health-Care Organization from a Management Perspective." *International Journal for Quality in Health Care* 19 (6): 341–348.

Leonard, M., S. Graham, and D. Bonacum. 2004. "The Human Factor: The Critical Importance of Effective Teamwork and Communication in Providing Safe Care." *Quality & Safety in Health Care* 13: 85–90.

Useful Websites

http://www.ahrq.gov/downloads/pub/advances2/vol3/advances-dingley_14.pdf

http://www.ibtimes.com/quality-crisis-gm-worst-year-recalls-2004-1588125

http://www.modernhealthcare.com/article/20140507/NEWS/305079939

http://www.qualityforum.org

http://www.qualitymeasures.ahrq.gov

INDEX

Page references followed by *fig* indicate an illustrated figure; followed by *t* indicate a table.